The Health Care Handbook

The Health Care Handbook

Editor: Delilah Kinsley

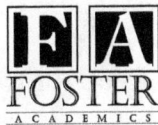

FA
FOSTER
ACADEMICS

www.fosteracademics.com

www.fosteracademics.com

FA FOSTER
ACADEMICS

Cataloging-in-Publication Data

The health care handbook / edited by Delilah Kinsley.
   p. cm.
Includes bibliographical references and index.
ISBN 978-1-63242-673-4
   1. Medical care. 2. Public health. 3. Health services administration.
4. Health planning. I. Kinsley, Delilah.
RA776.5 .H43 2019
613.2--dc23

Foster Academics,
118-35 Queens Blvd., Suite 400,
Forest Hills, NY 11375, USA

ISBN 978-1-63242-673-4 (Hardback)

Contents

Permissions

List of Contributors

Index

Preface

It is often said that books are a boon to mankind. They document every progress and pass on the knowledge from one generation to the other. They play a crucial role in our lives. Thus I was both excited and nervous while editing this book. I was pleased by the thought of being able to make a mark but I was also nervous to do it right because the future of students depends upon it. Hence, I took a few months to research further into the discipline, revise my knowledge and also explore some more aspects. Post this process, I begun with the editing of this book.

Health care refers to the maintenance of health by preventing, diagnosing and treating illnesses and injuries in humans. Health professionals are the ones who deliver health care. They may be operating and dealing within all branches of health care. Some of the common branches of health care are nursing, surgery, pharmacy, optometry, midwifery, audiology, dentistry and psychology. Healthcare practitioners usually include physicians, pharmacists, surgeons, nurses, dietitians, therapists, paramedics, surgeon's assistant and naturopaths. The leadership, administration and management of a hospital, health care system, hospital network and public health system is known as healthcare management. This book studies, analyzes and upholds the pillars of health care and its utmost significance in modern times. It covers in detail some existing theories and innovative concepts revolving around health care. Doctors, researchers and students actively engaged in this field will find this book full of crucial and unexplored concepts.

I thank my publisher with all my heart for considering me worthy of this unparalleled opportunity and for showing unwavering faith in my skills. I would also like to thank the editorial team who worked closely with me at every step and contributed immensely towards the successful completion of this book. Last but not the least, I wish to thank my friends and colleagues for their support.

Editor

Citizen Science and Community Engagement in Tick Surveillance—A Canadian Case Study

Julie Lewis, Corinne R. Boudreau, James W. Patterson, Jonathan Bradet-Legris and Vett K. Lloyd *

Department. Biology, Mount Allison University, Sackville, NB E4L 1G7, Canada; jlewis@mta.ca (J.L.); crboudreau@mta.ca (C.R.B.); jpatterson@mta.ca (J.W.P.); jhbradetlegris@mta.ca (J.B.-L.)

* Correspondence: vlloyd@mta.ca

Abstract: Lyme disease is the most common tick-borne disease in North America and Europe, and on-going surveillance is required to monitor the spread of the tick vectors as their populations expand under the influence of climate change. Active surveillance involves teams of researchers collecting ticks from field locations with the potential to be sites of establishing tick populations. This process is labor- and time-intensive, limiting the number of sites monitored and the frequency of monitoring. Citizen science initiatives are ideally suited to address this logistical problem and generate high-density and complex data from sites of community importance. In 2014, the same region was monitored by academic researchers, public health workers, and citizen scientists, allowing a comparison of the strengths and weaknesses of each type of surveillance effort. Four community members persisted with tick collections over several years, collectively recovering several hundred ticks. Although deviations from standard surveillance protocols and the choice of tick surveillance sites makes the incorporation of community-generated data into conventional surveillance analyses more complex, this citizen science data remains useful in providing high-density longitudinal tick surveillance of a small area in which detailed ecological observations can be made. Most importantly, partnership between community members and researchers has proven a powerful tool in educating communities about of the risk of tick-vectored diseases and in encouraging tick bite prevention.

Keywords: tick surveillance; Lyme disease; citizen science; community partnership; crowdsourcing; public health

1. Introduction

Lyme borreliosis, also known as Lyme disease, is the most common tick-borne disease in North America and Europe [1,2]. The disease is initiated by an infection with a member of at least 19 species of bacteria in the *Borrelia* genus known as the Lyme borreliosis group or *Borrelia burgdorferi sensu lato* [3,4]. If undetected and untreated, Lyme borreliosis can cause debilitating and, in some cases, fatal, multisystem symptoms [5–7].

In North America, *Ixodes scapularis* is the primary vector in the eastern and central parts of the continent, and *Ixodes pacificus* is prevalent in in the western regions, although *Ixodes cookei*, *Ixodes angustus*, and *Ixodes muris* have also been found to be vectors, and other species are potential vectors [8–11]. In Europe, the *Ixodes ricinus* species group is the primary vector [1,3]. Tick populations are expanding their range in response to climate change in North America, and this has brought them to Canada [12]. However, the prediction of new areas of population expansion is challenging because of the constant seeding of adventitious ticks introduced by migratory birds and mammals [13–16]. The survival of these ticks in either transient or small local populations, only some of which may proliferate into large, established "endemic" tick populations, is difficult to detect, yet important, as even small and transient populations pose a health risk to those living in those areas.

As ticks are expanding their range, the risk to public health has mobilized considerable resources to generate Lyme borreliosis risk maps and models [17–19]. These maps and models draw, in various measures, upon passive tick surveillance—ticks collected on companion animals and humans—or field collection of ticks, also known as active surveillance or tick dragging. In addition, case reports from humans, environmental factors such as climate, biogeography, distribution of the wildlife species needed to sustain tick and *Borrelia* populations, and canine Lyme seropositivity studies have been used to predict the risk of Lyme borreliosis [18]. While these risk models aim to predict areas where tick populations may establish, with the attendant evaluated risk of tick-vectored diseases, these models all require field validation, most frequently by active surveillance. Active surveillance, collecting ticks on a cloth dragged through potential tick habitat, is widely recognized to suffer from being a low-sensitivity method of tick detection. For example, Koffi et al. (2012) [19] reported that only 60% of the predicted tick high-risk areas yielded ticks upon field sampling. Similarly, a retrospective study of active surveillance of areas that subsequently became endemic showed only 50% sensitivity [20]. Thus, the low sensitivity of this form of surveillance is useful when defining tick endemic areas, large areas with high tick density, but is not well suited for identifying areas where tick populations are emerging. Additionally, field sampling is a logistically complex and expensive process, and, as a result, field teams generally only visit a site once. If the weather, day, time, or any of a host of other factors is not suitable, ticks may not be recovered. It is here that citizen science can play an important role by mobilizing citizens to monitor their own neighbourhoods and regions.

Citizen science involves engaging members of the general community in order to "crowdsource" data acquisition. The value of citizen science for researchers lies in the capacity for a tremendous expansion in data acquisition capacity. Universities are well positioned to engage in such community-centered research initiatives as many already have active community-engagement policies and practices; the same rational applies to public health researchers. From the community perspective, citizen science allows members of the public to not only explore an intrinsic interest in the natural world, but also engage in research relevant to their own health and that of their families and community members. When individuals are engaged in scientific research, as they are in citizen science projects, there is a heightened trust in science leading to personal empowerment, which underlies changes in behaviour that are needed to adapt to the changing environmental risk. The value of the citizen science approach has been appreciated, and citizen science has been extensively incorporated into ecological studies, but much less so in public health initiatives [21,22].

Passive tick surveillance involves members of the public, veterinary or humanmedical professionals submitting ticks for study. This type of "crowdsourcing" of ticks is highly effective for surveillance [17,23] as well as in providing ticks for a tick bank, bioclimatic modeling, or other purposes, as exemplified by the study of Laaksonen et al. (2017) [23], in which nearly 20,000 crowdsourced ticks were used to map changed tick distributions and new tick-vectored pathogens in Finland. If such initiatives return the results of tick pathogen testing to the donor, both partners benefit. However, with increased community involvement, even greater engagement and mutual benefit is achieved [21,22,24].

One way to increase community participation is by partnering with community volunteers in active tick surveillance. Members of the public are in a position to intensively monitor the same site, for example a backyard, favorite park, or school playground, over one or many seasons. For example, Seifert et al. (2016) [24] described the success of a program of tick education implemented in rural high schools, a tribal school, and a correctional facility that involved training volunteers in active tick surveillance. This project demonstrated that this active participation increased student knowledge of tick biology, awareness of tick bite prevention strategies, recognition of common signs and symptoms of Lyme disease, and student interest in science. All of these outcomes are highly desirable from the public health, medical, and societal perspectives. On a national scale, Garcia-Marti et al. (2017) [25] reported on the impressive results of a large study in Holland. In this project, trained volunteers conducted active surveillance, producing extensive and detailed collection records composed of over 3000 observations at 15 sites over nine years. This large and comprehensive dataset allowed geographic and spaciotemporal mapping of tick populations and pathogens at the national level. While traditional public health active surveillance initiatives are constructed around a standardized research methodology, as demonstrated by Garcia-Marti et al. (2017) [25], the variability in collection methodology implicit in citizen science initiatives is still compatible with highly effective public health surveillance.

The research question addressed here focuses on the relative strengths and advantages of academic, public health, and community-driven tick surveillance efforts. We approached this question by comparing the outcomes of each of these surveillance approaches, conducted during the same time period and in the same region. The volunteer community surveillance initiatives generated the greatest number of ticks, over a period of several years, at virtually no cost. While non-conventional and diverse methodology was used, these community tick collections provide detailed information on tick seasonal activity, abundance, density, infection rate, ability to overwinter, and similar biological factors, data not otherwise readily attainable. Most importantly, this initiative resulted in extensive community-based peer education efforts. Thus, partnerships between community volunteers and researchers promotes both research and education on the health risk posed by ticks.

2. Materials and Methods

2.1. Tick Collection—Academic Researchers

Field collection of ticks was performed by "tick dragging". A piece of animal scent-treated (wet dog or sheep) flannel, sourced from a thrift store, one square meter in dimension with solid wooden rods at each end and a rope at the front for pulling, was slowly dragged on the ground at a pace of approximately 8.6 m/min. Every ten paces, the sheets were checked for ticks. Each site was sampled for approximately 3 person-hours. Field workers wore protective clothing and performed tick checks. The choice of the surveillance locations was determined on the basis of records from passive tick surveillance initiatives (Lewis and Lloyd, unpublished) and canine seroprevalence studies [26], and of information on tick encounters from community leaders, veterinarians, and Lyme advocacy groups. Tick dragging sites generally included tall grass, areas with leaf litter, and broken woods. Ticks removed from the tick drags or the field workers were placed in a labeled container for same-day transport to the laboratory where species identification and DNA extraction took place. No animal care or environmental certification was required for these collections.

2.2. Tick Collection—Public Health

Although the criteria for site selection differed from the academic study, field tick collection was performed in essentially the same manner. Each site was sampled once by the same researcher, sites were 10,000 m^2 in size, and ticks were collected by dragging a one-meter flannel through vegetation, as described by Gabriele-Rivet et al. (2015) [27].

2.3. Tick Collection—Community Members

For the recruitment of community volunteer researchers, members of the community or municipal leaders contacted the senior author of this study for information on tick surveillance. Tick collections by community members were in some cases conducted with the academic researchers, using a standard approach. Those citizen scientists who joined the tick drags were instructed on personal protective clothing and in how to do tick checks. In other cases, tick collection was conducted independently and varied in time spent, area surveyed, and method employed. The same information on tick repellents, suitable clothing, and tick checks was conveyed to those collectors who approached the academic researchers with pre-existing tick collections. The Nova Scotia collection was obtained by fairly conventional flagging, although the time spent at each site was not standardized. The St. John collection was obtained by a combination of active and passive surveillance; ticks were obtained by flagging backyard vegetation with a white hand towel, removing ticks from flowers harvested in the backyard, and collecting ticks from the household cat. The Rothesay and Hampton collections were obtained by passive surveillance; ticks were removed from household pets and humans following daily inspections after exposure to the same backyard or neighbourhood areas. Information on the number of site visits and number of sites is provided in Tables 1 and 2. Environmental, landscape, and wildlife tick control measures were not in use in any of the regions surveyed. No ethics approval was required as the role of the humans in this study was to provide access to the ticks and information about ticks and humans were not the focus of the research.

2.4. Comparison of Tick Surveillance Strategies

Comparisons were made between the community, academic, and public health site visits that occurred between May 1 and September 30, 2014 in the greater St. John region which includes the communities of St. John, Rothesay, Quispamsis, and Hampton in southwestern New Brunswick, a Canadian Atlantic province. This region spans approximately 40×40 km and is within the Fundy coastal ecoregion, so it experiences similar climate, geography, and wildlife throughout its territory.

2.5. Tick Species Identification

Upon arrival in the laboratory, ticks were morphologically identified as species according to Keirans and Litwak (1989) [28], then stored frozen at $-20\,°C$ for molecular analysis to assess the presence of *Borrelia* DNA. The results of this testing were returned to the tick donors.

2.6. DNA Extraction and Nested PCR

DNA extraction was performed in a biological safety cabinet in a room separate from PCR and DNA analyses as described by Patterson et al. (2017) [29]. The detection of *Borrelia* in ticks was based on the amplification of two *B. burgdorferi* genes, *Flagellin B* (*FlagB*) and *Outer surface protein A* (*OspA*) by nested PCR, as described by Patterson et al. (2017) [29]. The primers used were: *OspA*outR: 5′-CAACTGCTGACCCCTCTAAT-3′, *OspA*outF: 5′-CTTGAAGTTTTCAAAGAAGAT-3′, *OspA*inR: 5′-TTGGTGCCATTTGAGTCGTA-3′, *OspA*inF: 5′-ACTTGATTAGCCTGCGCAAT-3′, *Flag*BoutR: 5′-TTCAATCAGGTAACGGCACA-3′, *Flag*BoutF: 5′-ACTTGATTAGCCTGCGCAAT-3′, *Flag*BinR: 5′-AGCTGAAGAGCTTGGAATGC-3′, *Flag*BinF: 5′-TCATTGCCATTGCAGATTGT-3′. The annealing temperatures were $55\,°C$ and $58\,°C$ for the first and second rounds, respectively, for both genes.

3. Results

During the spring and summer of 2014 (May–September), public health, academic, and citizen science tick surveillance projects were conducted in New Brunswick, Canada (Table 1). Initially, academic researchers already engaged in active tick surveillance were approached by community members interested in monitoring their local areas for ticks, and community members joined the academic researchers for 16 of the 66 academic tick drags conducted across the province. Additionally, some community members chose to monitor ticks independently and simply used academic researchers as resources for tick identification and testing. During the same period, a public health surveillance project was conducted in the province.

Some of the community-initiated surveillance efforts were discontinued after one or a few field collections (Table 1—health center, recreational, forestry lot collections). However, four of the community-initiated surveillance efforts continued over multiple years and encompassed many individual collections (Table 1—St. John, Nova Scotia, Hampton, Rothesay). Of these surveillance initiatives, three of the community collections (St. John, Hampton, Rothesay) overlapped spatially and temporally with a subset of the academic and public health site visits, offering the opportunity to compare surveillance strategies and tick recoveries (Table 2).

Table 1. Tick recoveries from academic and community-initiated surveillance efforts.

Collection	Collection Type	Year	Location	Number of Sites	Number of Site Visits	Collection Method	*Ixodes scapularis*					Other Ticks
							Larvae	Nymph	Adult Female	Adult Male	Total	
Mt. Allison	academic	2014	NB	66	1	active	0	0	6	3	9	
Sackville Health Center	community/academic	2014	Sackville, NB	1	1	active	0	0	0	0	0	*I. cookei* (3 adults)
Recreational	community/academic	2014	Kejimkujik Park, NS	1	3	active	0	0	0	0	0	*Dermacentor variabilis* (6 adults)
NB Forestry	community/academic	2015	Fredericton, NB	7	1	active	0	0	0	0	0	*D. variabilis* (4 adults)
St. John	citizen	2014	Millidgeville, NB	1	38	passive	33	82	2	0	117	
		2015		1	53		13	108	11	1	133	
		2016		1	26		1	137	2	0	140	
Nova Scotia	citizen	2015	Lunenburg, NS	2	6	active	0	0	93	73	166	*D. variabilis* not enumerated
		2016		2	12		0	1	304	220	525	
		2017		2	16		0	0	388	328	716	
Hampton	citizen	2012	Hampton, NB	1	200 [a]	passive	0	0	13	0	13	
		2013		1	200 [a]		0	0	12	0	12	
		2014		1	200 [a]		0	0	15	0	15	
		2016		1	200 [a]		0	0	3	0	3	
Rothesay	citizen	2014	Rothesay, NB	1	6	passive	0	0	3	3	6	
		2016		1	8		0	0	5	9	14	

[a] Estimated number of site visits.

Table 2. Comparison of effectiveness of tick recovery per site visit by different groups performing tick surveillance in the same area during the same time period.

Collection	Total of Ticks Recovered [a]	Number of Sites [b]	Number of Visits/Site	Average Tick/Site Visit
Public Health	0	8	1	0
Academic	7	38	1	0.2
Citizen (St. John)	94	1	38	2.5
Citizen (Hampton)	15	1	100 [c]	0.15
Citizen (Rothesay)	6	1	8	0.75

[a] Ticks recovered from May 1 to September 30, 2014 from collections within the St. John regional area in southwestern New Brunswick, Canada; [b] a site is defined as a location separated by >200 m from another location; [c] Estimated number of site visits.

The community-initiated efforts differed from the academic and public health surveillance efforts in a number of ways, including the criteria for surveillance location, the area surveyed, the number of site visits, the sampling effort, and the sampling methodology. While research teams sampled each location only once for 3 person-hours per site, in some cases (St. John and Hampton collections) the same site was sampled by the same collector daily or every few days from early spring to late fall over the course of three years. The Nova Scotia and Rothesay collections involved a broader opportunistic approach where different "likely" regions within convenient distance of the collector's home were sampled on a daily, weekly, or biweekly schedule (Nova Scotia), or on a less frequent schedule (Rothesay). The areas selected for surveillance by the citizen scientist tick collectors were areas of concern for the collectors, their families, or communities, whereas academic or public health researchers tend to select sites to answer specific research questions. Research surveillance seeks to standardize search effort, area surveyed, and tick collector expertise. In contrast, these parameters varied for the citizen science collectors depending on the weather, terrain, prior recoveries, collector interest, collector visual acuity, collector health, and many other variables. Nevertheless, these collections all have value. These collections generate ticks that are themselves of value (Table 1), they generate data on the presence of ticks (Table 2, Figure 1), and they promote greater community awareness of ticks (Figure 2).

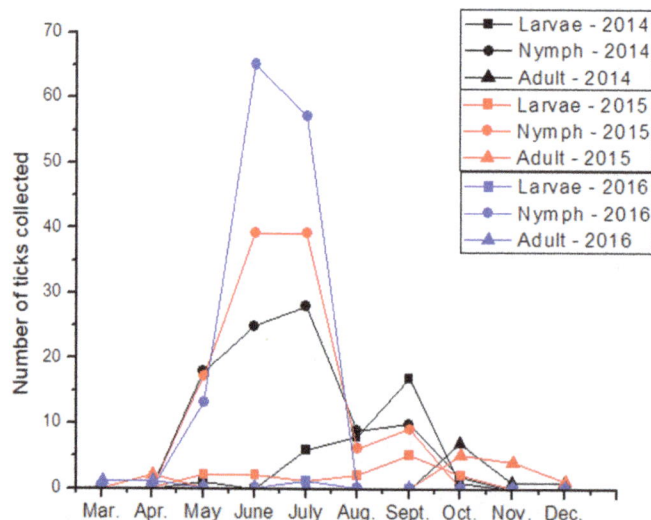

Figure 1. Monthly totals of *Ixodes scapularis* recoveries from the St. John collection, collected from one backyard site by passive surveillance every 2–3 days between 2014 and 2016.

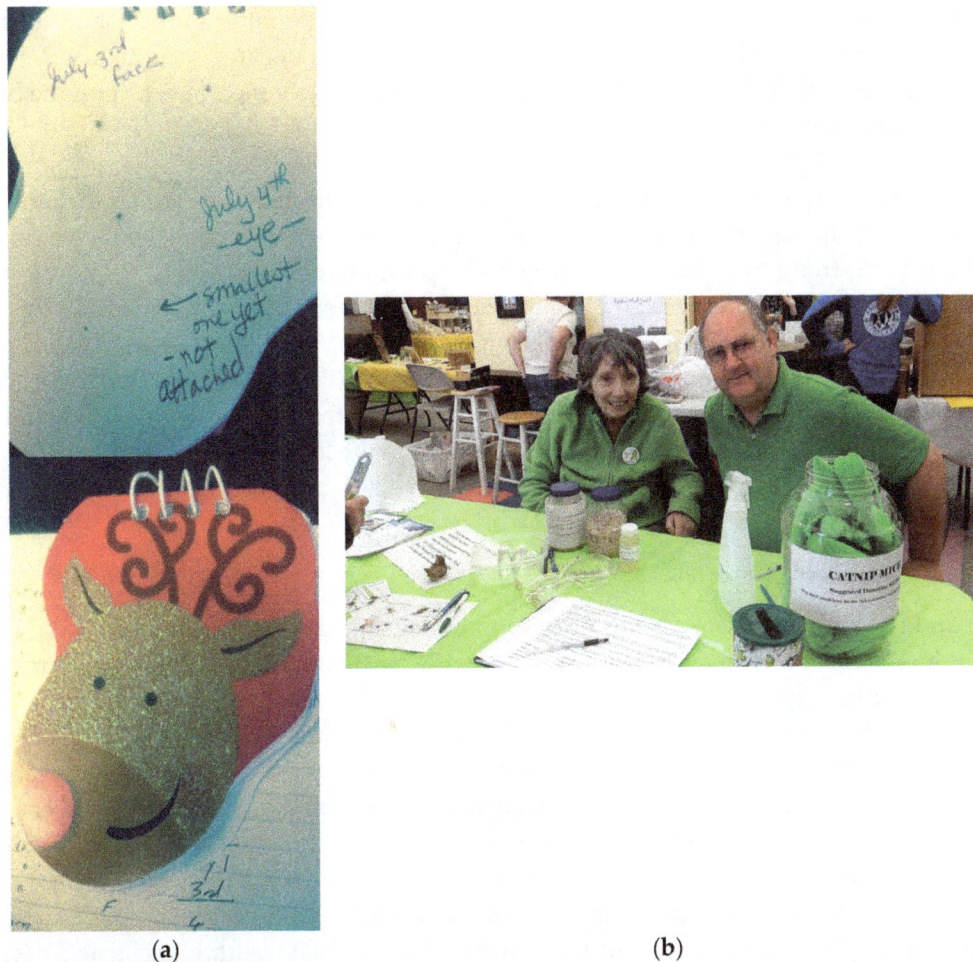

(a)   (b)

Figure 2. Community-initiated tick bite prevention education. (**a**) Ticks collected by a community member, taped to a notebook for display in schools (St. John collection); (**b**) Community members Brenda Sterling-Goodwin and Steve Goodwin at a Lyme awareness–tick education table at the New Glasgow, Nova Scotia, farmer's market in 2015. The containers in the center of the table contain ticks of different species and life stages obtained from two of the community-initiated tick surveillance collections described here (Nova Scotia and Hampton collections).

The St. John collection is remarkable for the very careful and frequent monitoring of a small site (family backyard) which allowed recovery of ticks at multiple life stages, including larval and nymphal ticks, as well as adults. This intensive sampling of one location also allowed the mapping of seasonal emergence of the different life stages (Figure 1), information that is generally not available from surveillance efforts using standard methodology. This type of intensive one-site sampling also lends itself to analysis of climactic factors, as described by Garcia-Marti et al. [25]. The region sampled in this collection, and the other sustained collections, were considered endemic or suspected endemic and so would not otherwise be eligible for surveillance by regional public health officials. Interestingly, tick abundance increased over the three years of intensive monitoring (Figure 1). Although this might represent improved tick surveillance methodology, the number of ticks in this collection and the recovery of larvae each year suggest that the surveillance was meticulous. This may suggest that the risk of tick-vectored disease is dynamic, even in endemic areas. The Nova Scotia collection is remarkable for the sheer number of ticks collected, although primarily adults were selected for collection. This collection also features careful notes on microclimate and vegetation conducive to tick recovery (data not shown), which is of considerable practical interest to residents of the area.

A subset of the ticks recovered from the university surveillance efforts, the St. John, Nova Scotia, Hampton, and Rothesay collections were tested for *B. burgdorferi* infection by nested PCR. From the university collection, 0/6 (0%) tested positive for both genes (*OspA* and *FlagB*). From the St. John, Nova Scotia, Hampton, and Rothesay collections, 2/13 (15%), 6/20 (30%), 5/70 (7%), and 0/27 (0%) were positive, respectively, for both genes (*OspA* and *FlagB*).

In addition to providing collected ticks and associated collection data to researchers, two of the community members have been very active in displaying their collections in their community and all have been strong local advocates for tick bite preventative behaviours, helping the public appreciate the presence, abundance and small size of ticks, hence the need for careful tick checks of children, adults, and pets. These activities have included showing the collected ticks at schools, farmer's markets, and other community and social gatherings (Figure 2). By having these activities initiated within the community by trusted community members, these initiatives are a powerful means to raise public awareness of the risk of tick-borne diseases in the local area.

4. Discussion

4.1. Advantages of Citizen Science and Community–Researcher Partnerships for Tick Surveillance

As part of a broader academic mandate to support and engage with communities, academic tick researchers partnered with community members for both joint and independent tick collection. Some of these community members joined the academic tick drags to observe the standard surveillance methodology, while others chose to monitor ticks based on a methodology of convenience or obtained from internet resources, and simply used academic researchers as a resource for identification and testing. Of these citizen science initiatives, relatively few were sustained, as reported by others, even in the context of a very well supported citizen science tick surveillance program in Holland [25]. However, four community collectors continued to monitor ticks over a multi-year period, one performing a remarkable 146 submission days (St. John collection) and another recovering over 1400 ticks (Nova Scotia collection). During the spring and summer of 2014, public health officials and designates also conducted active surveillance in New Brunswick [27]. As some of these collections overlapped geographically and temporally, this allowed the comparison of the relative outcomes of each type of collection approach (Table 2).

The public health and academic surveillance projects both used very similar methodologies: active surveillance by a standardized 3 person-hours tick dragging at each site, but with only one site visit. This approached recovered 0–0.2 ticks/site (Table 2). Within the same region, the citizen science tick collectors found 0.15–2.5 ticks per site visit (Table 2). Despite the range in tick recoveries, which could be due to geography or collector experience and skill, the community surveillance efforts clearly outperformed both the academic and public health tick surveillance initiatives in numbers of ticks recovered, both in total ticks recovered and per site visit.

The enhanced tick recovery by the community members could be due to any of the differences in methodology between community tick collectors and academic or public health researchers. One likely contribution to enhanced recovery is repeated site visits. Recovery of ticks by active surveillance is well known to be inefficient and dependent on a host of variables, both abiotic and biotic [19,20]. Multiple field samplings can mitigate the effect of these variables. Repeated site visits is an approach favoured by citizen scientists for its convenience and responsiveness to local concerns, but it is an approach that is logistically challenging for research and public health surveillance. In addition to repeated site visits, the community tick collections described here used primarily passive rather than active tick surveillance. However, even if passive surveillance is the reason for the enhanced recovery by the citizen scientists, both approaches had zero recovery days suggesting that it is the repeated visits that make these citizen collections so effective. The repeated site visits are also what makes these collections so valuable.

Access to the high-density, local scale, longitudinal tick surveillance data provided by community-based active tick surveillance is not otherwise readily available. This type of data allows investigation of interplay between local microclimate, local reservoir species abundance, and the variety of other biotic and abiotic factors that affect tick populations but are not well understood. This work, Seifert et al. (2016) [24],, and Garcia-Marti et al. (2017) [25] all document the microheterogeneity of tick recoveries: simultaneous tick drags conducted only a few meters apart or conducted only a few days apart can yield very different recoveries. Yet, as demonstrated by Garcia-Marti et al. (2017) [25], the high-density longitudinal data generated by volunteer community members can generate valuable data that can start to address these questions and even provide sufficient data for the construction of a model that can predict daily tick activity at a national level.

The ticks recovered are also a research resource in themselves; the ticks recovered by the community surveillance initiatives described here have been used for a variety of research projects ranging from novel tick diagnostics to tick microbiome analysis [30]. Further, with the exception of one larva recovered in the public health surveillance initiative [27], the St. John collection yielded the most plentiful supply of immature ticks. As the immature life stages are often of prime interest to researchers, this demonstrates the value of the meticulous and intensive tick surveillance conducted by community members.

Finally, the most important advantage of tick surveillance is the increased community awareness and commitment to tick bite prevention practices, which would be expected to result in decreased risk of tick borne disease in that community (Figure 2). The educational value of researcher – community partnership is demonstrated by Seifert et al. (2016) [24] who quantified the increased awareness of tick bite prevention strategies, consisting in tick checks, the use of protective clothing and repellents, and the awareness of signs of early infection, in high school students engaged in citizen science tick surveillance. Resistance or indifference to conventional public health messaging is an ongoing problem that can be effectively and inexpensively circumvented by partnering with trusted community leaders [31]. A public health poster on a doctor's office wall can easily be ignored; your neighbour showing you a tick retrieved from the head of their child will have much greater emotional impact. This seems not only intuitively reasonable, but also strongly suggested by anecdotal evidence as shown in Figure 2. Finally, the low rate of tick recoveries during many tick drags can also be useful in countering "tickophobia" and provide an increased sense of personal security outdoors and empowerment that can lead to increased use of outdoor areas for recreation [24].

4.2. Disadvantages

Community members provided much more extensive and detailed tick collections, with attendant high-density information, than either recourse-limited academic or public health tick surveillance initiatives (Tables 1 and 2). However, despite the value of this dataset and the other important advantages of community engagement in tick surveillance through citizen science, there are disadvantages to this approach. In this study, all of the sustained collections were by individuals who used their own methodology for tick collection rather than a standard methodology. Whether this is coincidental or due to trained researchers having a higher tolerance for the tedium intrinsic to the standard methodology is unclear. Seifert et al. (2016) [24] also noted that the generation of innovative approaches increased tick recovery, and that this innovation was coupled to engagement in the surveillance initiative. Unsuccessful citizen science initiatives are characterized by a top-down attempt to get community members to perform activities to research standards. After an initial phase of enthusiasm, community engagement evaporates under pressure from the daily demands of life [31]. In contrast, successful citizen science projects are collaborative, often iterative, in adapting a methodology to volunteers' need, interest, and time. In this study, their average per site tick recovery and the recoveries of immature stages by the different community tick collectors varied more than tenfold. The different recoveries of adults and immature stages presumably reflect a combination of geographic considerations, sampling effort, and collector ability. The latter may have a very strong influence on the recoveries of the immature stages, considering that all sites surveyed were endemic, thus including all life stages, and were surveyed throughout the year. However, it is important to note that this is not a weakness restricted to citizen scientist collectors; academic and public health researchers also had limited recovery of the immature stages. Regardless of the cause of this variation, variation in data collection methodologies and quality is a normal aspect of many studies that can be managed through the introduction of appropriate internal quality control monitoring and post-collection data analysis. Using the number of site visits and of immatures stages recovered as indicators of collection integrity and quality would be convenient and obvious internal quality assessment measures. Garcia-Marti (2017) et al. [25] successfully used citizen science-generated data to generate a nation-wide predictive model for tick abundance by using such internal quality control steps, although at the cost of discarding data from many of their collections. Similarly, Kampen et al. (2015) [32] and Bates et al. (2015) [33] noted similar considerations in their citizen science invertebrate surveillance studies. The participation of community members greatly increases the scope of the surveillance efforts as long as project design and analysis are adaptive and a strong communication with community members is maintained. Indeed, the use of different methodologies by different investigators working on the same problem is the norm in science and does not prevent the comparison of results or scientific progress, so this aspect of citizen science, while requiring some effort on the part of the research partners, does not negate the value of the data generated by citizen science projects or the associated value of these initiatives.

A related consideration, although specific only to this study, is that the two most productive collections were from areas already identified as endemic and the other two from suspected endemic areas. The focus of researcher-initiated surveillance efforts is on regions of expanding and newly establishing tick populations so, in this sense, surveillance is only useful when directed at areas where tick populations are not endemic. In contrast, local concerns tend to be high in areas of high tick density—in these areas, people are more likely to encounter ticks, and concerns as to whether playing in a backyard or school playground is safe for children are a very immediate and powerful motivator (Figure 3). Additionally, collecting in endemic areas provides a greater "reward" in that the probability of finding ticks is greater. However, the risk to human health is greatest in endemic areas so, while research and community motivations are disparate, they do overlap and the outcomes of both community-based and public health- and academic-based surveillance efforts overlap considerably and yield valuable information (Figure 3).

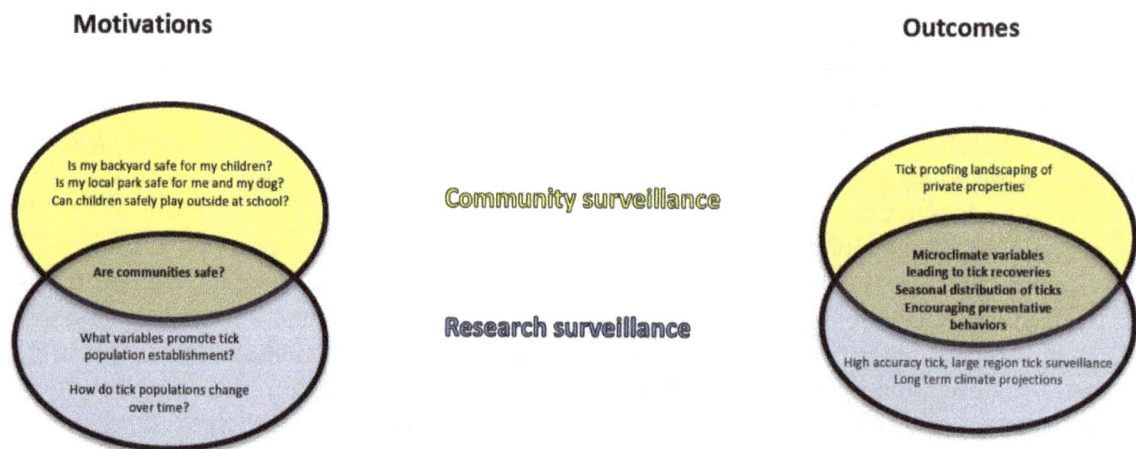

Figure 3. Overlap in motivations and outcomes of community- and research-initiated tick surveillance efforts. Community- and research-initiated efforts differ in the scale and expense of their investigation but, as both are designed to enhance community safety, research and community outcomes are highly overlapping.

4.3. Benefits and Applications of Citizen Science Tick Surveillance Projects

In addition to the overlapping motivations and outcomes of tick surveillance, tick surveillance lends itself to community–researcher partnerships; repeated sampling of small sites is too expensive for academic or public health researchers, but the molecular analysis required to assess the infection status of the ticks requires sophisticated molecular genetic expertise not otherwise available to community members. Citizen science projects such as the community–academic tick surveillance partnerships described here lay the foundation for transmission of scientific knowledge to the public and allow communities can act on this information. A collaborative partnership between academic partners and schools was effective in encouraging students to practice tick bite prevention strategies, as described by Seifert et al. (2016) [24]. Various patient advocacy groups, for example the Global Lyme Alliance, working in partnership with educators has designed teaching modules focusing on tick awareness education for students of all ages (globallymealliance.org) which could be readily introduced into educational programs. Further, the high-density data generated by these partnerships can be used to model seasonal, even daily, tick activity estimates, as described by Garcia-Marti (2017) et al. [25]. This information could be used to inform those using wilderness areas recreationally or working in forested areas of the local and seasonal risk of tick encounters, in much the same way that forest fire risk is advertised, or flu season activity is publicly posted. Park maintenance activities, such as mowing and watering, could also be seasonally modified to reduce public risk. The Dutch citizen science website Tekenradar [Tick radar] (www.tekenradar.nl) posts tick risk maps, as does the Tick Encounter Resource Center, an initiative of the University of Rhode Island that actively engages the public in tick awareness and monitoring (www.tickencounter.org). Thus, the success of the community-driven tick surveillance efforts documented here emphasizes the value of partnering with community members in citizen science tick surveillance.

5. Conclusions

By adapting our tick surveillance methodology to incorporate contributions and participation from community volunteers in response to local and individual interests and needs, we have maintained useful submissions over a multi-year period. Community-initiated tick surveillance provides information complementary to that from standardized tick surveillance, and can be thus used to address research questions not otherwise accessible from broad-scale surveillance. Most importantly, citizen science initiatives are ideally suited to promote local knowledge, foster trust, and translate this knowledge into effective preventative behaviours needed to protect the public in the face of the increased risk of tick-vectored diseases.

Acknowledgments: The Lloyd lab would like to thank the community members who participated in the field collection of ticks, including the New Brunswick Lyme disease support groups, and particularly Brenda and Steve Goodwin, Elizabeth McNutt, Robert Murray, Bonnie Adams, and Kristina Stanley. We also thank all the members of the Lloyd lab for discussion and the two anonymous reviewers for insightful comments, and K. Harris, A. Kirby, and C. Filiaggi for *Borrelia* testing of some of the ticks included in this work. This work was supported by CanLyme (101327) and NSERC (2015-04426) to VKL.

Author Contributions: James Patterson, Corinne Boudreau, Jonathan Bradet-Legris, and Vett Lloyd collected ticks and trained volunteers. Community tick collections were curated by Vett Lloyd, and *Borrelia* testing was performed by Julie Lewis. The manuscript was written by Vett Lloyd and Julie Lewis.

References

1.   Sperling, J.L.; Sperling, F.A. Lyme borreliosis in Canada: Biological diversity and diagnostic complexity from an entomological perspective. *Can. Entomol.* **2009**, *141*, 521–549. [CrossRef]

2.   Borgermans, L.; Goderis, G.; Vandevoorde, J.; Devroey, D. Relevance of chronic lyme disease to family medicine as a complex multidimensional chronic disease construct: A systematic review. *Int. J. Fam. Med.* **2014**, *2014*. [CrossRef] [PubMed]

3.   Rudenko, N.; Golovchenko, M.; Grubhoffer, L.; Oliver, J.H., Jr. Updates on *Borrelia burgdorferi* sensu lato complex with respect to public health. *Ticks Tick Borne Dis.* **2011**, *2*, 123–128. [CrossRef] [PubMed]

4.   Tappe, J.; Jordan, D.; Janecek, E.; Fingerle, V.; Strube, C. Revisited: *Borrelia burgdorferi* sensu lato infections in hard ticks (*Ixodes ricinus*) in the city of Hanover (Germany). *Parasit. Vectors* **2014**, *7*, 441. [CrossRef] [PubMed]

5.   Marcus, L.C.; Steere, A.C.; Duray, P.H.; Anderson, A.E.; Mahoney, E.B. Fatal pancarditis in a patient with coexistent lyme disease and babesiosis. Demonstration of spirochetes in the myocardium. *Ann. Intern. Med* **1985**, *103*, 374–376. [CrossRef] [PubMed]

6.   Reimers, C.D.; de Koning, J.; Neubert, U.; Preac-Mursic, V.; Koster, J.G.; Muller-Felber, W.; Pongratz, D.E.; Duray, P.H. *Borrelia burgdorferi* myositis: Report of eight patients. *J. Neurol.* **1993**, *240*, 278–283. [CrossRef] [PubMed]

7.   Muehlenbachs, A.; Bollweg, B.C.; Schulz, T.J.; Forrester, J.D.; DeLeon, C.M.; Molins, C.; Ray, G.S.; Cummings, P.M.; Ritter, J.M.; Blau, D.M.; et al. Cardiac tropism of *Borrelia burgdorferi*: An autopsy study of sudden cardiac death associated with lyme carditis. *Am. J. Pathol.* **2016**, *186*, 1195–1205. [CrossRef] [PubMed]

8.   Hall, J.E.; Amrine, J.W., Jr.; Gais, R.D.; Kolanko, V.P.; Hagenbuch, B.E.; Gerencser, V.F.; Clark, S.M. Parasitization of humans in West Virginia by *Ixodes cookei* (acari: Ixodidae), a potential vector of lyme borreliosis. *J. Med. Entomol.* **1991**, *28*, 186–189. [CrossRef] [PubMed]

9.   Dolan, M.C.; Lacombe, E.H.; Piesman, J. Vector competence of *Ixodes muris* (acari: Ixodidae) for *Borrelia burgdorferi*. *J. Med. Entomol.* **2000**, *37*, 766–768. [CrossRef] [PubMed]

10. Peavey, C.A.; Lane, R.S.; Damrow, T. Vector competence of *Ixodes angustus* (acari: Ixodidae) for *Borrelia burgdorferi* sensu stricto. *Exp. Appl. Acarol.* **2000**, *24*, 77–84. [CrossRef] [PubMed]

11. Scott, J.; Clark, K.; Anderson, J.; Foley, J.; Young, M. Lyme disease Bacterium, *Borrelia burgdorferi* sensu lato, detected in multiple tick species at Kenora, Ontario, Canada. *J. Bact. Parasitol.* **2017**, *8*. [CrossRef]

12. Ogden, N.H.; Maarouf, A.; Barker, I.K.; Bigras-Poulin, M.; Lindsay, L.R.; Morshed, M.G.; O'Callaghan, C.J.; Ramay, F.; Waltner-Toews, D.; Charron, D.F. Climate change and the potential for range expansion of the Lyme disease vector *Ixodes scapularis* in Canada. *Int. J. Parasitol.* **2006**, *36*, 63–70. [CrossRef] [PubMed]

13. Ogden, N.H.; Lindsay, L.R.; Hanincova, K.; Barker, I.K.; Bigras-Poulin, M.; Charron, D.F.; Heagy, A.; Francis, C.M.; O'Callaghan, C.J.; Schwartz, I. Role of migratory birds in introduction and range expansion of *Ixodes scapularis* ticks and of *Borrelia burgdorferi* and *Anaplasma phagocytophilum* in Canada. *Appl. Environ. Microbiol.* **2008**, *74*, 1780–1790. [CrossRef] [PubMed]

14. Scott, J.D.; Anderson, J.F.; Durden, L.A. Widespread dispersal of *Borrelia burgdorferi*-infected ticks collected from songbirds across Canada. *J. Parasitol.* **2012**, *98*, 49–59. [CrossRef] [PubMed]

15. Ogden, N.H.; Barker, I.K.; Francis, C.M.; Heagy, A.; Lindsay, L.R.; Hobson, K.A. How far north are migrant birds transporting the tick *Ixodes scapularis* in Canada? Insights from stable hydrogen isotope analyses of feathers. *Ticks Tick Borne Dis.* **2015**, *6*, 715–720. [CrossRef] [PubMed]

16. Scott, J.D. Studies abound on how far north *Ixodes scapularis* ticks are transported by birds. *Ticks Tick Borne Dis.* **2016**, *7*, 327–328. [CrossRef] [PubMed]

17. Ogden, N.H.; Bouchard, C.; Kurtenbach, K.; Margos, G.; Lindsay, L.R.; Trudel, L.; Nguon, S.; Milord, F. Active and passive surveillance and phylogenetic analysis of *Borrelia burgdorferi* elucidate the process of Lyme disease risk emergence in Canada. *Environ. Health Perspect* **2010**, *118*, 909–914. [CrossRef] [PubMed]

18. Mead, P.; Goel, R.; Kugeler, K. Canine serology as adjunct to human Lyme disease surveillance. *Emerg. Infect. Dis.* **2011**, *17*, 1710–1712. [CrossRef] [PubMed]

19. Koffi, J.K.; Leighton, P.A.; Pelcat, Y.; Trudel, L.; Lindsay, L.R.; Milord, F.; Ogden, N.H. Passive surveillance for *I. scapularis* ticks: Enhanced analysis for early detection of emerging Lyme disease risk. *J. Med. Entomol.* **2012**, *49*, 400–409. [CrossRef] [PubMed]

20. Ogden, N.H.; Koffi, J.K.; Lindsay, L.R. Assessment of a screening test to identify lyme disease risk. In *Canada Communicable Disease Report*; Public Health Agency of Canada, Government of Canada: Ottawa, ON, Canada, 6 March 2014.

21. Dickinson, J.L.; Shirk, J.; Bonter, D.; Bonney, R.; Crain, R.L.; Martin, J.; Phillips, T.; Purcell, K. The current state of citizen science as a tool for ecological research and public engagement. *Front. Ecol. Environ.* **2012**, *10*, 291–297. [CrossRef]

22. Ranard, B.L.; Ha, Y.P.; Meisel, Z.F.; Asch, D.A.; Hill, S.S.; Becker, L.B.; Seymour, A.K.; Merchant, R.M. Crowdsourcing—Harnessing the masses to advance health and medicine, a systematic review. *J. Gen. Intern. Med.* **2014**, *29*, 187–203. [CrossRef] [PubMed]

23. Laaksonen, M.; Sajanti, E.; Sormunen, J.J.; Penttinen, R.; Hanninen, J.; Ruohomaki, K.; Saaksjarvi, I.; Vesterinen, E.J.; Vuorinen, I.; Hytonen, J.; et al. Crowdsourcing-based nationwide tick collection reveals the distribution of *Ixodes ricinus* and *I. persulcatus* and associated pathogens in Finland. *Emerg. Microbes Infect.* **2017**, *6*, e31. [CrossRef] [PubMed]

24. Seifert, V.A.; Wilson, S.; Toivonen, S.; Clarke, B.; Prunuske, A. Community partnership designed to promote Lyme disease prevention and engagement in citizen science. *J. Microbiol. Biol. Educ.* **2016**, *17*, 63–69. [CrossRef] [PubMed]

25. Garcia-Marti, I.; Zurita-Milla, R.; van Vliet, A.J.H.; Takken, W. Modelling and mapping tick dynamics using volunteered observations. *Int. J. Health Geogr.* **2017**, *16*, 41. [CrossRef] [PubMed]

26. Bjurman, N.K.; Bradet, G.; Lloyd, V.K. Lyme disease risk in dogs in New Brunswick. *Can. Vet. J.* **2016**, *57*, 981–984. [PubMed]

27. Gabriele-Rivet, V.; Arsenault, J.; Badcock, J.; Cheng, A.; Edsall, J.; Goltz, J.; Kennedy, J.; Lindsay, L.R.; Pelcat, Y.; Ogden, N.H. Different ecological niches for ticks of public health significance in Canada. *PLoS ONE* **2015**, *10*, e0131282. [CrossRef] [PubMed]

28. Keirans, J.E.; Litwak, T.R. Pictorial key to the adults of hard ticks, family ixodidae (ixodida: Ixodoidea), east of the Mississippi River. *J. Med. Entomol.* **1989**, *26*, 435–448. [CrossRef] [PubMed]

29. Patterson, J.; Duncan, A.M.; McIntyre, K.C.; Lloyd, V. Evidence for genetic hybridization between *Ixodes scapularis* and Ixodes cookei. *Can. J. Zool.* **2017**, *95*, 527–537. [CrossRef]

30. Sperling, J.L.; Silva-Brandao, K.L.; Brandao, M.M.; Lloyd, V.K.; Dang, S.; Davis, C.S.; Sperling, F.A.H.; Magor, K.E. Comparison of bacterial *16S rRNA* variable regions for microbiome surveys of ticks. *Ticks Tick Borne Dis.* **2017**, *8*, 453–461. [CrossRef] [PubMed]

31. Newman, G.; Wiggins, A.; Crall, A.; Graham, E.; Newman, S.; Crowston, K. The future of citizen science: Emerging technologies and shifting paradigms. *Front. Ecol. Environ.* **2012**, *10*, 298–304. [CrossRef]

32. Kampen, H.; Medlock, J.M.; Vaux, A.G.; Koenraadt, C.J.; van Vliet, A.J.; Bartumeus, F.; Oltra, A.; Sousa, C.A.; Chouin, S.; Werner, D. Approaches to passive mosquito surveillance in the EU. *Parasit. Vectors* **2015**, *8*, 9. [CrossRef] [PubMed]

33. Bates, A.J.; Fraser, P.L.; Robinson, L.; Tweddle, J.C.; Sadler, J.P.; West, S.E.; Norman, S.; Batson, M.; Davies, L. The OPAL bugs count survey: Exploring the effects of urbanisation and habitat characteristics using citizen science. *Urban Ecosyst.* **2015**, *18*, 1477–1497. [CrossRef]

2

The Link between Posttraumatic Stress Disorder and Functionality among United States Military Service Members Psychiatrically Hospitalized Following a Suicide Crisis

Sissi Palma Ribeiro [1] [iD], Jessica M. LaCroix [1], Fernanda De Oliveira [1], Laura A. Novak [1], Su Yeon Lee-Tauler [1], Charles A. Darmour [1], Kanchana U. Perera [1], David B. Goldston [2], Jennifer Weaver [3], Alyssa Soumoff [4] and Marjan Ghahramanlou-Holloway [1,*]

[1] Suicide Care, Prevention, and Research Initiative, Department of Medical & Clinical Psychology, Uniformed Services University, Bethesda, MD 20814, USA; spribeiro3@gmail.com (S.P.R.); jessica.lacroix.ctr@usuhs.edu (J.M.L.); fernanda.de-oliveira@usuhs.edu (F.D.O.); laura.novak.ctr@usuhs.edu (L.A.N.); su-yeon.lee-tauler.ctr@usuhs.edu (S.Y.L.-T.); charles.darmour.ctr@usuhs.edu (C.A.D.); kanchana.perera.ctr@usuhs.edu (K.U.P.)
[2] Department of Psychiatry, Duke University, Durham, NC 27708, USA; david.goldston@duke.edu
[3] Inpatient Psychiatry, Fort Belvoir Community Hospital, VA 22060, USA; jennifer.j.weaver6.civ@mail.mil
[4] Department of Psychiatry, Walter Reed National Military Medical Center, Bethesda, MD 20889, USA; alyssa.a.soumoff.mil@mail.mil
*   Correspondence: marjan.holloway@usuhs.edu

Abstract: Posttraumatic stress disorder (PTSD) is one of the most commonly diagnosed psychiatric disorders in the United States and has been linked to suicidal thoughts and behaviors, yet the role of a PTSD diagnosis on functional impairment among suicidal individuals remains unknown. This study examined the association between PTSD status and functional impairment among military psychiatric inpatients admitted for acute suicide risk ($N = 166$) with a lifetime history of at least one suicide attempt. Measures of functionality included: (1) alcohol use; (2) sleep quality; (3) social problem-solving; and (4) work and social adjustment. Thirty-eight percent of the sample met criteria for PTSD. Women were more likely than men to meet criteria for PTSD ($p = 0.007$), and participants who met PTSD criteria had significantly more psychiatric diagnoses ($p < 0.001$). Service members who met PTSD criteria reported more disturbed sleep ($p = 0.003$) and greater difficulties with work and social adjustment ($p = 0.004$) than those who did not meet PTSD criteria. However, functionality measures were not significantly associated with PTSD status after controlling for gender and psychiatric comorbidity. Gender and number of psychiatric comorbidities other than PTSD were significant predictors of PTSD in logistic regression models across four functionality measures. Future studies should assess the additive or mediating effect of psychiatric comorbidities in the association between impaired functioning and PTSD. Clinicians are encouraged to assess and address functionality during treatment with suicidal individuals, paying particular attention to individuals with multiple psychiatric diagnoses.

Keywords: PTSD; functionality; suicide; comorbidity; military; inpatient

1. Introduction

Posttraumatic stress disorder (PTSD) and suicide are serious health concerns among U.S. military service members and veterans. In a recent meta-analysis by Fulton and colleagues [1], the overall prevalence of PTSD among Operation Enduring Freedom (OEF)/Operation Iraqi Freedom (OIF)

veterans was estimated at 23%. Among over 100,000 returning Iraq and Afghanistan veterans, 25% received at least one mental health diagnosis, and more than half of those were diagnosed with PTSD (52%) [2]. The link between PTSD and suicidal thoughts and behaviors is well-documented among military samples [3–7], and suicide is currently a leading cause of death among active duty U.S. military personnel [8]. According to the most recent Department of Defense Suicide Event Report (DoDSER) [9], PTSD was among the most common psychiatric diagnoses for individuals with a history of suicide attempt; two-thirds of active duty personnel with a documented suicide attempt received at least one mental health diagnosis, 20% of whom received a PTSD diagnosis.

One potential mechanism by which PTSD and suicide may be linked is through impaired functioning. The diathesis-stress model has been applied to several psychiatric diagnoses when describing how biological, historical, and environmental factors impact functionality before and after adverse events. Specifically, the diathesis-stress model has been used to conceptualize the development of psychiatric disorders, such as PTSD and Major Depressive Disorder (MDD), as the result of events and circumstances that surpass the individual's ability to cope [10]. Previous research among civilians diagnosed with PTSD indicate that functional impairment may manifest in the forms of disrupted sleep patterns [11], poor social support [12], and increased likelihood of divorce [13]. Functional impairment may in turn be associated with increased risk for suicide. For instance, among individuals who had planned or attempted suicide, 82% reported severe or extreme life impairment, compared to 70% among individuals who had suicide ideation, and 37% among individuals with no suicide ideation [14].

Similar links between PTSD and functioning related to social domains, alcohol use, and sleep difficulties have been found in military samples. One longitudinal study found a strong predictive relationship between PTSD and decreased social support over time, suggesting that interpersonal functioning difficulties associated with PTSD symptoms may erode the quality and quantity of social support resources [15]. Among individuals with PTSD, interpersonal difficulties may come about when social support networks are perceived as dangerous and unreliable [16]. As support networks are viewed with frustration, members are deemed unsafe, and social interactions may reintroduce elements of the traumatic exposure [17]. Over time, trauma-exposed individuals may avoid social relationships to increase perceived safety, thereby negatively affecting their social bonds. Additionally, in an analysis of data collected from veterans diagnosed with PTSD, researchers found evidence that those who reported no available social support networks were at greater risk of suicidal ideation and behaviors [18]. Thus, the relation between PTSD symptoms and interpersonal difficulties, including social problem-solving difficulties and social support, may indicate an individual's limited functionality.

Alcohol use among military members diagnosed with PTSD is common and potentially problematic, with excess alcohol consumption often leading to military service related occupational and legal issues [19]. In a study of 596 combat veterans, problematic alcohol use was estimated in approximately 39% of the sample [20]. A study of 205 OEF/OIF combat veterans indicated that alcohol-related consequences partially mediated the association between PTSD and quality of life [21]. Moderate to high alcohol use over 30 years of follow-up period was associated with adverse structural brain outcomes including hippocampal atrophy [22]. Cognitive impairment associated with alcohol misuse may impede recovery from alcohol or PTSD treatment, due to reduced ability to comprehend treatment materials or not being able to fully practice the strategies learned for treatment success [23].

In military service members, sleep disturbances are common and are often the result of rotating work schedules, work stress, and deployment related events [24]. Sleep problems are also a feature of PTSD [25] and may contribute to the maintenance of PTSD symptomatology [26]. Sleep deprivation is thought to affect basic arousal systems such as the limbic system [27] and prevent extinction of conditioned fear learning [28]. These disturbances may indicate decreased functionality and performance in a host of cognitive and emotional areas [29,30], which may prevent treatment, hinder work and life balance, and put the service member at risk for other taxing outcomes such as additional psychiatric diagnoses.

Overall, several researchers have stressed the importance of identifying correlates related to functionality [31,32]. Despite the recent influx of literature on PTSD, we continue to lack understanding on the association between functional impairment and PTSD among individuals at elevated risk of suicide. One important question that remains unexplored is whether functional impairment among military service members with acute suicide risk have greater likelihood of having a PTSD diagnosis, regardless of gender and number of psychiatric comorbidities.

The current study sought to examine the association between PTSD status and functional impairment among military psychiatric inpatients admitted for a recent suicide crisis and at least one lifetime suicide attempt. Functionality was explored using a functional measure for work and social adjustment, as well as proxy measures investigating alcohol use, sleep quality, and social problem-solving abilities. We hypothesized that individuals who met criteria for PTSD would report greater alcohol use, more sleep problems, greater social problem-solving difficulties, and more work and social impairments, compared to individuals who did not meet PTSD criteria.

2. Materials and Methods

2.1. Participants and Procedures

Participants were military personnel, at least 18 years of age, who were psychiatrically hospitalized at an inpatient military treatment facility following a suicide crisis (i.e., a recent suicide attempt or suicide ideation requiring admission to an inpatient unit; $N = 166$). Participants were recruited within 72 h of admission. All participants had a history of at least one lifetime suicide attempt defined as "a potentially self-injurious behavior with a nonfatal outcome for which there is evidence, either explicit or implicit, that the individual intended to kill himself or herself" [33]. Data were collected as part of an ongoing randomized controlled trial evaluating the efficacy of Post-Admission Cognitive Therapy (PACT) to reduce suicide risk among psychiatric inpatients [34,35]. Participants were voluntarily admitted to the inpatient unit, able to provide informed consent, cognitively capable of completing psychological assessments, able to communicate in English, and were cleared by the inpatient treatment team to participate. Cross-sectional baseline data were used for this study.

2.2. Measures

All measures used in this study were administered as part of the baseline assessment for the larger randomized controlled trial. Self-report measures were administered by a bachelor's or master's level research case manager. Clinician-administered measures were administered by a doctoral-level research clinician. The current study used a functional measure for work and social adjustment, the Work and Social Adjustment Scale (WSAS), as well as proxy measures of functionality to assess alcohol use, sleep quality, and social problem-solving abilities. These measures were added as proxy measures of functionality given the association of increased alcohol use [36,37], poor sleep quality [38], and social problem-solving difficulties [39] with PTSD symptomatology and functioning deficits.

2.2.1. Alcohol Use Disorders Identification Test (AUDIT)

The AUDIT is a 10-item, clinician-administered measure that screens for excessive drinking. Items are rated on a 5-point Likert scale, with higher total scores indicating greater alcohol use and greater alcohol-related impairment. The AUDIT has been tested in a variety of settings and populations and has demonstrated high internal consistency and test-retest reliability. The internal consistency of the AUDIT for the current sample showed a Cronbach's α of 0.89 [40].

2.2.2. Columbia Suicide Severity Rating Scale (C-SSRS)

The C-SSRS is a clinician-administered measure of lifetime intensity of suicide ideation and behavior. Assessed behaviors include preparatory behavior and interrupted, aborted, and actual suicide attempts based on definitions by the Centers for Disease Control and Prevention [41].

2.2.3. Mini International Neuropsychiatric Screen and Interview (MINI)

The MINI is a brief, structured, clinician-administered assessment of psychiatric disorders corresponding to the Diagnostic and Statistical Manual, Fourth Edition, Text Revision (DSM-IV-TR), including PTSD (Module I) [42]. The PTSD module is composed of six dichotomous questions (I1 through I6) which explore current and past experiences of traumatic events according to the DSM-IV-TR criteria. PTSD criteria were assessed based on questions pertaining to lifetime and primarily current (i.e., past month) experience of PTSD symptoms. A "Yes/No" coding was assigned to each participant based on whether they met criteria for a current PTSD diagnosis. Note that the MINI does not provide information regarding PTSD symptom severity [43].

2.2.4. Pittsburgh Sleep Quality Index (PSQI)

The PSQI is a 19-item self-report measure that assesses overall sleep quality and patterns within the past month. Higher scores indicate more impaired sleep. The PSQI has demonstrated high internal consistency (Cronbach's $\alpha = 0.83$), global score test-retest reliability, and good sensitivity and specificity in distinguishing between good and poor sleepers [44].

2.2.5. Social Problem-Solving Inventory-Revised, Short Form (SPSI-R:S)

The SPSI-R:S is a 25-item self-report measure that assesses participants' problem-solving abilities. Questions are rated on a 5-point Likert scale, with responses ranging from 0 ("not at all true of me") to 4 ("extremely true of me"). Lower scores on the SPSI-R:S indicate worse problem-solving abilities. For the current study, the SPSI-R:S demonstrated a Cronbach's α of 0.67 [45].

2.2.6. Work and Social Adjustment Scale (WSAS)

The WSAS is a 5-item self-report questionnaire that measures the impact of an individual's mental health on their ability to work and perform daily tasks effectively. Items are rated on a 9-point Likert scale ranging from 0 ("not at all impaired") to 8 ("severely impaired"). Higher scores on the WSAS indicate greater impairment in work and social adjustment. The WSAS demonstrated good internal consistency with the current sample (Cronbach's $\alpha = 0.86$) [46].

2.3. Statistical Analysis

Initial analyses were conducted using between-subjects t-tests and chi-square tests to compare participants who did and did not meet PTSD criteria on demographic variables and functional outcomes of interest. Additionally, Cohen's d was computed to provide another form of presenting the association between functionality measures and PTSD. Logistic regression analyses were then conducted to further explore the association between functional measures and PTSD status adjusting for data-driven covariates (i.e., gender and psychiatric comorbidities).

3. Results

3.1. Demographic Characteristics

Detailed demographic information is presented in Table 1. Participants were predominately male (65%), and Caucasian (65%), and nearly half were married (43%). The average age was 29.8 years old ($SD = 8.8$). All participants had a history of at least one lifetime suicide attempt, and 62% reported a lifetime history of multiple suicide attempts. Overall, 38% ($n = 63$) of participants met criteria for PTSD.

Women were more likely than men to meet criteria for PTSD (52% vs. 48%; $p = 0.007$), and participants who met PTSD criteria had significantly more psychiatric diagnoses than those who did not meet PTSD criteria ($M = 6.37$, $SD = 2.30$ vs. $M = 3.66$, $SD = 2.30$).

Table 1. Demographic and military service characteristics of military psychiatric inpatients hospitalized following a suicide crisis ($N = 166$).

Characteristic	N	%
Age (*M*, *SD*), Years	29.8	8.8
Gender		
Male	108	65.1
Female	58	34.9
Race		
American Indian or Alaska Native	3	1.8
Asian	10	6.0
Black or African American	31	18.7
Native Hawaiian or Other Pacific Islander	2	1.2
White or Caucasian	107	64.5
Two or More Races	12	7.2
Other	1	0.6
Marital Status		
Single	62	37.3
Married	72	43.4
Separated/Divorced	22	19.2
Service Branch		
Air Force	17	10.2
Army	75	45.2
Coast Guard	1	0.6
Marine Corps	30	18.1
Navy	43	25.9
Rank		
E-1–E-4	74	44.6
E-5–E-8	66	39.8
O-1–O-5	17	10.2
W-2–W-3	3	1.8
Cadet/Midshipmen	6	3.6
Deployment History		
No	79	47.6
Yes	85	51.2
Combat Deployment		
No	26	15.7
Yes	58	34.9
Not Applicable	79	47.6

3.2. Functional Differences

A series of *t*-tests using Bonferroni adjusted α levels of 0.0125 per test (i.e., 0.05/4) were conducted to investigate between-group differences on each of the functionality measures. Participants who met criteria for PTSD had significantly higher level of impaired sleep as measured by PSQI ($p = 0.003$), and significantly greater impairment in work and social adjustment as measured by the WSAS ($p = 0.004$), compared to participants who did not meet the criteria for PTSD. No statistically significant differences between groups were found on the AUDIT or the SPSI-R:S (Table 2).

Table 2. Mean difference in functional impairment measures across participants with lifetime suicide attempt histories who did or did not meet PTSD criteria.

Measures	N	M (SD)		Cohen's d	t	p
		Met PTSD Criteria n = 63	Did Not Meet PTSD Criteria n = 103			
Alcohol Use Disorders Identification Test (AUDIT)	166	8.33 (9.00)	6.82 (7.86)	−0.18	1.14	0.255
Pittsburgh Sleep Quality Index (PSQI)	165	13.74 (3.42)	11.80 (4.30)	−0.49	3.03	0.003
Social Problem-Solving Inventory-Revised, Short Form (SPSI-R:S) [1]	166	95.49 (16.59)	94.51 (17.70)	−0.06	0.35	0.724
Work and Social Adjustment Scale (WSAS)	166	28.29 (8.16)	23.76 (10.47)	−0.47	2.93	0.004

[1] SPSI-R:S: age adjusted scores.

3.3. Logistic Regression Results

Logistic regression analyses were conducted to assess for the effects of functional measures on the odds of participants meeting the PTSD criteria after controlling for gender and number of additional psychiatric disorders. Results indicated that higher scores on any functional measures were not associated with meeting the PTSD criteria after controlling for gender and number of additional psychiatric disorders (Table 3). Female gender significantly predicted meeting criteria for PTSD in all four models. Similarly, a greater number of additional psychiatric diagnoses was predictive of meeting PTSD criteria in all models.

Table 3. The odds of meeting PTSD criteria by functional measures (i.e., alcohol, sleep, social problem-solving, and work and social adjustment) adjusting for gender and number of other psychiatric diagnoses.

Measures	OR	95% CI	p
Alcohol Use Disorders Identification Test (AUDIT)			
AUDIT Total Score	0.992	1	0.748
Male (Reference = female)	0.378	1	0.018
n other psychiatric diagnoses	1.636	1	<0.001
Pittsburgh Sleep Quality Index (PSQI)			
PSQI Total Score	1.045	1	0.378
Male (Reference = female)	0.352	1	0.008
n other psychiatric diagnoses	1.578	1	<0.001
Social Problem-Solving Inventory-Revised, Short Form (SPSI-R:S) [1]			
SPSI-R:S Total Score	1.023	1	0.050
Male (Reference = female)	0.363	1	0.010
n other psychiatric diagnoses	1.690	1	<0.001
Work and Social Adjustment Scale (WSAS)			
WSAS Total Score	1.011	1	0.622
Male (Reference = female)	0.374	1	0.013
n other psychiatric diagnoses	1.604	1	<0.001

[1] SPSI-R:S: age adjusted scores.

4. Discussion

The current study examined the extent to which functionality was associated with meeting diagnostic criteria for PTSD (versus not meeting PTSD criteria) in a sample of psychiatric inpatients with an acute suicide crisis and at least one lifetime attempted suicide. We found that more than one third (38%) of the sample of patients psychiatrically hospitalized for acute suicide ideation or attempt met criteria for PTSD. Women and patients with higher psychiatric comorbidities were more likely to meet PTSD criteria. While individuals with PTSD had greater impairment in sleep and work and social adjustment, the associations between functional measures and PTSD were no longer significant when adjusting for gender and number of psychiatric diagnoses. Number of psychiatric comorbidities and gender were significant predictors of meeting PTSD criteria for all four of our functionality measures.

4.1. Demographics

While it is estimated that between 14% and 16% percent of deployed veterans and military personnel have been diagnosed with PTSD [47], little is known about the prevalence of PTSD in military inpatient settings. The current study found that 97% of participants met criteria for at least one psychiatric diagnosis (separate analysis) and over a third of them met criteria for PTSD. This result corroborates previous data reporting the occurrence of PTSD and psychiatric comorbidities [2,48–50]. Notably, this finding supports current concerns about a lack of trauma-focused services offered to high-risk individuals, such as those with a history of a suicide attempt and psychiatric comorbidities [51]. Historically, most clinical trials testing the efficacy of evidence-based treatments for PTSD, such as Cognitive Processing Therapy (CPT) and Prolonged Exposure (PE) therapy, have been known to exclude participants with suicidal thoughts and behaviors, resulting in a dearth of knowledge on how to best treat individuals at high-risk of suicide with PTSD [52].

Additionally, the current study found that women were more likely than men to meet PTSD criteria, corroborating the findings of previous studies [53]. A study by Kang and colleagues [54] reported that, while women in the military generally have lower rates of combat exposure, they report higher rates of military sexual trauma, which has been shown to have a strong association with the development of PTSD. Similarly, a meta-analysis of 290 studies found that women are more likely than men to meet criteria for PTSD despite being less likely to experience potentially traumatic events, with the exception of sexual assault or abuse [53]. While the current study did not take a particular focus on gender differences or the types of trauma reported by participants, it is important to consider that the results could be associated with extraneous factors, such as that women are more likely to seek help for mental health-related disorders [55] and are more willing to disclose distressing information to others [56]. On the other hand, mental health stigma is generally higher among men, especially for those who have been sexually assaulted, thus increasing the chances of underreporting trauma [57].

4.2. PTSD, Functionality and Comorbidity

Initial analyses demonstrated that, compared to participants who did not meet criteria for PTSD, participants who met criteria for PTSD were significantly more likely to report sleep difficulties and greater impairment in work and social adjustment. The significant association of PTSD criteria and functional deficits in sleep and work and social adjustment has been robustly supported in previous studies [15,58]. We did not find significant differences on alcohol use or social problem-solving abilities across PTSD status. Because our sample was characterized by both high suicide risk and psychiatric comorbidities, functionality measures such as alcohol use and social problem-solving skills may not have been noticeably different between those with and without PTSD.

After controlling for gender and psychiatric comorbidity, however, there was no significant association between the measures of functional impairment and the outcome of PTSD status. Instead, female gender and increased psychiatric comorbidities were associated with higher likelihood of meeting criteria for PTSD. Further analyses are necessary to determine if psychiatric comorbidities are stronger predictors of PTSD status or if psychiatric comorbidities mediate or moderate the association between functional measures and PTSD.

Psychiatric comorbidity is common among people who die by suicide [58,59]. While depressive and substance use disorders have the strongest association with increased suicide risk, PTSD, insomnia, poor sleep quality, and nightmares have also been found to increase risk of suicide in multiple studies [60,61]. Veterans who screened positive for PTSD and two or more psychiatric diagnoses were significantly more likely to endorse suicidal ideation than veterans with PTSD alone [5]. Further, a case-control analysis of 5.4 million citizens in Denmark found that those diagnosed with PTSD and depression showed additive risk for suicide compared to those diagnosed with either disorder alone [61], and studies on alcohol use disorder have found similar results [62]. This study and our findings highlight the importance of psychiatric comorbidity in relation to PTSD status, above and beyond functionality among individuals with heightened suicide risk.

4.3. Limitations and Strengths

Several limitations should be considered when interpreting results. First, this study presents baseline data analysis of a larger study assessing the efficacy of the PACT treatment for suicide thoughts and behaviors that was not originally intended to assess functionality in relation to PTSD status. The WSAS was the only measure in this study specifically designed to assess functionality, and is a short, 5-item self-report measure that is not considered a gold standard assessment of functionality. The AUDIT, PSQI, and SPSI-R:S are measures for investigating important clinical domains that have a functional impact on the overall well-being of a patient but were not intentionally designed to assess functional domains. Previous studies have used the Outcome Questionnaire-45 (OQ-45) [63] and the 36-Item Short Form Health Survey [64] when investigating functional outcomes. Both measures are valid, reliable, and easy to administer in a clinical or research setting. Functionality has been mostly studied for other psychiatric diagnoses, such as MDD and bipolar disorder [65–67].

Furthermore, the strengths of associations in our current study may have be limited due to restricting our study to a high-risk, highly comorbid inpatient sample with elevated functional impairments. As previously mentioned, all participants in the current study were presented to the inpatient psychiatric unit following a suicide-related crisis and had a lifetime history of at least one suicide attempt. Results and interpretations should not be extended to those without a lifetime history of suicide attempt. Similarly, the results of the current study should not be extended to all members of the United States military as only a subset of the military population has acute suicide risk. In addition, our use of cross-sectional data from an RCT study made it impossible to assess causality between PTSD status and functional impairment.

The current study benefited from the inclusion of a widely used, reliable, clinician-administered diagnostic measure, the MINI. Many studies rely on retrospective chart reviews or self-report assessments to determine psychiatric diagnoses, which, particularly in settings where the individual's full psychiatric history is not accessible (e.g., emergency departments, inpatient facilities, and other settings outside of an individual's usual mental health care network), may lead to inaccurate data. The MINI is one of the most widely used assessment tools for the screening of psychiatric diagnoses and has been found to have good validity and reliability [42]. This assessment allowed for more standardized data gathering. However, it is important to note that the MINI was developed to be administered as a screener, acting as a decision support tool, and is meant to be used in conjunction with a clinical interview and other diagnostic tools.

Despite these limitations, findings from the current study may inform assessment and treatment of individuals psychiatrically hospitalized following a suicide-related crisis and have implications for future research on the link between functionality and PTSD among individuals with acute suicidal thoughts and behaviors.

4.4. Implications

It is important for clinicians to assess functionality throughout treatment. For over thirty years, the American Psychiatric Association has included a section in the Diagnostic and Statistical Manual (DSM) entirely focused on the assessment of one's functionality, called the Global Assessment of Functioning Scale (GAF; Axis V) [43]. In 2013, the new DSM dropped the multiaxial organization, along with the separate section for the assessment of functioning, opting instead for the recommendation that providers consider a new tool, the World Health Organization Disability Assessment Schedule 2.0 (WHODAS 2.0). As Gold described in her recent review [68], this new measure makes a conceptual distinction between medical and mental health conditions, and the disabilities resulting from them.

This was found to be a notable improvement with important clinical implications, bringing more focus to mental health conditions and better assessment of important functional variables when assessing a patient's quality of life. Clinicians and patients can benefit from the implementation of functional assessments in clinical and research settings. The current study adds to a growing body of literature examining functional domains in relation to PTSD and suicide thoughts and behaviors.

4.5. Recommendations for Future Research

In addition to addressing the limitations described above, future studies should consider assessing additive or mediating effects of psychiatric comorbidity on PTSD and suicidal thoughts and behaviors. As mentioned previously, veterans with PTSD who screened positive for two other diagnoses were 5.7 times more likely to endorse suicide ideation than those with a PTSD diagnosis alone [5]. This comorbidity, in turn, may place the individual at a higher risk of suicide. For individuals with comorbid psychiatric conditions, it is important to investigate the role of each psychiatric diagnosis and the combinations of psychiatric comorbidities in increasing functional impairments and suicide risk.

Furthermore, future studies should assess whether specific types of functional impairments (in addition to the ones investigated in this study) are associated with PTSD and increased risk for suicide. For example, PTSD has been shown to have an indirect effect on suicidal ideation through increased interpersonal conflict, apprehension, and decreased perceived family support [69]. Functional impairments should also be considered during the development and administration of psychotherapy by monitoring comprehensive constructs of functionality and addressing functionality as a mechanism to improve patients' well-being.

5. Conclusions

The current study provides further evidence on the notable rates of PTSD and psychiatric comorbidity in a sample of psychiatric inpatients with at least one lifetime suicide attempt. Psychiatrically hospitalized individuals with a history of suicide attempt who met criteria for PTSD reported more disturbed sleep and greater difficulty in the ability to work and perform daily activities effectively. However, the association between functionality and PTSD status was no longer significant after adjusting for gender and psychiatric comorbidity. Notably, the vast majority of the sample met criteria for at least one psychiatric diagnosis and those with a greater number of psychiatric comorbidities demonstrated higher likelihood of meeting PTSD criteria. Future studies should consider investigating the causal pathways in which multiple medical and psychiatric comorbidities are associated with functional deterioration and PTSD outcomes.

Author Contributions: The opinions expressed are those of the authors and do not necessarily reflect the views of the Uniformed Services University of the Health Sciences or the United States Department of Defense. S.P.R., F.D.O., and J.M.L. conceived and designed the current study based on existing data collected as part of a randomized controlled trial; M.G.H. applied for and received funding for the randomized controlled trial as Principal Investigator; M.G.H trained and hired research personnel, prepared and obtained regulatory board approvals, delivered risk management services, and provided daily oversight for the implementation of the study as well data collection, interpretation, and write-up; K.P.U. set up the database for the study and K.P.U. and J.M.L. performed data analyses; S.P.R., F.D.O. and L.A.N. prepared draft reports for internal reviewers; S.P.R., F.D.O., S.Y.L.-T., J.M.L., K.P.U., L.A.N., C.A.D. and M.G.H. wrote and edited this paper; and D.B.G., J.W. and A.S. served as site Principal Investigators for Duke University, Fort Belvoir Community Hospital, and Walter Reed National Military Medical Center, respectively, and contributed to conceptualization of original randomized controlled trial as well as risk management, protocol development, and implementation.

Funding: This research was funded by the United States Army Medical Research and Material Command, Military Operational Medicine Research Program (MOMRP) grant number W81XWH-11-2-0106 provided to Principal Investigator, Dr. Marjan Ghahramanlou-Holloway.

Ethical Statement: All participants provided informed consent for inclusion prior to official study enrollment. The study was conducted in accordance with the Declaration of Helsinki, and the protocol was approved by the Institutional Review Boards (protocol number 367775) at the Uniformed Services University of the Health Sciences, Walter Reed National Military Medical Center, Fort Belvoir Community Hospital, and the Washington, DC VA Medical Center.

References

1. Fulton, J.J.; Calhoun, P.S.; Wagner, H.R.; Schry, A.R.; Hair, L.P.; Feeling, N.; Beckham, J.C. The prevalence of posttraumatic stress disorder in Operation Enduring Freedom/Operation Iraqi Freedom (OEF/OIF) veterans: A meta-analysis. *J. Anxiety Disord.* **2015**, *31*, 98–107. [CrossRef] [PubMed]

2. Seal, K.H.; Bertenthal, D.; Miner, C.R.; Sen, S.; Marmar, C.R. Mental health disorders among 103,788 US veterans returning from Iraq and Afghanistan seen at Department of Veterans Affairs facilities. *Arch. Intern. Med.* **2007**, *167*, 476–482. [CrossRef] [PubMed]

3. Bryan, C.J.; Corso, K.A. Depression, PTSD, and suicidal ideation among active duty veterans in an integrated primary care clinic. *Psychol. Serv.* **2011**, *8*, 94–103. [CrossRef]

4. Guerra, V.S.; Calhoun, P.S. Examining the relation between posttraumatic stress disorder and suicidal ideation in an OEF/OIF veteran sample. *J. Anxiety Disord.* **2011**, *25*, 12–18. [CrossRef] [PubMed]

5. Jakupcak, M.; Cook, J.; Imel, Z.; Rosenheck, R.; McFall, M. PTSD as a Risk Factor for Suicidal Ideation in Iraq and Afghanistan War Veterans. *J. Trauma Stress* **2009**, *22*, 303–306. [CrossRef] [PubMed]

6. Pietrzak, R.H.; Goldstein, M.B.; Malley, J.C.; Rivers, A.J.; Johnson, D.C.; Southwick, S.M. Risk and protective factors associated with suicidal ideation in veterans of Operations Enduring Freedom and Iraqi Freedom. *J. Affect. Disord.* **2010**, *123*, 102–107. [CrossRef] [PubMed]

7. Ramsawh, H.J.; Fullerton, C.S.; Mash, H.H.; Ng, T.H.; Kessler, R.C.; Stein, M.B.; Ursano, R.J. Risk for suicidal behaviors associated with PTSD, depression, and their comorbidity in the U.S. Army. *J. Affect. Disord.* **2014**, *161*, 116–122. [CrossRef] [PubMed]

8. Armed Forces Health Surveillance Center (AFHSC). Surveillance snapshot: Manner and cause of death, active component, US Armed Forces, 1998–2013. *MSMR* **2014**, *21*, 21.

9. Pruitt, L.D.; Smolenski, D.J.; Bush, N.E.; Skopp, N.A.; Hoyt, T.V.; Grady, B.J. Department of Defense Suicide Event Report (DoDSER) Calendar Year 2015 Annual Report. Available online: http://t2health.dcoe.mil/programs/dodser (accessed on 31 July 2018).

10. McKeever, V.M.; Huff, M.E. A diathesis-stress model of posttraumatic stress disorder: Ecological, biological, and residual stress pathways. *Rev. Gen. Psychol.* **2003**, *7*, 237–250. [CrossRef]

11. Dell'Osso, L.; Massimetti, G.; Conversano, C.; Bertelloni, C.A.; Carta, M.G.; Ricca, V.; Carmassi, C. Alterations in circadian/seasonal rhythms and vegetative functions are related to suicidality in DSM-5 PTSD. *BMC Psychiatry* **2014**, *14*, 352. [CrossRef] [PubMed]

12. Kotler, M.; Iancu, I.; Efroni, R.; Amir, M. Anger, impulsivity, social support, and suicide risk in patients with posttraumatic stress disorder. *J. Nerv. Ment. Dis.* **2001**, *189*, 162–167. [CrossRef] [PubMed]

13. Maia, D.B.; Marmar, C.R.; Metzler, T.; Nóbrega, A.; Berger, W.; Mendlowicz, M.V.; Coutinho, E.S.; Figueira, I. Post-traumatic stress symptoms in an elite unit of Brazilian police officers: Prevalence and impact on psychosocial functioning and on physical and mental health. *J. Affect. Disord.* **2007**, *97*, 241–245. [CrossRef] [PubMed]

14. Tarrier, N.; Gregg, L. Suicide risk in civilian PTSD patients: Predictors of suicidal ideation, planning and attempts. *Soc. Psychiatry. Epidemiol.* **2004**, *39*, 655–661. [CrossRef] [PubMed]

15. King, D.W.; Taft, C.; King, L.A.; Hammond, C.; Stone, E.R. Directionality of the association between social support and posttraumatic stress disorder: A longitudinal investigation. *J. Appl. Soc. Psychol.* **2006**, *36*, 2980–2992. [CrossRef]

16. Ehlers, A.; Clark, D.M. A cognitive model of posttraumatic stress disorder. *Behav. Res. Ther.* **2000**, *38*, 319–345. [CrossRef]

17. Price, M.; Gros, D.F.; Strachan, M.; Ruggiero, K.J.; Acierno, R. The role of social support in exposure therapy for Operation Iraqi Freedom/Operation Enduring Freedom veterans: A preliminary investigation. *Psychol. Trauma* **2013**, *5*, 93. [CrossRef] [PubMed]

18. Jakupcak, M.; Vannoy, S.; Imel, Z.; Cook, J.W.; Fontana, A.; Rosenheck, R.; McFall, M. Does PTSD moderate the relationship between social support and suicide risk in Iraq and Afghanistan War Veterans seeking mental health treatment? *Depress. Anxiety* **2010**, *27*, 1001–1005. [CrossRef] [PubMed]

19.   Stahre, M.A.; Brewer, R.D.; Fonseca, V.P.; Naimi, T.S. Binge drinking among US active-duty military personnel. *Am. J. Prev. Med.* **2009**, *36*, 208–217. [CrossRef] [PubMed]

20.   Eisen, S.V.; Schultz, M.R.; Vogt, D.; Glickman, M.E.; Elwy, A.R.; Drainoni, M.; Martin, J. Mental and physical health status and alcohol and drug use following return from deployment to Iraq or Afghanistan. *Am. J. Public Health* **2012**, *102*, S66–S73. [CrossRef] [PubMed]

21.   Angkaw, A.C.; Haller, M.; Pittman, J.E.; Nunnink, S.E.; Norman, S.B.; Lemmer, J.A.; Baker, D.G. Alcohol-related consequences mediating PTSD symptoms and mental health-related quality of life in OEF/OIF combat veterans. *Mil. Med.* **2015**, *180*, 670–675. [CrossRef] [PubMed]

22.   Topiwala, A.; Allan, C.L.; Valkanova, V.; Zsoldos, E.; Filippini, N.; Sexton, C.; Mahmood, A.; Fooks, P.; Singh-Manoux, A.; Mackay, C.E.; et al. Moderate alcohol consumption as risk factor for adverse brain outcomes and cognitive decline: Longitudinal cohort study. *BMJ* **2017**, *357*, j2353. [CrossRef] [PubMed]

23.   Allen, D.N.; Goldstein, G.; Seaton, B.E. Cognitive rehabilitation of chronic alcohol abusers. *Neuropsychol. Rev.* **1997**, *7*, 21–39. [CrossRef] [PubMed]

24.   Peterson, A.L.; Goodie, J.L.; Satterfield, W.A.; Brim, W.L. Sleep disturbance during military deployment. *Mil. Med.* **2008**, *173*, 230–235. [CrossRef] [PubMed]

25.   American Psychiatric Association. *Diagnostic and Statistical Manual of Mental Disorders: DSM-5*, 5th ed.; American Psychiatric Association: Washington, DC, USA, 2013.

26.   Gilbert, K.S.; Kark, S.M.; Gehrman, P.; Bogdanova, Y. Sleep disturbances, TBI and PTSD: Implications for treatment and recovery. *Clin. Psychol. Rev.* **2015**, *40*, 195–212. [CrossRef] [PubMed]

27.   Rauch, S.L.; Whalen, P.J.; Shin, L.M.; McInerney, S.C.; Macklin, M.L.; Lasko, N.B.; Pitman, R.K. Exaggerated amygdala response to masked facial stimuli in posttraumatic stress disorder: A functional MRI study. *Biol. Psychiatry* **2000**, *47*, 769–776. [CrossRef]

28.   Wessa, M.; Flor, H. Failure of extinction of fear responses in posttraumatic stress disorder: Evidence from second-order conditioning. *Am. J. Psychiatry* **2007**, *164*, 1684–1692. [CrossRef] [PubMed]

29.   Killgore, W.D.; Balkin, T.J.; Wesensten, N.J. Impaired decision making following 49 h of sleep deprivation. *J. Sleep Res.* **2006**, *15*, 7–13. [CrossRef] [PubMed]

30.   Pilcher, J.J.; Huffcutt, A.J. Effects of sleep deprivation on performance: A meta-analysis. *Sleep* **1996**, *19*, 318–326. [CrossRef] [PubMed]

31.   Pietrzak, R.H.; Johnson, D.C.; Goldstein, M.B.; Malley, J.C.; Rivers, A.J.; Morgan, C.A.; Southwick, S.M. Psychosocial buffers of traumatic stress, depressive symptoms, and psychosocial difficulties in veterans of Operations Enduring Freedom and Iraqi Freedom: The role of resilience, unit support, and postdeployment social support. *J. Affect. Disord.* **2010**, *120*, 188–192. [CrossRef] [PubMed]

32.   Thomas, J.L.; Wilk, J.E.; Riviere, L.A.; McGurk, D.; Castro, C.A.; Hoge, C.W. Prevalence of mental health problems and functional impairment among Active Component and National Guard soldiers 3 and 12 months following combat in Iraq. *Arch. Gen. Psychiatry* **2010**, *67*, 614–623. [CrossRef] [PubMed]

33.   O'Carroll, P.W.; Berman, A.L.; Maris, R.W.; Moscicki, E.K.; Tanney, B.L.; Silverman, M.M. Beyond the tower of Babel: A nomenclature for suicidology. *Suicide Life Threat Behav.* **1996**, *26*, 237–252. [CrossRef] [PubMed]

34.   Ghahramanlou-Holloway, M.; Cox, D.; Greene, F. Post-admission cognitive therapy: A brief intervention for psychiatric inpatients admitted after a suicide attempt. *Cogn. Behav. Pract.* **2012**, *19*, 233–244. [CrossRef]

35.   Ghahramanlou-Holloway, M.; Neely, L.L.; Tucker, J. A cognitive behavioral strategy for preventing suicide. *Curr. Psychiatry* **2014**, *13*, 18–25.

36.   Grossbard, J.R.; Hawkins, E.J.; Lapham, G.T.; Williams, E.C.; Rubinsky, A.D.; Simpson, T.L.; Seal, K.H.; Kivlahan, D.R.; Bradley, K.A. Follow-up care for alcohol misuse among OEF/OIF veterans with and without alcohol use disorders and posttraumatic stress disorder. *J. Subst. Abuse Treat.* **2013**, *45*, 409–415. [CrossRef] [PubMed]

37.   Sannibale, C.; Teesson, M.; Creamer, M.; Sitharthan, T.; Bryant, R.A.; Sutherland, K.; Taylor, K.; Bostock-Matusko, D.; Visser, A.; Peek-O'Leary, M. Randomized controlled trial of cognitive behaviour therapy for comorbid post-traumatic stress disorder and alcohol use disorders. *Addiction* **2013**, *108*, 1397–1410. [CrossRef] [PubMed]

38.   Mohr, D.; Vedantham, K.; Neylan, T.; Metzler, T.J.; Best, S.; Marmar, C.R. The mediating effects of sleep in the relationship between traumatic stress and health symptoms in urban police officers. *Psychosom. Med.* **2003**, *65*, 485–489. [CrossRef] [PubMed]

39. Hofmann, S.G.; Litz, B.T.; Weathers, F.W. Social anxiety, depression, and PTSD in Vietnam veterans. *J. Anxiety Disord.* **2003**, *17*, 573–582. [CrossRef]

40. Babor, T.F.; Higgins-Biddle, J.C.; Saunders, J.B.; Monteiro, M.G.; World Health Organization (WHO). The Alcohol Use Disorders Identification Test: Guidelines for Use in Primary Care. Available online: http://apps.who.int/iris/bitstream/handle/10665/67205/WHO_MSD_MSB_01.6a.pdf;jsessionid= 46F1535BD74886CCD130D5E5FDE9B3BF?sequence=1 (accessed on 7 July 2018).

41. Posner, K.; Brown, G.K.; Stanley, B.; Brent, D.A.; Yershova, K.V.; Oquendo, M.A.; Currier, G.W.; Melvin, G.A.; Greenhill, L.; Shen, S.; et al. The Columbia–Suicide Severity Rating Scale: Initial validity and internal consistency findings from three multisite studies with adolescents and adults. *Am. J. Psychiatry* **2011**, *168*, 1266–1277. [CrossRef] [PubMed]

42. American Psychiatric Association. *DSM-IV-TR: Diagnostic and Statistical Manual of Mental Disorders, Text Revision*, 4th ed.; American Psychiatric Association: Washington, DC, USA, 2000.

43. Sheehan, D.V.; Lecrubier, Y.; Sheehan, K.H.; Janavs, J.; Weiller, E.; Keskiner, A.; Schinka, J.; Knapp, E.; Sheehan, M.F.; Dunbar, G.C. The validity of the Mini International Neuropsychiatric Interview (MINI) according to the SCID-P and its reliability. *Eur. Psychiatry* **1997**, *12*, 232–241. [CrossRef]

44. Buysse, D.J.; Reynolds, C.F.; Monk, T.H.; Berman, S.R.; Kupfer, D.J. The Pittsburgh Sleep Quality Index: A new instrument for psychiatric practice and research. *Psychiatry Res.* **1989**, *28*, 193–213. [CrossRef]

45. D'Zurilla, T.J.; Nezu, A.M.; Maydeu-Olivares, A. *Social Problem-Solving Inventory—Revised (SPSI-R)*; Multi-Health Systems: North Tonawanda, NY, USA, 2002.

46. Mundt, J.C.; Marks, I.M.; Shear, M.K.; Greist, J.M. The Work and Social Adjustment Scale: A simple measure of impairment in functioning. *Br. J. Psychiatry* **2002**, *180*, 461–464. [CrossRef] [PubMed]

47. Gates, M.A.; Holowka, D.W.; Vasterling, J.J.; Keane, T.M.; Marx, B.P.; Rosen, R.C. Posttraumatic stress disorder in veterans and military personnel: Epidemiology, screening, and case recognition. *Psychol. Serv.* **2012**, *9*, 361–382. [CrossRef] [PubMed]

48. Stein, M.B.; McQuaid, J.R.; Pedrelli, P.; Lenox, R.; McCahill, M.E. Posttraumatic stress disorder in the primary care medical setting. *Gen. Hosp. Psychiatry* **2000**, *22*, 261–269. [CrossRef]

49. Brown, P.J.; Stout, R.L.; Mueller, T. Substance use disorder and posttraumatic stress disorder comorbidity: Addiction and psychiatric treatment rates. *Psychol. Addict. Behav.* **1999**, *13*, 115–122. [CrossRef]

50. Kessler, R.C.; Sonnega, A.; Bromet, E.; Hughes, M.; Nelson, C.B. Posttraumatic stress disorder in the National Comorbidity Survey. *Arch. Gen. Psychiatry* **1995**, *52*, 1048–1060. [CrossRef] [PubMed]

51. Bryan, C.J.; Clemans, T.A.; Hernandez, A.M.; Mintz, J.; Peterson, A.L.; Yarvis, J.S.; Resick, P.A. Evaluating potential iatrogenic suicide risk in trauma-focused group cognitive behavioral therapy for the treatment of PTSD in active duty military personnel. *Depress. Anxiety* **2016**, *33*, 549–557. [CrossRef] [PubMed]

52. Bakalar, J.L.; Carlin, E.A.; Blevins, C.L.; Ghahramanlou-Holloway, M. Generalizability of evidence-based PTSD psychotherapies to suicidal individuals: A review of the Veterans Administration and Department of Defense clinical practice guidelines. *Mil. Psychol* **2016**, *28*, 331–343. [CrossRef]

53. Tolin, D.F.; Foa, E.B. Sex differences in trauma and posttraumatic stress disorder: A quantitative review of 25 years of research. *Psychol. Bull.* **2006**, *132*, 959. [CrossRef] [PubMed]

54. Kang, H.; Dalager, N.; Mahan, C.; Ishii, E. The role of sexual assault on the risk of PTSD among Gulf War veterans. *Ann. Epidemiol.* **2005**, *15*, 191–195. [CrossRef] [PubMed]

55. Wang, P.S.; Aguilar-Gaxiola, S.; Alonso, J.; Angermeyer, M.C.; Borges, G.; Bromet, E.J.; Bruffaerts, R.; De Girolamo, G.; De Graaf, R.; Gureje, O.; et al. Use of mental health services for anxiety, mood, and substance disorders in 17 countries in the WHO world mental health surveys. *Lancet* **2007**, *370*, 841–850. [CrossRef]

56. Ward, M.; Tedstone Doherty, D.; Moran, R. *It's Good to Talk: Distress Disclosure and Psychological Wellbeing*; Health Research Board: Dublin, Ireland, 2007.

57. Vogel, D.L.; Wade, N.G. Stigma and help-seeking. *Psychologist* **2009**, *22*, 20–23.

58. Babson, K.A.; Feldner, M.T. Temporal relations between sleep problems and both traumatic event exposure and PTSD: A critical review of the empirical literature. *J. Anxiety Disord.* **2010**, *24*, 1–15. [CrossRef] [PubMed]

59. Conner, K.R.; Bohnert, A.S.; McCarthy, J.F.; Valenstein, M.; Bossarte, R.; Ignacio, R.; Lu, N.; Ilgen, M.A. Mental disorder comorbidity and suicide among 2.96 million men receiving care in the Veterans Health Administration health system. *J. Abnorm. Psychol.* **2013**, *122*, 256–263. [CrossRef] [PubMed]

60. Ribeiro, J.D.; Pease, J.L.; Gutierrez, P.M.; Silva, C.; Bernert, R.A.; Rudd, M.D.; Joiner, T.E. Sleep problems outperform depression and hopelessness as cross-sectional and longitudinal predictors of suicidal ideation and behavior in young adults in the military. *J. Affect. Disord.* **2012**, *136*, 743–750. [CrossRef] [PubMed]

61. Gradus, J.L.; Qin, P.; Lincoln, A.K.; Miller, M.; Lawler, E.; Sørensen, H.T.; Lash, T.L. Posttraumatic stress disorder and completed suicide. *Am. J. Epidemiol.* **2010**, *171*, 721–727. [CrossRef] [PubMed]

62. Flensborg-Madsen, T.; Knop, J.; Mortensen, E.L.; Becker, U.; Sher, L.; Grønbæk, M. Alcohol use disorders increase the risk of completed suicide—Irrespective of other psychiatric disorders. A longitudinal cohort study. *Psychiatry Res.* **2009**, *167*, 123–130. [CrossRef] [PubMed]

63. Lambert, M.J.; Burlingame, G.M.; Umphress, V.; Hansen, N.B.; Vermeersch, D.A.; Clouse, G.C.; Yanchar, S.C. The reliability and validity of the Outcome Questionnaire. *Clin. Psychol. Psychother.* **1996**, *3*, 249–258. [CrossRef]

64. Ware, J.E., Jr.; Sherbourne, C.D. The MOS 36-item short-form health survey (SF-36): I. Conceptual framework and item selection. *Med. Care* **1992**, *30*, 473–483. [CrossRef] [PubMed]

65. Reznik, A.E.; Sudharshan, L.; Stephens, J.M.; Shelbaya, A.; Pappadopulos, E.; Haider, S.; Lin, I.; Gao, C. Impact of Major depressive Disorder on Patient functionality and work performance in Emerging Markets. *Value Health* **2015**, *18*, A123. [CrossRef]

66. Prelipceanu, D.; Purnichi, T.; Marinescu, V.; Matei, V. The daily functionality in a major depressive episode cohort of Romanian patients—A non-interventional study. *Maedica* **2015**, *10*, 39. [PubMed]

67. Esposito-Smythers, C.; Goldstein, T.; Birmaher, B.; Goldstein, B.; Hunt, J.; Ryan, N.; Keller, M. Clinical and psychosocial correlates of non-suicidal self-injury within a sample of children and adolescents with bipolar disorder. *J. Affect. Disord.* **2010**, *125*, 89–97. [CrossRef] [PubMed]

68. Gold, L.H. DSM-5 and the assessment of functioning: The World Health Organization Disability Assessment Schedule 2.0 (WHODAS 2.0). *J. Am. Acad. Psychiatry Law Online* **2014**, *42*, 173–181.

69. Dutton, C.E.; Rojas, S.M.; Badour, C.L.; Wanklyn, S.G.; Feldner, M.T. Posttraumatic stress disorder and suicidal behavior: Indirect effects of impaired social functioning. *Arch. Suicide Res.* **2016**, *20*, 567–579. [CrossRef] [PubMed]

3

A Systematic Review on Healthcare Analytics: Application and Theoretical Perspective of Data Mining

Md Saiful Islam [1], Md Mahmudul Hasan [1], Xiaoyi Wang [1], Hayley D. Germack [1,2,3] and Md Noor-E-Alam [1,*] [iD]

[1] Mechanical and Industrial Engineering, Northeastern University, Boston, MA 02115, USA; islam.m@husky.neu.edu (M.S.I.); hasan.mdm@husky.neu.edu (M.M.H.); wang.xiaoyi@husky.neu.edu (X.W.); hayley.germack@yale.edu (H.D.G.)

[2] National Clinician Scholars Program, Yale University School of Medicine, New Haven, CT 06511, USA

[3] Bouvé College of Health Sciences, Northeastern University, Boston, MA 02115, USA

* Correspondence: mnalam@neu.edu

Abstract: The growing healthcare industry is generating a large volume of useful data on patient demographics, treatment plans, payment, and insurance coverage—attracting the attention of clinicians and scientists alike. In recent years, a number of peer-reviewed articles have addressed different dimensions of data mining application in healthcare. However, the lack of a comprehensive and systematic narrative motivated us to construct a literature review on this topic. In this paper, we present a review of the literature on healthcare analytics using data mining and big data. Following Preferred Reporting Items for Systematic Reviews and Meta-Analyses (PRISMA) guidelines, we conducted a database search between 2005 and 2016. Critical elements of the selected studies—healthcare sub-areas, data mining techniques, types of analytics, data, and data sources—were extracted to provide a systematic view of development in this field and possible future directions. We found that the existing literature mostly examines analytics in clinical and administrative decision-making. Use of human-generated data is predominant considering the wide adoption of Electronic Medical Record in clinical care. However, analytics based on website and social media data has been increasing in recent years. Lack of prescriptive analytics in practice and integration of domain expert knowledge in the decision-making process emphasizes the necessity of future research.

Keywords: healthcare; data analytics; data mining; big data; healthcare informatics; literature review

1. Introduction

Healthcare is a booming sector of the economy in many countries [1]. With its growth, come challenges including rising costs, inefficiencies, poor quality, and increasing complexity [2]. U.S. healthcare expenditures increased by 123% between 2010 and 2015—from $2.6 trillion to $3.2 trillion [3]. Inefficient—non-value added tasks (e.g., readmissions, inappropriate use of antibiotics, and fraud)—constitutes 21–47% of this enormous expenditure [4]. Some of these costs were associated with low quality care—researchers found that approximately 251,454 patients in the U.S. die each year due to medical errors [5]. Better decision-making based on available information could mitigate these challenges and facilitate the transition to a value-based healthcare industry [4]. Healthcare institutions are adopting information technology in their management system [6]. A large volume of data is collected through this system on a regular basis. Analytics provides tools and techniques to extract information from this complex and voluminous data [2] and translate it into information to assist decision-making in healthcare.

Analytics is the way of developing insights through the efficient use of data and application of quantitative and qualitative analysis [7]. It can generate fact-based decisions for "planning, management, measurement, and learning" purposes [2]. For instance, the Centers for Medicare and Medicaid Services (CMS) used analytics to reduce hospital readmission rates and avert $115 million in fraudulent payment [8]. Use of analytics—including data mining, text mining, and big data analytics—is assisting healthcare professionals in disease prediction, diagnosis, and treatment, resulting in an improvement in service quality and reduction in cost [9]. According to some estimates, application of data mining can save $450 billion each year from the U.S. healthcare system [10]. In the past ten years, researchers have studied data mining and big data analytics from both applied (e.g., applied to pharmacovigilance or mental health) and theoretical (e.g., reflecting on the methodological or philosophical challenges of data mining) perspectives.

In this review, we systematically organize and summarize the published peer-reviewed literature related to the applied and theoretical perspectives of data mining. We classify the literature by types of analytics (e.g., descriptive, predictive, prescriptive), healthcare application areas (i.e., clinical decision support, mental health), and data mining techniques (i.e., classification, sequential pattern mining); and we report the data source used in each review paper which, to our best knowledge, has never done before.

Motivation and Scope

There is a large body of recently published review/conceptual studies on healthcare and data mining. We outline the characteristics of these studies—e.g., scope/healthcare sub-area, timeframe, and number of papers reviewed—in Table 1. For example, one study reviewed awareness effect in type 2 diabetes published between 2001 and 2005, identifying 18 papers [11]. This current review literature is limited—most of the papers listed in Table 1 did not report the timeframe and/or number of papers reviewed (expressed as N/A).

Table 1. Characteristics of existing review/conceptual studies on the related topics.

Paper	Scope	Timeframe Considered	Number of Papers Reviewed
[11]	Awareness effect in type 2 diabetes	2001–2005	18
[12]	Fraud detection	N/A	N/A
[13]	Data mining techniques and guidelines for clinical medicine	N/A	N/A
[14]	Text mining, Ontologies	N/A	N/A
[15]	Challenges and future direction	N/A	N/A
[16]	Data mining algorithm, their performance in clinical medicine	1998–2008	84
[17]	Clinical medicine	N/A	N/A
[18]	Skin diseases	N/A	N/A
[19]	Clinical medicine	N/A	84
[20]	Algorithms, and guideline	N/A	N/A
[9]	Data mining process and algorithms	N/A	N/A
[21]	Algorithms for locally frequent disease in healthcare administration, clinical care and research, and training	N/A	N/A
[7]	Electronic Medical Record (EMR) and Visual analytics	N/A	N/A
[10]	Big data, Level of data usage	N/A	N/A

Table 1. *Cont.*

Paper	Scope	Timeframe Considered	Number of Papers Reviewed
[22]	MapReduce architectural framework based big data analytics	2007–2014	32
[23]	Big data analytics and its opportunities	N/A	N/A
[24]	Big data analytics in image processing, signal processing, and genomics	N/A	N/A
[25]	Social media data mining to detect Adverse Drug Reaction, Natural language processing techniques (NLP)	2004–2014	39
[26]	Text mining, Adverse Drug Reaction detection	N/A	N/A
[8]	Big data analytics in critical care	N/A	N/A
[27]	Methodology of big data analytics in healthcare	N/A	N/A
Our study	**Application and theoretical perspective of data mining and big data analytics in whole healthcare domain**	**2005–2016**	**117**

N/A represents Not Reported.

There is no comprehensive review available which presents the complete picture of data mining application in the healthcare industry. The existing reviews (16 out of 21) are either focused on a specific area of healthcare, such as clinical medicine (three reviews) [16,17,19], adverse drug reaction signal detection (two reviews) [25,26], big data analytics (four reviews) [8,10,22,24], or the application and performance of data mining algorithms (five reviews) [9,13,14,20,21]. Two studies focused on specific diseases (diabetes [11], skin diseases [18]). To the best of our knowledge, none of these studies present the universe of research that has been done in this field. These studies are also limited in the rigor of their methodology except for four articles [11,16,22,25], which provide key insights including the timeframe covered in the study, database search, and literature inclusion or exclusion criteria, but they are limited in their scope of topics covered (see Table 1).

Beyond condensing the applied literature, our review also adds to the body of theoretical reviews in the analytics literature. Current theoretical reviews are limited to methodological challenges and techniques to overcome those challenges [15,16,27] and application and impact of big data analytics in healthcare [23]. In summary, the current reviews listed in Table 1 lacks in (1) width of coverage in terms of application areas, (2) breadth of data mining techniques, (3) assessment of literature quality, and (4) systematic selection and analysis of papers. In this review, we aim to fill the above-mentioned gaps. We add to this literature by covering the applied and theoretical perspective of data mining and big data analytics in healthcare with a more comprehensive and systematic approach.

2. Methodology

The methodology of our review followed the checklist proposed by the Preferred Reporting Items for Systematic Reviews and Meta-Analyses (PRISMA) [28]. We assessed the quality of the selected articles using JBI Critical Appraisal Checklist for analytical cross sectional studies [29] and Critical Appraisal Skills Programme (CASP) qualitative research checklist [30].

2.1. Input Literature

Selected literature and their selection process for the review are described in this section. Initially a two phase advance keyword search was conducted on the database Web of Science and one phase (Phase 2) search in PubMed and Google Scholar with time filter 1 January 2005 to 31 December 2016 in "All Fields". Journal articles written in English was added as additional filters. Keywords listed in Table 2 were used in different phases. The complete search procedure was conducted using the following procedure:

- Inclusion criteria: The phase 1 search resulted in thousands of articles which was then narrowed down using the phase 2 keywords within the initial search space. Second phase resulted in 129 articles in Web of Science, and 5255 articles in PubMed. Search in Google Scholar search engine was conducted with phase 2 keywords which resulted in 700 articles. The title, abstract, and keywords of those articles were screened and those *discussing the application of data mining and big data in the healthcare decision-making process* were retained for full-text review. To make the screening process efficient, duplicate articles were removed at the eligibility phase instead of screening phase of the PRISMA review process (Figure 1).

- Exclusion criteria: This included articles reporting on results of: *qualitative study, survey, focus group study, feasibility study, monitoring device, team relationship measurement, job satisfaction, work environment, "what-if" analysis, data collection technique, editorials or short report, merely mention data mining, and articles not published in international journals.* Duplicates were removed (33 articles). Finally, 117 articles were retained for the review. Figure 1 provides a PRISMA [28] flow diagram of the review process and Supplementary Information File S1 (Table S1) provides the PRISMA checklist.

Table 2. Keywords for database search.

Phase	Keyword 1 (OR [1])		Keyword 2 (OR [1])
1	Healthcare, Health care	AND	Data analysis
2	Healthcare, Health care, Cancer [2], Disease, Genomics		Data mining, Big data

[1] A logical operator used between the keywords during database search. [2] Cancer was listed independently because other dominant associations have the word "disease" associated with them (i.e., heart disease, skin disease, mental disease etc.).

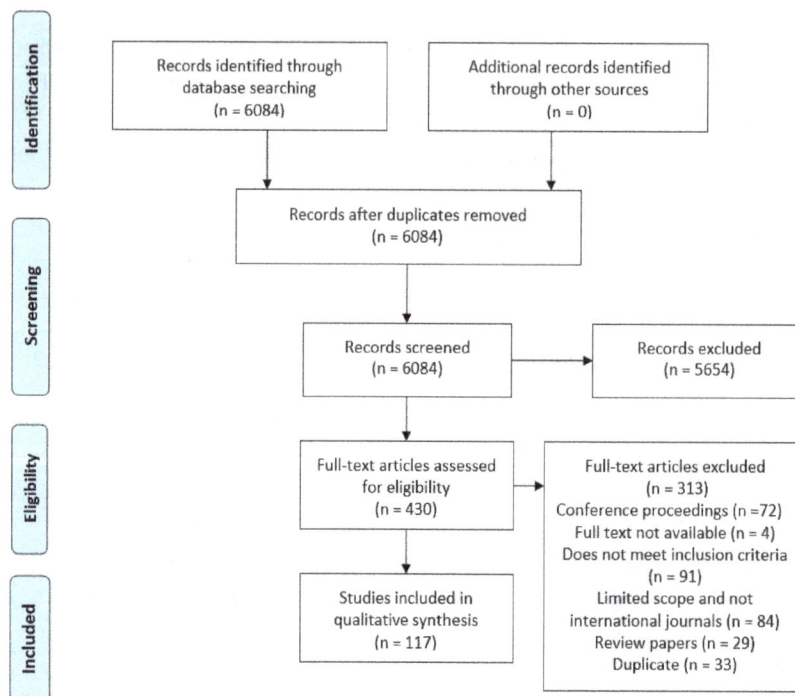

Figure 1. Preferred Reporting Items for Systematic Reviews and Meta-Analyses (PRISMA) flow chart [28] illustrating the literature search process.

2.2. Quality Assessment and Processing Steps

The full text of each of the 117 articles was reviewed separately by two researchers to eliminate bias [28]. To assess the quality of the cross sectional studies, we applied the JBI Critical Appraisal

Checklist for Analytical Cross Sectional Studies [29]. For theoretical papers, we applied the Critical Appraisal Skills Programme (CASP) qualitative research checklist [30]. We modified the checklist items, as not all items specified in the JBI or CASP checklists were applicable to studies on healthcare analytics (Supplementary Materials Table S2). We evaluated each article's quality based on inclusion of: (1) clear objective and inclusion criteria; (2) detailed description of sample population and variables; (3) data source (e.g., hospital, database, survey) and format (e.g., structured Electronic Medical Record (EMR), International Classification of Diseases code, unstructured text, survey response); (4) valid and reliable data collection; (5) consideration of ethical issues; (6) detailed discussion of findings and implications; (7) valid and reliable measurement of outcomes; and (8) use of an appropriate data mining tool for cross-sectional studies and (1) clear statement of aims; (2) appropriateness of qualitative methodology; (3) appropriateness of research design; (4) clearly stated findings; and (5) value of research for the theoretical papers. Summary characteristics from any study fulfilling these criteria were included in the final data aggregation (Supplementary Materials Table S3).

To summarize the body of knowledge, we adopted the three-step processing methodology outlined by Levy and Ellis [31] and Webster and Watson [32] (Figure 2). During the review process, information was extracted by identifying and defining the problem, understanding the solution process and listing the important findings ("Know the literature"). We summarized and compared each article with the articles associated with the similar problems ("Comprehend the literature"). This simultaneously ensured that any irrelevant information was not considered for the analysis. The summarized information was stored in a spreadsheet in the form of a concept matrix as described by Webster and Watson [32]. We updated the concept matrix periodically, after completing every 20% of the articles which is approximately 23 articles, to include new findings ("Apply"). Based on the concept matrix, we developed a classification scheme (see Figure 3) for further comparison and contrast. We established an operational definition (see Table 3) for each class and same class articles were separated from the pool ("Analyze and Synthesis"). We compared classifications between researchers and we resolved disagreements (on six articles) by discussion. The final classification provided distinguished groups of articles with summary, facts, and remarks made by the reviewers ("Evaluate").

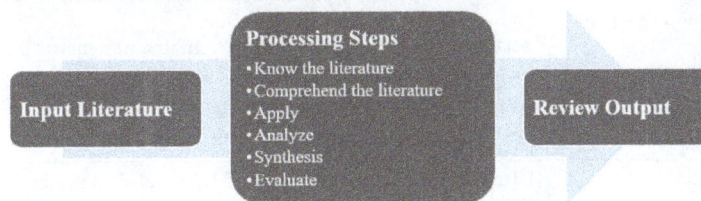

Figure 2. Three stages of effective literature review process, adapted from Levy and Ellis [31].

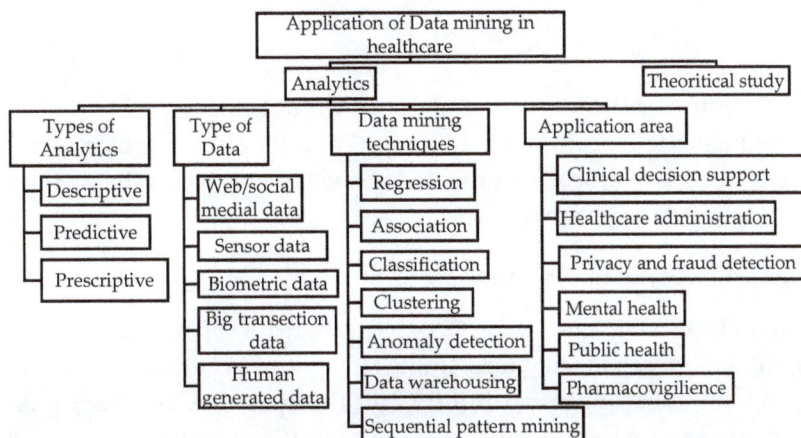

Figure 3. Classification scheme of the literature.

Table 3. Operational definition of the classes.

Class	Operational Definition *
Analytics	Knowledge discovery by analyzing, interpreting, and communicating data
3A. Types of Analytics	Data Interpretation and Communication method
• Descriptive	Exploration and discovery of information in the dataset [33]
• Predictive	Prediction of upcoming events based on historical data [22]
• Prescriptive	Utilization of scenarios to provide decision support [22]
3B. Types of Data	Type or nature of data used in the study
• Web/social media data (WS)	Data extracted from websites, blogs, social media like Facebook, Twitter, LinkedIn [23]
• Sensor data (SD)	Readings from medical devices and sensors [23]
• Biometric data (BM)	"Finger prints, genetics, handwriting, retinal scans, X-ray and other medical images, blood pressure, pulse and pulse-oximetry readings, and other similar types of data" [23]
• Big transection data (BT)	Healthcare bill, insurance claims and transections [23]
• Human generated data (HG)	Semi-structured and unstructured documents like prescription, Electronic Medical Record (EMR), notes and emails [23]
3C. Data mining techniques	Techniques applied to extract and communicate information from the dataset
• Regression	Relationship estimation between variables
• Association	Finding relation between variables
• Classification	Mapping to predefined class based on shared characteristics
• Clustering	Identification of groups and categories in data
• Anomaly detection	Detection of out-of-pattern events or incidents
• Data warehousing	A large storage of data to facilitate decision-making
• Sequential pattern mining	Identification of statistically significant patterns in a sequence of data
3D. Application Area	Different areas in healthcare where data mining is applied for knowledge discovery and/or decision support
• Clinical decision support	Analytics applied to analyze, extract and communicate information about diseases, risk for clinical use
• Healthcare administration	Application of analytics to improve quality of care, reduce the cost of care and to improve overall system dynamics
• Privacy and fraud detection	Privacy: Protection of patient identity in the dataset; Fraud detection: Deceptive and unauthorized activity detection
• Mental health	Analytical decision support for psychiatric patients or patient with mental disorder
• Public health	Analysis of problems which affect a mass population, a region, or a country
• Pharmacovigilance	Post market monitoring of Adverse Drug Reaction (ADR)
3E. Theoretical study	Discusses impact, challenges, and future of data mining and big data analytics in healthcare

* Most of the definitions listed in this table are well established in literature and well know. Therefore, we did not use any specific reference. However, for some classes, specifically for types of analytics and data, varying definitions are available in the literature. We cited the sources of those definitions.

2.3. Results

The network diagram of selected articles and the keywords listed by authors in Figure 4 represents the outcome of the methodological review process. We elaborate on the resulting output in the subsequent sections using the structure of the developed classification scheme (Figure 3). We also report the potential future research areas.

2.3.1. Methodological Quality of the Studies

Out of 117 papers included in this review, 92 applied analytics and 25 were qualitative/conceptual. The methodological quality of the analytical studies (92 out of 117) were evaluated by a modified version of 8 yes/no questions suggested in JBI Critical Appraisal Checklist for Analytical Cross Sectional Studies [29]. Each question contains 1 point (1 if the answer is Yes or 0 for No). The score achieved by each paper is provided in the final column of Supplementary Materials Table S3. On average, each paper applying analytics scored 7.6 out of 8, with a range of 6–8 points. Major drawbacks were the absence of data source and performance measure of data mining algorithms. Out of 92 papers, 23 did not evaluate or mention the performance of the applied algorithms and eight did not mention the source of the data. However, all the papers in healthcare analytics had a clear objective and a detailed discussion of sample population and variables. Data used in each paper was either de-identified/anonymized or approved by institute's ethical committee to ensure patient confidentiality.

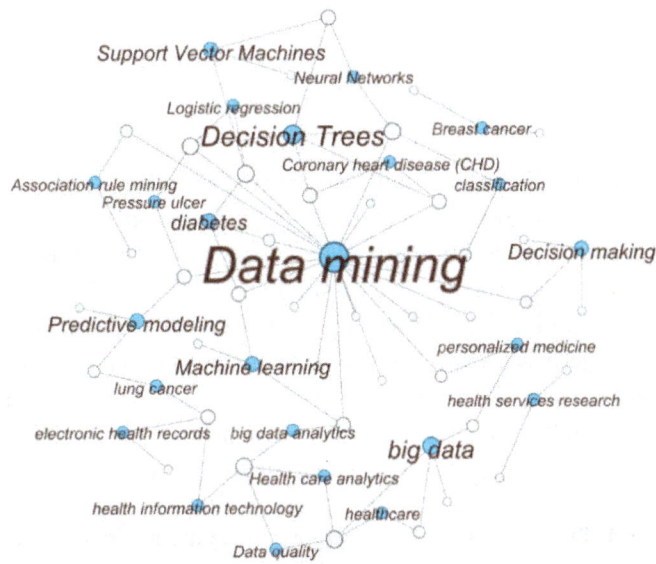

Figure 4. Visualization of high-frequency keywords of the reviewed papers. The white circles symbolize the articles and the blue circles represent keywords. The keywords that occurred only once are eliminated as well as the corresponding articles. The size of the blue circles and the texts represent how often that keyword is found. The size of the white circles is proportional to the number of keywords used in that article. The links represents the connections between the keywords and the articles. For example, if a blue circle has three links (e.g., Decision-Making) that means that keyword was used in three articles. The diagram is created with the open source software Gephi [34].

We applied the Critical Appraisal Skills Programme (CASP) qualitative research checklist [30] to evaluate the quality of the 25 theoretical papers. Five questions (out of ten) in that checklist were not applicable to the theoretical studies. Therefore, we evaluated the papers in this section in a five-point scale (1 if the answer is Yes or 0 for No). Papers included in this review showed high methodological quality as 21 papers (out of 25) scored 5. The last column in the Supplementary Materials Table S3 provides the score achieved by individual papers.

2.3.2. Distribution by Publication Year

The distribution of articles published related to data mining and big data analytics in healthcare across the timeline of the study (2005–2016) is presented in Figure 5. The distribution shows an upward trend with at least two articles in each year and more than ten articles in the last four years. Additionally, this trend represents the growing interest of government agencies, healthcare practitioners, and academicians in this interdisciplinary field of research. We anticipate that the use of analytics will continue in the coming years to address rising healthcare costs and need of improved quality of care.

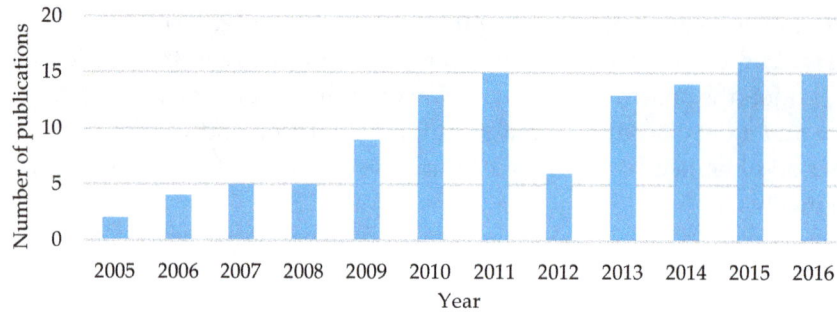

Figure 5. Distribution of publication by year (117 articles).

2.3.3. Distribution by Journal

Articles published in 74 different journals were included in this study. Table 4 lists the top ten journals in terms of number of papers published. *Expert System with Application* was the dominant source of literature on data mining application in healthcare with 7 of the 117 articles. Journals were interdisciplinary in nature and spanned computational journals like *IEEE Transection on Information Technology in Biomedicine* to policy focused journal like *Health Affairs*. Articles published in *Expert System with Application, Journal of Medical Systems, Journal of the American Medical Informatics Association, Healthcare Informatics Research* were mostly related to analytics applied in clinical decision-making and healthcare administration. On the other hand, articles published in *Health Affairs* were predominantly conceptual in nature addressing policy issues, challenges, and potential of this field.

Table 4. Top 10 journals on application of data mining in healthcare.

	Journal	Number of Articles
1.	Expert Systems with Applications	7
2.	IEEE Transection on Information Technology in Biomedicine	6
3.	Journal of Medical Internet Research	5
4.	Journal of Medical Systems	4
5.	Journal of the American Medical Informatics Association	4
6.	Health Affairs	4
7.	Journal of Biomedical Informatics	4
8.	Healthcare Informatics Research	3
9.	Journal of Digital Imaging	3
10.	PLoS ONE	3

3. Healthcare Analytics

Out of 117 articles, 92 applied analytics for decision-making in healthcare. We discuss the types of analytics, the application area, the data, and the data mining techniques used in these articles and summarize them in Supplementary Materials Table S4.

3.1. Types of Analytics

We identified three types of analytics in the literature: descriptive (i.e., exploration and discovery of information in the dataset), predictive (i.e., prediction of upcoming events based on historical data) and prescriptive (i.e., utilization of scenarios to provide decision support). Five of the 92 studies employed both descriptive and predictive analytics. In Figure 6, which displays the percentage of healthcare articles using each analytics type, we show that descriptive analytics is the most commonly used in healthcare (48%). Descriptive analytics was dominant in all the application areas except in clinical decision support. Among the application areas, pharmacovigilance studies only used descriptive analytics as this application area is focused on identifying an association between adverse drug effects with medication. Predictive analytics was used in 43% articles. Among application areas, clinical decision support had the highest application of predictive analytics as many studies in this area are involved in risk and morbidity prediction of chest pain, heart attack, and other diseases. In contrast, use of prescriptive analytics was very uncommon (only 9%) as most of these studies were focused on either a specific population base or a specific disease scenario. However, some evidence of prescriptive analytics was found in public healthcare, administration, and mental health (see Supplementary Materials Table S4). These studies create a data repository and/or analytical platform to facilitate decision-making for different scenarios.

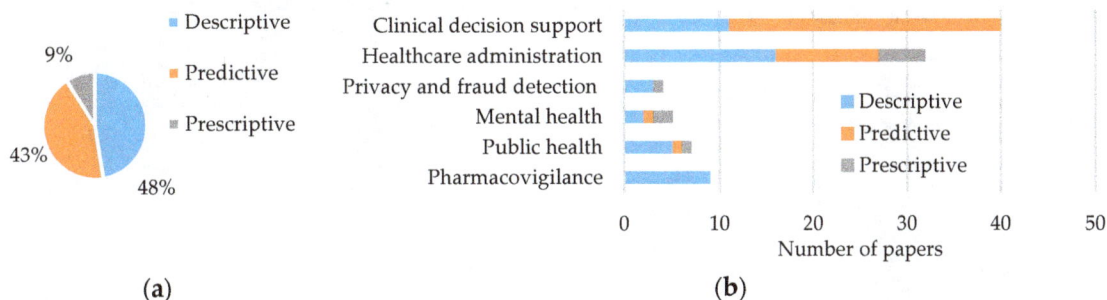

Figure 6. Types of analytics used in literature. (**a**) Percentage of analytics type; (**b**) Analytics type by application area.

3.2. Types of Data

To identify types of data, we adopted the classification scheme identified by Raghupathi and Raghupathi [23] which takes into account the nature (i.e., text, image, number, electronic signal), source, and collection method of data together. Table 3 provides the operational definitions of taxonomy adopted in this paper. Figure 7a presents the percentage of data type used and Figure 7b, the number of usage by application area. As expected, human generated (HG) data, including EMR, Electronic Health Record (HER), and Electronic Patient Record (EPR), is the most commonly (77%) used form. Web or Social media (WS) data is the second dominant (11%) type of data, as increasingly more people are using social media now and ongoing digital revolution in the healthcare sector [35]. In addition, recent development in Natural Language Processing (NLP) techniques is making the use of WS data easier than before [36]. The other three types of data (SD, BT, and BM) consist of only about 12% of total data usage, but popularity and market growth of wearable personal health tracking devices [37] may increase the use of SD and BM data.

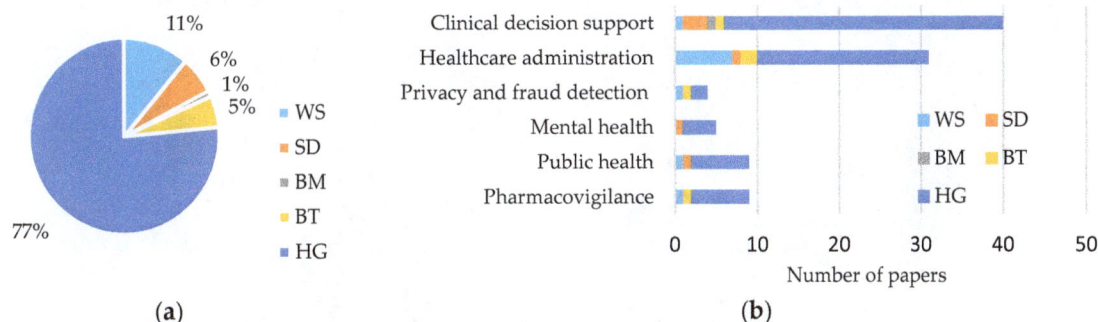

Figure 7. Percentage of data type used (**a**) and type of data used by application area (**b**).

3.3. Data Mining Techniques

Data mining techniques used in the articles reviewed include classification, clustering, association, anomaly detection, sequential pattern mining, regression, and data warehousing. While elaborate description of each technique and available algorithms is out of scope of this review, we report the frequency of each technique and its sector wise distribution in Figure 8a,b, respectively. Among the articles included in the review, 57 used classification techniques to analyze data. Association and clustering were used in 21 and 18 articles, respectively. Use of other techniques was less frequent.

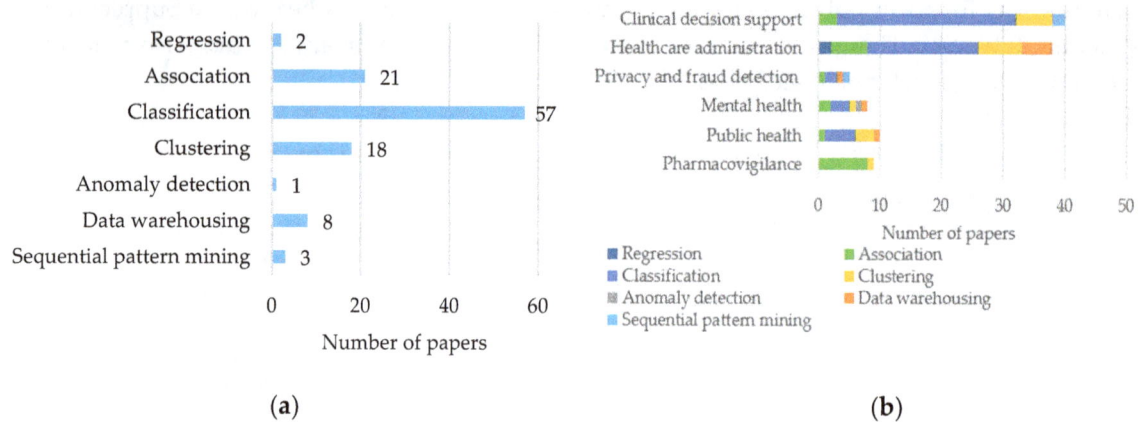

(a)   **(b)**

Figure 8. Utilization of data mining techniques, (**a**) by percentage and (**b**) by application area.

A high proportion (8 out of 9) of pharmacovigilance papers used association. Use of classification was dominant in every sector except pharmacovigilance (Figure 8b). Data warehousing was mostly used in healthcare administration (Figure 8b).

We delved deeper into classification as it was utilized in the majority (57 out of 92) of the papers. There are a number of algorithms used for classification, which we present in a word cloud in Figure 9. Support Vector Machine (SVM), Artificial Neural Network (ANN), Logistic Regression (LR), Decision Tree (DT), and DT based algorithms were the most commonly used. Random Forest (RF), Bayesian Network and Fuzzy-based algorithms were also often used. Some papers (three papers) introduced novel algorithms for specific applications. For example, Yeh et al. [38] developed discrete particle swarm optimization based classification algorithm to classify breast cancer patients from a pool of general population. Self-organizing maps and K-means were the most commonly used clustering algorithm in healthcare. Performance (e.g., accuracy, sensitivity, specificity, area under the ROC curve, positive predictive value, negative predictive value etc.) of each of these algorithms varied by application and data type. We recommend applying multiple algorithms and choosing the one which achieves the best accuracy.

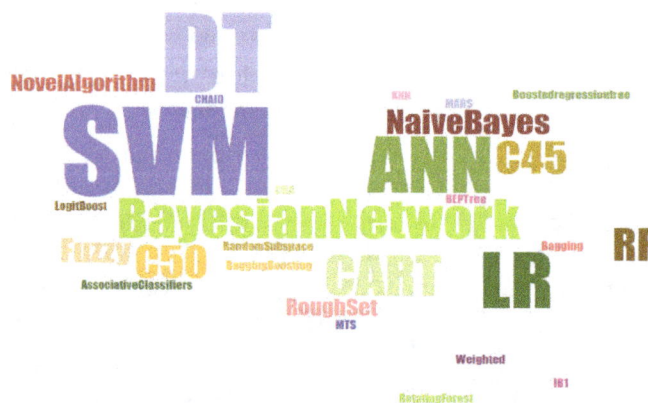

Figure 9. Word cloud [39] with classification algorithms.

4. Application of Analytics in Healthcare

Table 3 provides the operational definitions of the six application areas (i.e., clinical decision support, healthcare administration, privacy and fraud detection, mental health, public health, and pharmacovigilance) identified in this review. Figure 10 shows the percentage of articles in each area. Among different classes in healthcare analytics, data mining application is mostly applied in clinical decision support (42%) and administrative purposes (32%). This section discusses the application of data mining in these areas and identifies the main aims of these studies, performance gaps, and key features.

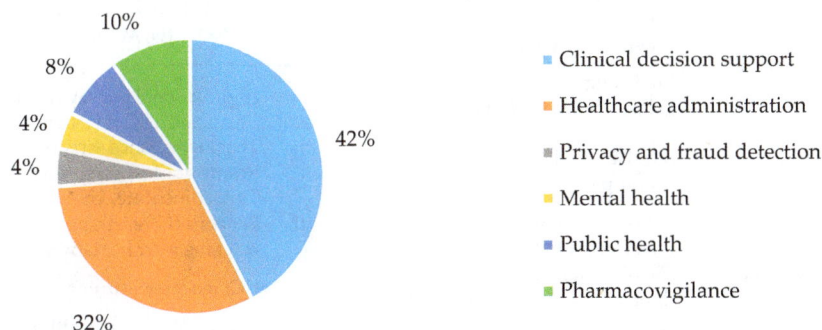

Figure 10. Percentage of papers utilized healthcare analytics by application area (92 articles out of 117).

4.1. Clinical Decision Support

Clinical decision support consists of descriptive and/or predictive analysis mostly related to cardiovascular disease (CVD), cancer, diabetes, and emergency/critical care unit patients. Some studies developed novel data mining algorithms which we review. Table 5 describes the topics investigated and data sources used by papers using clinical decision-making, organized by major diseases category.

Table 5. Topics and data sources of papers using clinical decision-making, organized by major disease category.

Reference	Major Disease	Topic Investigated	Data Source
[40]		Risk factors associated with Coronary heart disease (CHD)	Department of Cardiology, at the Paphos General Hospital in Cyprus
[41]		Diagnosis of CHD	Invasive Cardiology Department, University Hospital of Ioannina, Greece
[42]	Cardiovascular disease (CVD)	Classification of uncertain and high dimensional heart disease data	UCI machine learning laboratory repository
[43]		Risk prediction of Cardiovascular adverse event	U.S. Midwestern healthcare system
[44]		Cardiovascular event risk prediction	HMO Research Network Virtual Data Warehouse
[45]		Mobile based cardiovascular abnormality detection	MIT BIH ECG database
[46]		Management of infants with hypoplastic left heart syndrome	The University of Iowa Hospital and Clinics

Table 5. *Cont.*

Reference	Major Disease	Topic Investigated	Data Source
[47]		Identification of pattern in temporal data of diabetic patients	Synthetic and real world data (not specified)
[48]		Exploring the examination history of Diabetic patients	National Health Center of Asti Providence, Italy
[49]	Diabetes	Important factors to identify type 2 diabetes control	The Ulster Hospital, UK
[50]		Comparison of classification accuracy of algorithms for diabetes	Iranian national non-communicable diseases risk factors surveillance
[51]		Type 2 diabetes risk prediction	Independence Blue Cross Insurance Company
[52]		Evaluation of HTCP algorithm in classifying type 2 diabetes patients from non-diabetic patient	Olmsted Medical Center and Mayo Clinic in Rochester, Minnesota, USA
[53]		Predicting and risk diagnosis of patients for being affected with diabetes.	1991 National Survey of Diabetes data
[54]		Survival prediction of prostate cancer patients	The Surveillance, Epidemiology, and End Results (SEER) Program of the National Cancer Institute, USA
[38]		Classification of breast cancer patients with novel algorithm	Wisconsin Breast cancer data set, UCI machine learning laboratory repository
[42]	Cancer	Classification of uncertain and high dimensional breast cancer data	UCI machine learning laboratory repository
[55]		Visualization tool for cancer	Taiwan National Health Insurance Database
[56]		Lung cancer survival prediction with the help of a predictive outcome calculator	SEER Program of the National Cancer Institute, USA
[57]	Emergency Care	Classification of chest pain in emergency department	Hospital (unspecified) emergency department EMR
[58]		Grouping of emergency patients based on treatment pattern	Melbourne's teaching metropolitan hospital
[59]	Intensive care	Mortality rate of ICU patients	University of Kentucky Hospital
[60]		Prediction of 30 day mortality of ICU patients	MIMIC-II database
[61]		Treatment plan in respiratory infection disease	Various health center throughout Malaysia
[62]		Pressure ulcer prediction	Cathy General Hospital (06–07), Taiwan
[63]		Pressure ulcer risk prediction	Military Nursing Outcomes Database (MilNOD), US
[64]		Association of medication, laboratory and problem	Brigham and Women's Hospital, US
[65]		Chronic disease (asthma) attack prediction	Blue Angel 24 h Monitoring System, Tainan; Environmental Protection Administration Executive, Yuan; Central Weather Bureau Tainan, Taiwan
[66]		Personalized care, predicting future disease	No specified
[67]		Correlation between disease	Sct. Hans Hospital
[68]	Other applications	Glaucoma prediction using Fundus image	Kasturba Medical college, Manipal, India
[69]		Reducing follow-up delay from image analysis	Department of Veterans Affairs health-care facilities
[70]		Disease risk prediction in imbalanced data	National Inpatient Sample (NIS) data, available at http://www.ahrq.gov by Healthcare Cost and Utilization Project (HCUP)
[71]		Survivalist prediction of kidney disease patients	University of Iowa Hospital and Clinics
[72]		Comparison surveillance techniques for health care associated infection	University of Alabama at Birmingham Hospital
[73]		Parkinson disease prediction based on big data analytics	Big data archive by Parkinson's Progression Markers Initiative (PPMI)
[74]		Hospitalization prediction of Hemodialysis patients	Hemodialysis center in Taiwan
[75]		5 year Morbidity prediction	Northwestern Medical Faculty Foundation (NMFF)
[76]		Algorithm development for real-time disease diagnosis and prognosis	Not specified

4.1.1. Cardiovascular Disease (CVD)

CVD is one of the most common causes of death globally [45,77]. Its public health relevance is reflected in the literature—it was addressed by seven articles (18% of articles in clinical decision support).

Risk factors related to Coronary Heart Disease (CHD) were distilled into a decision tree based classification system by researchers [40]. The authors investigated three events: Coronary Artery Bypass Graft Surgery (CABG), Percutaneous Coronary Intervention (PCI), and Myocardial Infarction (MI). They developed three models: CABG vs. non-CABG, PCI vs. non-PCI, and MI VS non-MI. The risk factors for each event were divided into four groups in two stages. The risk factors were separated into before and after the event at the 1st stage and modifiable (e.g., smoking habit or blood pressure) and non-modifiable (e.g., age or sex) at the 2nd stage for each group. After classification, the most important risk factors were identified by extracting the classification rules. The Framingham equation [78]—which is widely used to calculate global risk for CHD was used to calculate the risk for each event. The most important risk factors identified were age, smoking habit, history of hypertension, family history, and history of diabetes. Other studies on CHD show similar results [79–81]. This study had implications for healthcare providers and patients by identifying risk factors to specifically target, identify and in the case of modifiable factors, reduce CHD risk [40].

Data mining has also been applied to diagnose Coronary Artery Disease (CAD) [41]. Researchers showed that in lieu of existing diagnostic methods (i.e., Coronary Angiography (CA))—which are costly and require high technical skill—data mining using existing data like demographics, medical history, simple physical examination, blood tests, and noninvasive simple investigations (e.g., heart rate, glucose level, body mass index, creatinine level, cholesterol level, arterial stiffness) is simple, less costly, and can be used to achieve a similar level of accuracy. Researchers used a four-step classification process: (1) Decision tree was used to classify the data; (2) Crisp classification rules were generated; (3) A fuzzy model was created by fuzzifying the crisp classifier rules; and (4) Fuzzy model parameters were optimized and the final classification was made. The proposed optimized fuzzy model achieved 73% of prediction accuracy and improved upon an existing Artificial Neural Network (ANN) by providing better interpretability.

Traditional data mining and machine learning algorithms (e.g., probabilistic neural networks and SVM) may not be advanced enough to handle the data used for CVD diagnosis, which is often uncertain and highly dimensional in nature. To tackle this issue, researchers [42] proposed a Fuzzy standard additive model (SAM) for classification. They used adaptive vector quantization clustering to generate unsupervised fuzzy rules which were later optimized (minimized the number of rules) by Genetic Algorithm (GA). They then used the incremental form of a supervised technique, Gradient Descent, to fine tune the rules. Considering the highly time consuming process of the fuzzy system given large number of features in the data, the number of features was reduced with wavelet transformation. The proposed algorithm achieved better accuracy (78.78%) than the probabilistic neural network (73.80%), SVM (74.27%), fuzzy ARTMAP (63.46%), and adaptive neuro-fuzzy inference system (74.90%). Another common issue in cardiovascular event risk prediction is the censorship of data (i.e., the patient's condition is not followed up after they leave hospital and until a new event occurs; the available data becomes right-censored). Elimination and exclusion of the censored data create bias in prediction results. To address the censorship of the data in their study on CVD event risk prediction after time, two studies [43,44] used Inverse Probability Censoring Weighting (IPCW). IPCW is a pre-processing step used to calculate the weights on data which are later classified using Bayesian Network. One of these studies [43] provided an IPCW based system which is compatible with any machine learning algorithm.

Electrocardiography (ECG)—non-invasive measurement of the electrical activity of the heartbeat—is the most commonly used medical studies in the assessment of CVD. Machine learning offers potential optimization of traditional ECG assessment which requires decompressing before making any diagnosis. This process takes time and large space in computers. In one study, researchers [45] developed a framework for real-time diagnosis of cardiovascular abnormalities based on compressed ECG. To reduce diagnosis time—which is critical for clinical decision-making regarding appropriate and timely treatment—they proposed and tested a mobile based framework and applied it to wireless monitoring of the patient. The ECG was sent to the hospital server where the ECG signals were divided into normal and abnormal clusters. The system detected cardiac abnormality with 97% accuracy. The cluster information was sent to patient's mobile phone; and if any life-threatening abnormality was detected, the mobile phone alerted the hospital or the emergency personnel.

Data analytics have also been applied to more rare CVDs. One study [46] developed an intervention prediction model for Hypoplastic Left Heart Syndrome (HLHS). HLHS is a rare form of fatal heart disease in infants, which requires surgery. Post-surgical evaluation is critical as patient condition can shift very quickly. Indicators of wellness of the patients are not easily or directly measurable, but inferences can be made based on measurable physiological parameters including pulse, heart rhythm, systemic blood pressure, common atrial filling pressure, urine output, physical exam, and systemic and mixed venous oxygen saturations. A subtle physiological shift can cause death if not noticed and intervened upon. To help healthcare providers in decision-making, the researchers developed a prediction model by identifying the correlation between physiological parameters and interventions. They collected 19,134 records of 17 patients in Pediatric Intensive Care Units (PICU). Each record contained different physiological parameters measured by devices and noted by nurses. For each record, a wellness score was calculated by the domain experts. After classifying the data using a rough set algorithm, decision rules were extracted for each wellness score to aid in making intervention plans. A new measure for feature selection—Combined Classification Quality (CCQ)—was developed by considering the effect of variations in a feature values and distinct outcome each feature value leads to. Authors showed that higher value of CCQ leads to higher classification accuracy which is not always true for commonly used measure classification quality (CQ). For example, two features with CQ value of 1 leads to very different classification accuracy—35.5% and 75%. Same two features had CCQ value 0.25 and 0.40, features with 0.40 CCQ produced 75% classification accuracy. By using CCQ instead of CQ, researchers can avoid such inconsistency.

4.1.2. Diabetes

The disease burden related to diabetes is high and rising in every country. According to the World Health Organization's (WHO) prediction, it will become the seventh leading cause of death by 2030 [82]. Data mining has been applied to identify rare forms of diabetes, identify the important factors to control diabetes, and explore patient history to extract knowledge. We reviewed 7 studies that applied healthcare analytics to diabetes.

Researchers extracted knowledge about diabetes treatment pathways and identified rare forms and complications of diabetes using a three level clustering framework from examination history of diabetic patients [48]. In this three-level clustering framework, the first level clustered patients who went through regular tests for monitoring purposes (e.g., checkup visit, glucose level, urine test) or to diagnose diabetes-related complications (e.g., eye tests for diabetic retinopathy). The second level explored patients who went through diagnosis for specific or different diabetic complications only (e.g., cardiovascular, eye, liver, and kidney related complications). These two level produced 2939 outliers out of 6380 patients. At the third level, authors clustered these outlier patients to gain insight about rare form of diabetes or rare complications. A density based clustering algorithm, DBSCAN, was used for clustering as it doesn't require to specify the number of clusters apriori and is less sensitive to noise and outliers. This framework for grouping patients by treatment pathway can be utilized to evaluate treatment plans and costs. Another group of researchers [49] investigated the important factors related to type 2 diabetes control. They used feature selection via supervised model construction (FSSMC) to select the important factors with rank/order. They applied naïve bayes, IB1 and C4.5 algorithm with FSSMC technique to classify patients having poor or good diabetes control and evaluate the classification efficiency for different subsets of features. Experiments performed with physiological and laboratory information collected from 3857 patients showed that the classifier algorithms performed best (1–3% increase in accuracy) with the features selected by FSSMC. Age, diagnosis duration, and Insulin treatment were the top three important factors.

Data analytics have also been applied to identify patients with type 2 diabetes. In one study [52], using fragmented data from two different healthcare centers, researchers evaluated the effect of data fragmentation on a high throughput clinical phenotyping (HTCP) algorithm to identify patients at risk of developing type 2 diabetes. When a patient visits multiple healthcare centers during a study period, his/her data is stored in different EMRs and is called fragmented. In such cases, using HTPC algorithm can lead to improper classification. An experiment performed in a rural setting showed that using data from two healthcare centers instead of one decreased the false negative rate from 32.9% to 0%. In another study, researchers [51] utilized sparse logistic regression to predict type 2 diabetes risk from insurance claims data. They developed a model that outperformed the traditional risk prediction methods for large data sets and data sets with missing value cases by increasing the AUC value from 0.75 to 0.80. The dataset contained more than 500 features including demography, specific medical conditions, and comorbidity. And in another study, researchers [53] developed prediction and risk diagnosis model using a hybrid system with SVM. Using features like blood pressure, fasting blood sugar, two-hour post-glucose tolerance, cholesterol level along with other demographic and anthropometric features, the SVM algorithm was able to predict diabetes risk with 97% accuracy. One reason for achieving high accuracy compared to the study using insurance claims data [51] is the structured nature of the data which came from a cross-sectional survey on diabetes.

Different statistical and machine learning algorithms are available for classification purposes. Researchers [50] compared the performance of two statistical method (LR and Fisher linear discriminant analysis) and four machine learning algorithms (SVM (using radial basis function kernel), ANN, Random Forest, and Fuzzy C-mean) for predicting diabetes diagnosis. Ten features (age, gender, BMI, waist circumference, smoking, job, hypertension, residential region (rural/urban), physical activity, and family history of diabetes) were used to test the classification performance (diabetes or no diabetes). Parameters for ANN and SVM were optimized through Greedy search. SVM showed best performance in all performance measures. SVM was at least 5% more accurate than other classification techniques. Statistical methods performed similar to the other machine learning algorithms. This study was limited by a low prevalence of diabetes in the dataset, however, which can cause poor classification performance. Researchers [47] also proposed a novel pattern recognition algorithm by using convolutional nonnegative matrix factorization. They considered a patient as an entity and each of patients' visit to the doctor, prescriptions, test result, and diagnosis are considered as an event over time. Finding such patterns can be helpful to group similar patients, identify their treatment pathway as well as patient management. Though they did not compare the pattern recognition accuracy with existing methods like single value decomposition (SVD), the matrix-like representation makes it intuitive.

4.1.3. Cancer

Cancer is another major threat to public health [83]. Machine learning has been applied to cancer patients to predict survival, and diagnosis. We reviewed five studies that applied healthcare analytics to cancer.

Despite many advances in treatment, accurate prediction of survival in patients with cancer remains challenging considering the heterogeneity of cancer complexity, treatment options, and patient population. Survival of prostate cancer patients has been predicted using a classification model [54]. The model used a public database-SEER (Surveillance, Epidemiology, and End Result) and applied a stratified ten-fold sampling approach. Survival prediction among prostate cancer patients was made using DT, ANN and SVM algorithm. SVM outperformed other algorithms with 92.85% classification accuracy wherein DT and ANN achieved 90% and 91.07% accuracy respectively. This same database has been used to predict survival of lung cancer patients [56]. After preprocessing the 11 features available in the data set, authors identified two features (1. removed and examined regional lymph node count and 2. malignant/in-situ tumor count) which had the strongest predictive power. They used several supervised classification methods on the preprocessed data; ensemble voting of five decision tree based classifiers and meta-classifiers (J48 DT, RF, LogitBoost, Random Subspace, and Alternating DT) provided the best performance—74% for 6 months, 75% for 9 months, 77% for 1 year, 86% for 2 years, and 92% for 5 years survival. Using this technique, they developed an online lung cancer outcome calculator to estimate the risk of mortality after 6 months, 9 months, 1 year, 2 years and 5 years of diagnosis.

In addition to predicting survival, machine learning techniques have also been used to identify patients with cancer. Among patients with breast cancer, researchers [38] have proposed a new hybrid algorithm to classify breast cancer patient from patients who do not have breast cancer. They used correlation and regression to select the significant features at the first stage. Then, at the second stage, they used discrete Particle Swarm Optimization (PSO) to classify the data. This hybrid algorithm was applied to Wisconsin Breast Cancer Data set available at UCI machine learning repository. It achieved better accuracy (98.71%) compared to a genetic algorithm (GA) (96.14%) [84] and another PSO-based algorithm (93.4%) [85].

Machine learning has also been used to identify the nature of cancer (benign or malignant) and to understand demographics related to cancer. Among patients with breast cancer, researchers [42] applied the Fuzzy standard additive model (SAM) with GA (discussed earlier in relation to CVD)-predicting the nature of breast cancer (benign or malignant). They used a UCI machine learning repository which was capable of classifying uncertain and high dimensional data with greater accuracy (by 1–2%). Researchers have also used big data [55] to create a visualization tool to provide a dynamic view of cancer statistics (e.g., trend, association with other diseases), and how they are associated with different demographic variables (e.g., age, sex) and other diseases (e.g., diabetes, kidney infection). Use of data mining provided a better understanding of cancer patients both at demographic and outcome level which in terms provides an opportunity of early identification and intervention.

4.1.4. Emergency Care

The Emergency department (ED) is the primary route to hospital admission [58]. In 2011, 20% of US population had at least one or more visits to the ED [86]. EDs are experiencing significant financial pressure to increase efficiency and throughput of patients. Discrete event simulation (i.e., modeling system operations with sequence of isolated events) is a useful tool to understand and improve ED operations by simulating the behavior and performance of EDs. Certain features of the ED (e.g., different types of patients, treatments, urgency, and uncertainty) can complicate simulation. One way to handle the complexity is to group the patients according to required treatment. Previously, the "casemix" principle, which was developed by expert clinicians to groups of similar patients in case-specific settings (e.g., telemetry or nephrology units), was used, but it has limitations in the ED setting [58]. Researchers applied [58] data mining (clustering) to the ED setting to group the patients based on treatment pattern (e.g., full ward test, head injury observation, ECG, blood glucose, CT scan, X-ray). The clustering model was verified and validated by ED clinicians. These grouping data were then used in discrete event simulation to understand and improve ED operations (mainly length of stay) and process flows for each group.

Chest pain admissions to the ED have also been examined using decision-making framework. Researchers [57] proposed a three stage decision-making framework for classifying severity of chest pain as: AMI, angina pectoris, or other. At the first stage, lab tests and diagnoses were collected and the association between them were extracted. In the second stage, experts developed association rules between lab tests diagnosis to help physicians make quick diagnostic decisions based diagnostic tests and avoid further unnecessary lab tests. In the third stage, authors developed a classification tree to classify the chest pain diagnosis based on selected lab test, diagnosis and medical record. This hybrid model was applied to the emergency department at one hospital. They developed the classification system using 327 association rules to selected lab tests using C5.0, Neural Network (NN) and SVM. C5.0 algorithm achieved 94.18% accuracy whereas NN and SVM achieved 88.89% and 85.19% accuracy respectively.

4.1.5. Intensive Care

Intensive care units cater to patients with severe and life-threatening illness and injury which require constant, close monitoring and support to ensure normal bodily function. Death is a much more common event in an ICU compared to a general medical unit—one study showed that 22.4% of total death in hospitals occurred in the ICU [87]. Survival predictions and identification of important factors related to mortality can help healthcare providers plan care. We identified two papers [59,60] that developed prediction models for ICU mortality rate prediction. Using a large amount of ICU patient data (specifically from the first 24 h of the stay) collected from University of Kentucky Hospital from 1998 to 2007 (38,474 admissions), one group of researchers identified 15 out of 40 significant features using Pearson's Chi-square test (for categorical variables) and Student-t test (for continuous variable) [59]. The mortality rate was predicted by DT, ANN, SVM and APACHE III, a logistic regression based approach. Compared to the other methods applied, DT's AUC value was higher by 0.02. The study was limited, however, by only considering the first 24 h of admission to the ICU, which may not be enough to make prediction on mortality rate. Another team of researchers [60] applied a similarity metric to predict 30-day mortality prediction in 17,152 ICU admissions data extracted from MIMIC-II database [88]. Their analysis concluded that a large group of similar patient data (e.g., vital sign, laboratory test result) instead of all patient data would lead to slightly better prediction accuracy. The logistic regression model for mortality prediction achieved 0.83 AUC value when 5000 similar patients were used for training but, its performance declined to 0.81 AUC when all the available patient data were used.

4.1.6. Other Applications

In addition to CVD, diabetes, cancer, emergency care, and ICU care, data mining has been applied to various clinical decision-making problems like pressure ulcer risk prediction, general problem lists, and personalized medical care. To predict pressure ulcer formation (localized skin and tissue damage because of shear, friction, pressure or any combination of these factors), researchers [62] developed two classification-based predictive models. One included all 14 features (including age, sex, course, Anesthesia, body position during operation, and skin status) and another, reduced model, including significant features only (5 in DT model, 7 in SVM, LR and Mahalanobis Taguchi System model). Mahalanobis Taguchi System (MTS), SVM, DT, and LR were used for both classification and feature selection (in the second model only) purposes. LR and SVM performed slightly better when all the features were included, but MTS achieved better sensitivity and specificity in the reduced model (+10% to +15%). These machine learning techniques can provide better assistance in pressure ulcer risk prediction than the traditional Norton and Braden medical scale [62]. Though the study provides the advantages of using data mining algorithms, the data set used here was imbalanced as it only had 8 cases of pressure ulcer in 168 patients. Also among patients with pressure ulcers, another team of researchers [63] recommended a data mining based alternative to the Braden scale for prediction. They applied data mining algorithms to four years of longitudinal patient data to identify the most important factors related to pressure ulcer prediction (i.e., days of stay in the hospital, serum albumin, and age). In terms of C-statistics, RF (0.83) provided highest predictive accuracy over DT (0.63), LR (0.82), and multivariate adaptive regression splines (0.78).

For data mining algorithms, which often show poor performance with imbalanced (i.e., low occurrence of one class compared to other classes) data, researchers [70] developed a sub-sampling technique. They designed two experiments, one considered sub-sampling technique and another one did not. For a highly imbalanced data set, Random Forest (RF), SVM, and Bagging and Boosting achieved better classification accuracy with this sub-sampling technique in classifying eight diseases (male genital disease, testis cancer, encephalitis, aneurysm, breast cancer, peripheral atherosclerosis, and diabetes mellitus) that had less than 5% occurrences in the National Inpatient Sample (NIS) data of Healthcare Cost and Utilization Project (HCUP). Surprisingly, possibly due to balancing the dataset through sub-sampling, RF slightly outperformed (+0.01 AUC) the other two methods.

The patient problem list is a vital component of clinical medicine. It enables decision support and quality measurement. But, it is often incomplete. Researchers have [64] suggested that a complete list of problems leads to better quality treatment in terms of final outcome [64]. Complete problem lists enable clinicians to get a better understanding of the issue and influence diagnostic reasoning. One group of researchers proposed a data mining model to find an association between patient problems and prescribed medications and laboratory tests which can act as a support to clinical decision-making [64]. Currently, domain experts spend a large amount of time for this purpose but, association rule mining can save both time and other resources. Additionally, consideration of unstructured data like doctor's and/or nurse's written comments and notes can provide additional information. These association rules can aid clinicians in preventing errors in diagnosis and reduce treatment complexity. For example, a set of problems and medications can co-occur frequently. If a clinician has knowledge about this relation, he/she can prescribe similar medications when faced with a similar set of problems. One group of researchers [61] developed an approach which achieved 90% accuracy in finding association between medications and problems, and 55% accuracy between laboratory tests and problems. Among outpatients diagnosed with respiratory infection, 92.79% were treated with drugs. Physicians could choose any of the 100,013 drugs available in the inventory. Moreover, in an attempt to examine the treatment plan patterns, they identified the 78 most commonly used drugs which could be prescribed, regardless of patient's complaints and demography. The classification model used to identify the most common drugs achieved 74.73% accuracy and most importantly found variables like age, race, gender, and complaints of patients were insignificant.

Personalized medicine—tailored treatment based on a patient's predicted response or risk of disease—is another venue for data mining algorithms. One group of researchers [66] used a big data framework to create personalized care system. One patient's medical history is compared with other available patient data. Based on that comparison, possibility of a disease of an individual was calculated. All the possible diseases were ranked from high risk to low risk diseases. This approach is very similar to how online giants Netflix and Amazon suggest movies and books to the customer [66]. Another group of researchers [67] used the Electronic Patient Records (EPR), which contains structured data (e.g., disease code) and unstructured data (e.g., notes and comments made by doctors and nurses at different stages of treatment) to develop personalized care. From the unstructured text data, the researchers extracted clinical terms and mapped them to an ontology. Using this mapped codes and existing structured data (disease code), they created a phenotypic profile for each patient. The patients were divided into different clusters (with 87.78% precision) based on the similarity of their phenotypic profile. Correlation of diseases were captured by counting the occurrences of two or more diseases in patient phenotype. Then, the protein/gene structure associated with the diseases was identified and a protein network was created. From the sharing of specific protein structure by the diseases, correlation was identified.

Among patients with asthma, researchers [65] used environmental and patient physiological data to develop a prediction model for asthma attack to give doctors and patients a chance for prevention. They used data from a home-care institute where patients input their physical condition online; and environmental data (air pollutant and weather data). Their data mining model involved feature selection through sequential pattern mining and risk prediction using DT and association rule mining. This model can make asthma attack risk prediction with 86.89% accuracy. Real implementation showed that patients found risk prediction helpful to avoid severe asthma attacks.

Among patients with Parkinson's disease, researchers [73] introduced a comprehensive end-to-end protocol for complex and heterogeneous data characterization, manipulation, processing, cleaning, analysis and validation. Specifically, the researchers used a Synthetic Minority Over-sampling Technique (SMOTE) to rebalance the data set. Rebalancing the dataset using SMOTE improved SVM's classification accuracy from 76% to 96% and AdaBoost's classification accuracy from 96% to 99%. Moreover, the study found that traditional statistical classification approaches (e.g., generalized linear model) failed to generate reliable predictions but machine learning-based classification methods performed very well in terms of predictive precision and reliability.

Among patients with kidney disease, researchers [71] developed a prediction model to forecast survival. Data collected from four facilities of University of Iowa Hospital and Clinics contains 188 patients with over 707 visits and features like blood pressure measures, demographic variables, and dialysis solution contents. Data was transformed using functional relation (i.e., the similarity between two or more features when two features have same values for a set of patients, they are combined to form a single feature) between the features. The data set was randomly divided into eight sub-sets. Sixteen classification rules were generated for the eight sub-sets using two classification algorithms—Rough Set (RS) and DT. Classes represented survival beyond three years, less than three years and undetermined. To make predictions, each classification rule (out of 16) had one vote and the majority vote decided the final predictive class. Transformed data increased predictive accuracy by 11% than raw data and DT (67% accuracy) performed better than RS (56% accuracy). The researchers suggested that this type of predictive analysis can be helpful in personalized treatment selection, resource allocation for patients, and designing clinical study. Among patients on kidney dialysis, another group of researchers [74] applied temporal pattern mining to predict hospitalization using biochemical data. Their result showed that amount of albumin—a type of protein float in blood—is the most important predictor of hospitalization due to kidney disease.

Among patients over 50 years of age, researchers [75] developed a data mining model to predict five years mortality using the EHR of 7463 patients. They used Ensemble Rotating Forest algorithm with alternating decision tree to classify the patients into two classes of life expectancy: (1) less than five years and (2) equal or greater than five years. Age, comorbidity count, previous record of hospitalization record, and blood urea nitrogen were a few of the significant features selected by correlation feature selection along with greedy stepwise search method. Accuracy achieved by this approach (AUC 0.86) was greater than the standard modified Charlson Index (AUC 0.81) and modified Walter Index (AUC 0.78). Their study showed that age, hospitalization prior the visit, and highest blood urea nitrogen were the most important factors for predicting five years morbidity. This five-year morbidity prediction model can be very helpful to optimally use resources like cancer screening for those patients who are more likely to be benefit from the resources.

Another group of researchers [76] addressed the limitations of existing software technology for disease diagnosis and prognosis, such as inability to handle data stream (DT), impractical for complex and large systems (Bayesian Network), exhaustive training process (NN). To overcome these restriction, authors proposed a decision tree based algorithm called "Very Fast Decision Tree (VFDT)". Comparison with a similar system developed by IBM showed that VFDT utilizes lesser amount of system resources and it can perform real time classification.

Researchers have also used data mining to optimize the glaucoma diagnosis process [68]. Traditional approaches including Optical Coherence Tomography, Scanning Laser Polarimetry (SLP), and Heidelberg Retina Tomography (HRT) scanning methods are costly. This group used Fundus image data which is less costly and classified patient as either normal or glaucoma patient using SVM classifier. Before classification, authors selected significant features by using Higher Order Spectra (HOS) and Discrete Wavelet Transform (DWT) method combined and separately. Several kernel functions for SVM—all delivering similar levels of accuracy—were applied. Their approach produced 95% accuracy in glaucoma prediction. For diagnostic evaluation of chest imaging for suspicion for malignancy, researchers [69] designed trigger criteria to identify potential follow-up delays. The developed trigger predicted the patients who didn't require follow-up evaluation. The analysis of the experiment result indicated that the algorithm to identify patients' delays in follow-up of abnormal imaging is effective with 99% sensitivity and 38% specificity.

Data mining has also been applied to [72] compare three metrics to identify health care associated infections—Catheter Associated Bloodstream Infections, Catheter Associated Urinary Tract Infections and Ventilator Associated Pneumonia. Researchers compared traditional surveillance using National Healthcare Safety Network methodology to data mining using MedMined Data Mining Surveillance (CareFusion Corporation, San Diego, CA, USA), and administrative coding using ICD-9-CM. Traditional surveillance proved to be superior than data mining in terms of sensitivity, positive predictive value and rate estimation.

Data mining has been used in 38 studies of clinical decision-making CVD (7 articles), diabetes (seven articles), cancer (five articles), emergency care (two articles), intensive care (two articles), and other applications (16 articles). Most of the studies developed predictive models to facilitate decision-making and some developed decision support system or tools. Authors often tested their models with multiple algorithms; SVM was at the top of that list and often outperformed other algorithms. However, 15 [38,40,42,45,47,51,54,56,58,60,61,66,73,74,76] of the studies did not incorporate expert opinion from doctors, clinician, or appropriate healthcare personals in building models and interpreting results (see the study characteristics in Supplementary Materials Table S3). We also noted that there is an absence of follow-up studies on the predictive models, and specifically, how the models performed in dynamic decision-making situations, if doctors and healthcare professionals comfortable in using these predictive models, and what are the challenges in implementing the models if any exist? Existing literature does not focus on these salient issues.

4.2. Healthcare Administration

Data mining was applied to administrative purposes in healthcare in 32% (29 articles) of the articles reviewed. Researchers have applied data mining to: data warehousing and cloud computing; quality improvement; cost reduction; resource utilization; patient management; and other areas. Table 6 provides a list of these articles with major focus areas, problems analyzed and the data source.

Table 6. Problem analyzed and data sources in healthcare administration.

Reference	Focusing Area	Problem Analyzed	Data Source
[89]		Developing a platform to analyze the causes of readmission	Emory Hospital, US
[90]	Data warehousing and cloud computing	Development of a clinical data warehouse and analytical tools for traditional Chinese medicine	Traditional Chinese Medicine hospitals/wards
[91]		Cloud and big data analytics based cyber-physical system for patient-centric healthcare applications and services	Not specified
[92]		Repository of radiology reports	Not specified
[93]		Creation of large data repository and knowledge discovery with unsupervised learning	University of Virginia University Health System
[94]		Development of a mobile application to gather, store and provide data for rural healthcare	Not specified

Table 6. *Cont.*

Reference	Focusing Area	Problem Analyzed	Data Source
[95]		Treatment error prevention to improve quality and reduce cost	National Taiwan University Hospital
[96]		Healthcare cost prediction	US health insurance company
[97]		Healthcare resource utilization by lung cancer patients	Medicare beneficiaries for 1999, US
[98]		Length of stay prediction of Coronary Artery Disease (CAD)	Rajaei Cardiovascular Medical and Research Center, Tehran, Iran
[99]	Healthcare cost, quality and resource utilization	Methodology for structured development of monitoring systems and a primary HC network resource allocation monitoring model	National Institute of Public Health; Health Care Institute, Celje; Slovenian Social Security Database, and Slovenian Medical Chamber
[100]		Assess the ability of regression tree boosting to risk-adjust health care cost predictions	Thomson Medstat's Commercial Claims and Encounters database.
[101]		Evidence based recommendation in prescribing drugs	Dalhousie University Medical Faculty
[102]		Efficient pathology ordering system	Pathology company in Australia
[103]		Identifying people with or without insurance based on demographic and socio-economic factors	Behavioral Risk Factor Surveillance System 2004 Survey Data
[104]		Predicting care quality from patient experience	English National Health Service website
[105]		Scheduling of patients	A south-east rural U.S. clinic
[106]		Care plan recommendation system	A community hospital in the Mid-West U.S.
[107]	Patient management	Examination of risk factors to predict persistent healthcare frequent attendance	Tampere Health Centre, Finland
[108]		Forecasting number of patient visit for administrative task	Health care center in Jaen, Spain
[109]		Critical factors related to fall	1000 bed hospital in Taiwan
[110]		Verification of structured data, and codes in EMR of fall related injuries from unstructured data	Veterans Health Administration database, US
[111]		Relation between medical school training and practice	Center for Medicare and Medicaid Service (CMS)
[112]		Analysis of physician reviews from online platform	Good Doctor Online health community
[113]		Evaluation of Key Performance Indicator (KPIs) of hospital	Greek National Health Systems for the year of 2013
[114]	Other applications	Post market performance evaluation of medical devices	HCUPNet data (2002–2011)
[115]		Feasibility of measuring drug safety alert response from HC professional's information seeking behavior	UpToDate, an online medical resource
[116]		Influencing factors of home healthcare service outcome	U.S. home and hospice care survey (2000)
[117]		Compilation of various data types for tracing, and analyzing temporal events and facilitating the use of NoSQL and cloud computing techniques	Taiwan's National Health Insurance Research Database (NHIRD)

4.2.1. Data Warehousing and Cloud Computing

Data warehousing [90] and cloud computing are used to securely and cost-effectively store the growing volume of electronic patient data [1] and to improve hospital outcomes including readmissions. To identify cause of readmission, researchers [89] developed an open source software—Analytic Information Warehouse (AIW). Users can design a virtual data model (VDM) using this software. Required data to test the model can be extracted in terms of a temporal ontology from the data warehouse and analysis can be performed using any standard analyzing tool. Another group of researchers took a similar approach to develop a Clinical Data Warehouse (CDW) for traditional Chinese medicine (TCM). The warehouse contains clinical information (e.g., symptoms, disease, and treatment) for 20,000 inpatients and 20,000 outpatients. Data was collected in a structured way using pre-specified ontology in electronic form. CDW provides an interface for online data mining, online analytical processing (OLAP) and network analysis to discover knowledge and provide clinical decision support. Using these tools, classification, association and network analysis between symptoms, diseases and medications (i.e., herbs) can be performed.

Apart from clinical purposes, data warehouses can be used for research, training, education, and quality control purposes. Such a data repository was created using the basic idea of Google search engine [92]. Users can pull the radiology report files by searching keywords like a simple google search following the predefined patient privacy protocol. Another data repository was created as a part of collaborative study between IBM and University of Virginia and its partner, Virginia Commonwealth University Health System was created [93]. The repository contains 667,000 patient record with 208 attributes. HealthMiner—a data mining package for healthcare created by IBM—was used to perform unsupervised analysis like finding associations, pattern and knowledge discovery. This study also showed the research benefits of this type of large data repository. Researchers [91] proposed a framework based on cloud computing and big data to unify data collected from different sources like public databases and personal health devices. The architecture was divided into 3 layers. The first layer unified heterogeneous data from different sources, the second layer provided storage support and facilitated data processing and analytics access, and the third layer provided result of analysis and platform for professionals to develop analytical tools. Some researchers [94] used mobile devices to collect personal health data. Users took part in a survey on their mobile devices and got a diagnosis report based on their health parameters input in the survey. Each survey data were saved in a cloud-based interface for effective storage and management. From user input stored in cloud, interactive geo-spatial maps were developed to provide effective data visualization facility.

4.2.2. Healthcare Cost, Quality and Resource Utilization

Ten articles applied data mining to cost reduction, quality improvement and resource utilization issues. One group of researchers predicted healthcare costs using an algorithmic approach [96]. They used medical claim data of 800,000 people collected by an insurance company over the period of 2004–2007. The data included diagnoses, procedures, and drugs. They used classification and clustering algorithms and found that these data mining algorithms improve the absolute prediction error more than 16%. Two prediction models were developed, one using both cost and medical information and the other used only cost information. Both models had similar accuracy on predicting healthcare costs but performed better than traditional regression methods. The study also showed that including medical information does not improve cost prediction accuracy. Risk-adjusted health care cost predictions, with diagnostic groups and demographic variables as inputs, have also been assessed using regression tree boosting [100]. Boosted regression tree and main effects linear models were used and fitted to predict current (2001) and prospective (2002) total health care costs per patient. The authors concluded that the combination of regression tree boosting and a diagnostic grouping scheme are a competitive alternative to commonly used risk-adjustment systems.

A sizable amount ($37.6 billion) of healthcare costs is attributable to medical errors, 45% of which stems from preventable errors [95]. To aid in physician decision-making and reduce medical errors, researchers [95] proposed a data mining-based framework-Sequential Clustering Algorithm. They identified patterns of treatment plans, tests, medication types and dosages prescribed for specific diseases, and other services provided to treat a patient throughout his/her stay in the hospital. The proposed framework was based on cloud computing so that the knowledge extracted from the data could be shared among hospitals without sharing the actual record. They proposed to share models using Virtual Machine (VM) images to facilitate collaboration among international institutions and prevent the threat of data leakage. This model was implemented in two hospitals, one in Taiwan and another in Mongolia. To identify best practices for specific diseases and prevent medical errors, another group of researchers [101] proposed a decision support system using information extraction from online documents through text and data mining. They focused on evidence based management, quality control, and best practice recommendations for medical prescriptions.

Length of Stay (LOS) is another important indicator of cost and quality of care. Accurate prediction of LOS can lead to efficient management of hospital beds and resources. To predict LOS for CAD patients, researchers [98] compared multiple models—SVM, ANN, DT and an ensemble algorithm, combing SVM, C5.0, and ANN. Ensemble algorithm and SVM produced highest accuracy, 95.9% and 96.4% respectively. In contrast, ANN was least accurate with 53.9% accuracy wherein DT achieved 83.5% accuracy. Anticoagulant drugs, nitrate drugs, and diagnosis were the top three predictors along with diastolic blood pressure, marital status, sex, presence of comorbidity, and insurance status.

To predict healthcare quality, researchers [104] used sentiment analysis (computationally categorizing opinions into categories like positive, negative and neutral) on patients' online comments about their experience. They found above 80% agreement between sentiment analysis from online forums and traditional paper based surveys on quality prediction (e.g., cleanliness, good behavior, recommendation). Proposed approach can be an inexpensive alternative to traditional surveys and reports to measure healthcare quality.

Identification of influential factors in insurance coverage using data mining can aid insurance providers and regulators to design targeted service, additional service or proper allocation of resources to increase coverage rates. To develop a classification model to identify health insurance coverage, researchers [103] used data mining techniques. Based on 23 socio-economic, lifestyle and demographic factors, they developed a classification model with two classes, Insured and uninsured. The model was solved by ANN and DT. ANN provided 4% more accuracy than DT in predicting health insurance coverage. Among the factors, income, employment status, education, and marital status were the most important predictive factors of insurance coverage.

Among patients with lung cancer, researchers [97] investigated healthcare resource utilization (i.e., the number of visits to the medical oncologists) characteristics. They used DT, ANN and LR separately and an ensemble algorithm combining DT and ANN which resulted in the greatest accuracy (60% predictive accuracy). DT was employed to identify the important predictive features (among demographics, diagnosis, and other medical information) and ANN for classification. Data mining revealed that the utilization of healthcare resources by lung cancer patients is "supply-sensitive and patient sensitive" where supply represents availability of resources in certain region and patient represents patient preference and comorbidity. A resource allocation monitoring model for better management of primary healthcare network has also been developed [99]. Researchers considered the primary-care network as a collection of hierarchically connected modules given that patients could visit multiple physicians and physicians could have multiple care location, which is an indication of imbalanced resource distribution (e.g., number of physicians, care locations). The first level of the hierarchy consisted of three modules: health activities, population, and health resources. The second level monitored the healthcare provider availability and dispersion. The third level considered the actual visits, physicians and their availability, accessibility, and unlisted (i.e., without any assigned physician) patients. The top level of this network conducted an overall assessment of the network and made allocation accordingly. This hierarchical model was developed for a specific region in Slovenia, however, it could be easily adapted for any other region.

Overuse of screening and tests by physicians also contributes to inefficiencies and excess costs [102]. Current practice in pathology diagnosis is limited by disease focus. As an alternative to disease based system, researchers [102] used data mining in cooperation with case-based reasoning to develop an evidence based decision support system to decrease the use of unnecessary tests and reduce costs.

4.2.3. Patient Management

Patient management involves activities related to efficient scheduling and providing care to patients during their stay in a healthcare institute. Researchers [105] developed an efficient scheduling system for a rural free clinic in the United States. They proposed a hybrid system where data mining was used to classify the patients and association rule mining was used to assign a "no-show" probability. Results obtained from data mining were used to simulate and evaluate different scheduling techniques. On the other hand, these schedules could be divided into visits with administrative purposes and medical purposes. Researchers [108] suggested that patients who visit the health center for administrative purposes take less time than the patients with medical reasons. They proposed a predictive model to forecast the number of visits for administrative purposes. Their model improved the scheduling system with time saving of 21.73% (660,538 min). In contrast to administrative information/task seeking patients, some patients come for medical care very frequently and consume a large percentage of clinical workload [107]. Identifying the risk factors for frequent visit to health centers can help in reducing cost and resource utilization. A study among 85 working age "frequent attenders" identified the primary risk factors using Bayesian classification technique. The risk factors are, "high body mass index, alcohol abstinence, irritable bowel syndrome, low patient satisfaction, and fear of death" [107].

Improving publicly reported patient safety outcomes is also critical to healthcare institutions. Falls are one such outcome and are the most common and costly source of injury during hospitalization [110]. Researchers [109] analyzed the important factors related to patient falls during hospitalization. First, the authors selected significant features by Chi-square test (10 features out of 72 fall related variables were selected) and then applied ANN to develop a predictive model which achieves 0.77 AUC value. Stepwise logistic regression achieved 0.42 AUC value with 3 important variables. Both models showed that the fall assessment by nurses and use of anti-psychotic medication are associated with a lower risk of falls, and the use of diuretics is associated with an increased risk of falls. Another group of researchers [110] used fall related injury data to validate the structured information in EMR from clinical notes with the help of text mining. A group of nurses manually reviewed the electronic records to separate the correct documents from the erroneous ones which was considered as the basis of comparison. Authors employed both supervised (using a portion of manually labeled files as training set) and unsupervised technique (without considering the file labels) to classify and cluster the records. The unsupervised technique failed to separate the fare documents from the erroneous ones, wherein supervised technique performed better with 86% of fare documents in one cluster. This method can be applicable to semi-automate the EMR entry system.

4.2.4. Other Applications

Data mining has beed applied [111] to investigate the relationship between physician's training at specific schools, procedures performed, and costs of the procedure. Researchers explored this relationship at three level: (1) they explored the distribution of procedures performed; (2) the relationship between procedures performed by physician and their alma mater—the institute that a doctor attended or got his/her degree from; and (3) geographic distribution of amount billed and payment received. This study suggested that medical school training does relate to practice in terms of procedures performed and bill charged. Patients can also provide useful information about physicians and their performance. Another group of researchers [112] used topic modeling algorithm—Latent Dirichlet Allocation (LDA)—to understand patients' review of physicians and their concerns.

Data mining has also been applied [115] to analyze the information seeking behavior of health care professionals, and to assess the feasibility of measuring drug safety alert response from the usage logs of online medical information resources. Researchers analyzed two years of user log-in data in UpToDate website to measure the volume of searches associated with medical conditions and the seasonal distribution of those searches. In addition, they used a large collection of online media articles and web log posts as they characterized food and drug alert through the changes in UpToDate search activity compared to the general media activity. Some researchers [113] examined changes of key performance indicators (KPIs) and clinical workload indicators in Greek National Health System (NHS) hospitals with the help of data mining. They found significant changes in KPIs when necessary adjustments (e.g., workload) were made according to the diagnostic related group. The results remained for general hospitals like cancer hospitals, cardiac surgery as well as small health centers and regional hospitals. Their findings suggested that the assessment methodology of Greek NHS hospitals should be re-evaluated in order to identify the weaknesses in the system, and improve overall performance. And in home healthcare, another group of researchers [116] reviewed why traditional statistical analysis fails to evaluate the performance of home healthcare agencies. The authors proposed to use data mining to identify the drivers of home healthcare service among patients with heart failure, hip replacement, and chronic obstructive pulmonary disease using length of stay and discharge destination.

The relationship between epidemiological and genetic evidence and post market medical device performance has been evaluated using HCUPNet data [114]. This feasibility study explored the potential of using publicly accessible data for identifying genetic evidence (e.g., comorbidity of genetic factors like race, sex, body structure, and pneumothorax or fibrosis) related to devices. It focused on the ventilation-associated iatrogenic pneumothorax outcome in discharge of mechanical ventilation and continuous positive airway pressure (CPAP). The results demonstrated that genetic evidence-based epidemiologic analysis could lead to both cost and time efficient identification of predictive features. The literature of data mining applications in healthcare administration encompasses efficient patient management, healthcare cost reduction, quality of care, and data warehousing to facilitate analytics. We identified four studies that used cloud-based computing and analytical platforms. Most of the research proposed promising ideas, however, they do not provide the results and/or challenges during and after implementation. An ideal example of implementation could be the study of efficient appointment scheduling of patients [108].

4.3. Healthcare Privacy and Fraud Detection

Health data privacy and medical fraud are issues of prominent importance [118]. We reviewed four articles—displayed and described in Table 7—that discussed healthcare privacy and fraud detection.

Table 7. List of papers in healthcare privacy and fraud detection.

Reference	Problem Analyzed	Data Source
[119]	Cloud based big data framework to ensure data security	Not specified
[120]	Weakness in de-identification or anonymization of health data	MedHelp and Mp and Th1 (Medicare social networking sites)
[121]	Automatic and systematic detection of fraud and abuse	Bureau of National Health Insurance (BNHI) in Taiwan.
[122]	Novel algorithm to protect data privacy	Hong Kong Red Cross Blood Transfusion Service (BTS)

The challenges of privacy protection have been addressed by a group of researchers [122] who proposed a new anonymization algorithm for both distributed and centralized anonymization. Their proposed model performed better than K-anonymization model in terms of retaining data utility without losing much data privacy (for K = 20, the discernibility ratio—a normalized measure of data quality—of the proposed approach and traditional K-anonymization method were 0.1 and 0.4 respectively). Moreover, their proposed algorithm could handle large scale, high dimensional datasets. To address the limitations of today's healthcare information systems—EHR data systems limited by lack of inter-operability, data size, and security—a mobile cloud computing-based big data framework has been proposed [119]. This novel cloud-based framework proposed storing EHR data from different healthcare providers in an Internet provider's facility, offering providers and patients different levels of access and authority. Security would be ensured by using encryption algorithms, one-time passwords, or 2-factor authentication. Big data analytics would be handled using Google big query or MapReduce software. This framework could reduce cost, increase efficiency, and ensure security compared to the traditional technique which uses de-identification or anonymization technique. This traditional technique leaves healthcare data vulnerable to re-identification. In a case study, researchers demonstrated that hackers can make association between small pieces of information and can identify patients [120]. The case study made use of personal information provided in two Medicare social networking sites, MedHelp and Mp and Th1 to identify an individual.

Detection of fraud and abuse (i.e., suspicious care activity, intentional misrepresentation of information, and unnecessary repetitive visits) uses big data analytics. Using gynecological hospital data, researchers [121] developed a framework from two domain experts manually identifying features of fraudulent cases from a data pool of treatment plans doctors frequently follow. They applied this framework to Bureau of National Health Insurance (BNHI) data from Taiwan; their proposed framework detected 69% of the fraudulent cases, which improved the existing model that detected 63% of the fraudulent cases.

In summary, patient data privacy and fraud detection are of major concern given increasing use of social media and people's tendency to put personal information on social media. Existing data anonymization or de-identification techniques can become less effective if they are not designed considering the fact that a large portion of our personal information is now available on social media.

4.4. Mental Health

Mental illness is a global and national concern [123]. According to the National Survey on Drug Use and Health (NSDUH) data from 2010 to 2012, 52.2% of U.S. population had either mental illness, or substance abuse/dependence [124]. Additionally, nearly 30 million people in the U.S. suffer from anxiety disorders [125]. Table 8 summarizes the four articles we reviewed that apply data mining in analyzing, diagnosing, and treating mental health issues.

Table 8. List of data mining application in mental health with data sources.

Reference	Problem Analyzed	Data Source
[126]	Identification and intervention of developmental delay of children	Yunlin Developmental Delay Assessment Center
[125]	Personalized treatment for anxiety disorder	Volunteer participants
[127]	Abnormal behavior detection	Through experiment with human subject
[128]	Mental health diagnosis and exploration of psychiatrist's everyday practice	Queensland Schizophrenia Research center

To classify developmental delays of children based on illness, researchers [126] examined the association between illness diagnosis and delays by building a decision tree and finding association between cognitive, language, motor, and social emotional developmental delays. This study has implications for healthcare professionals to identify and intervene on delays at an early stage. To assist physicians in monitoring anxiety disorder, another group of researchers [125] developed a data mining based personalized treatment. The researchers used Context Awareness Information including static (personal information like, age, sex, family status etc.) and dynamic (stress, environmental, and symptoms context) information to build static and dynamic user models. The static model contained personal information and the dynamic model contained four treatment-supportive services (i.e., lifestyle and habits pattern detection service, context and stress level pattern detection service, symptoms and stress level pattern detection service, and stress level prediction service). Relations between different dynamic parameters were identified in first three services and the last service was used for stress level prediction under different scenarios. The model was validated using data from 27 volunteers who were selected by anxiety measuring test.

To predict early diagnosis for mental disorders (e.g., insomnia, dementia), researchers developed a model detecting abnormal physical activity recorded by a wearable device [127]. They performed two experiments to compare the development of a reference model using historical user physical movement data. In the first experiment, users wore the watch for one day and based on that day, a reference behavior model was developed. After 22 days, the same user used it again for a day and abnormality was detected if the user's activities were significantly different from the reference model. In the second experiment, users used the watch regularly for one month. Abnormality was detected with a fuzzy valuation function and validated with user's reported activity level. In both experiments, users manually reported their activity level, which was used as a validating point, only two out of 26 abnormal events were undetected. Through these two experiments, the researchers claimed that their model could be useful for both online and offline abnormal behavior detection as the model was able to detect 92% of the unusual events.

To classify schizophrenia, another study [128] used free speech (transcribed text) written or verbalized by psychiatric patients. In a pool of patients with schizophrenia and control subjects, using supervised algorithms (SVM and DT), they discriminated between patients with schizophrenia and normal control patients. SVM achieved 77% classification accuracy whereas DT achieved 78% accuracy. When they added patients with mania to the pool, they were unable to differentiate patients with schizophrenia.

Use of data analytics in diagnosing, analyzing, or treating mental health patients is quite different than applying analytics to predict cancer or diabetes. Context of data (static, dynamic, or unobservable environment) seemed more important than volume in this case [125], however, this is not always adopted in literature. A model without situational awareness (a context independent model) may lose predictive accuracy due to the confounding effect of surrounding environment [129].

4.5. Public Health

Seven articles addressed issues that were not limited to any specific disease or a demographic group, which we classified as public health problems. Table 9 contains the list of papers considering public health problems with data sources.

Table 9. List of data mining application in public health with data sources.

Reference	Problem Analyzed	Data Source
[130]	Designing preventive healthcare programs	World Health Organization (WHO)
[131]	Predicting the peak of health center visit due to influenza	Military Influenza case data provided by US Armed Forces Health Surveillance Center and Environmental data from US National Climate Data Center
[132]	Contrast patient and customer loyalty, estimating Customer lifetime value, and identifying the targeted customer	Iranian Public Hospital data extracted from Hospital information system
[133]	Understanding the information seeking behavior of public and professionals on infectious disease	National electronic Library of Infection and National Resource of Infection Control, Google Trends, and relevant media coverage (LexisNexis).
[134]	Knowledge extraction for non-expert user through automation of data mining process	Brazilian health ministry
[135]	Innovative use of data mining and visualization techniques for decision-making	Slovenian national Institute of Public Health
[136]	Real-time emergency response method using big data and Internet of Things	UCI machine learning repository

To make data mining accessible to non-expert users, specifically public health decision makers who manage public cancer treatment programs in Brazil, researchers [134] developed a framework for an automated data mining system. This system performed a descriptive analysis (i.e., identifying relationships between demography, expenditure, and tumor or cancer type) for public decision makers with little or no technical knowledge. The automation process was done by creating pre-processed database, ontology, analytical platform and user interface.

Analysis of disease outbreaks has also applied data analytics. [131,133] Influenza, a highly contagious disease, is associated with seasonal outbreaks. The ability to predict peak outbreaks in advance would allow for anticipatory public health planning and interventions to lessen the effect of the outbreaks. To predict peak influenza visits to U.S. military health centers, researchers [131] developed a method to create models using environmental and epidemiological data. They compared six classification algorithms—One-Classifier 1, One-Classifier 2 [137], a fusion of the One-Classifiers, DT, RF, and SVM. Among them, One-Classifier 1 was the most efficient with F-score 0.672 and SVM was second best with F-score 0.652. To examine the factors that drive public and professional search patterns for infectious disease outbreaks another group of researchers [133] used online behavior records and media coverage. They identified distinct factors that drive professional and layperson search patterns with implications for tailored messaging during outbreaks and emergencies for public health agencies.

To store and integrate multidimensional and heterogeneous data (e.g., diabetes, food, nutrients) applied to diabetes management, but generalizable to other diseases researchers [130] proposed an intelligent information management framework. Their proposed methodology is a robust back-end application for web-based patient-doctor consultation and e-Health care management systems with implications for cost savings.

A real-time medical emergency response system using the Internet of Things (networking of devices to facilitate data flow) based body area networks (BANs)—a wireless network of wearable computing devices was proposed by researchers [136]. The system consists of "Intelligent Building"—a data analysis model which processes the data collected from the sensors for analysis and decision. Though the author claims that the proposed system had the capability of efficiently processing wireless BAN data from millions of users to provide real-time response for emergencies, they did not provide any comparison with the state-of-the-art methods.

Decision support tools for regional health institutes in Slovenia [135] have been developed using descriptive data mining methods and visualization techniques. These visualization methods could analyze resource availability, utilization and aid to assist in future planning of public health service.

To build better customer relations management at an Iranian hospital, researchers [132] applied data mining techniques on demographic and transactions information. The authors extended the traditional Recency, Frequency, and Monetary (RFM) model by adapting a new parameter "Length" to estimate the customer life time value (CLV) of each patient. Patients were separated into classes according to estimated CLV with a combination of clustering and classification algorithms. Both DT and ANN performed similarly in classification with approximately 90% accuracy. This type of stratification of patient groups with CLV values would help hospitals to introduce new marketing strategies to attract new customers and retain existing ones.

The application of data mining to public health decision-making has become increasingly common. Researchers utilized data mining to design healthcare programs and emergency response, to identify resource utilization, patient satisfaction as well as to develop automated analytics tool for non-expert users. Continuation of this effort could lead to a patient-centered, robust healthcare system.

4.6. Pharmacovigilance

Pharmacovigilance involves post-marketing monitoring and detection of adverse drug reactions (ADRs) to ensure patient safety [138]. The estimated annual social cost of ADR events exceeds one billion dollars, making it an important part of healthcare system [139]. Characteristics of the nine papers addressing pharmacovigilance are displayed in Table 10.

Table 10. List of data mining application in pharmacovigilance with data sources.

Reference	Problem Analyzed	Data Source
[140]	Sentiment and network analysis based on social media data to find ADR signal	Cancer discussion forum websites
[138]	ADR signal detection from multiple data sources	Food and Drug Administration (FDA) database and publicly available electronic health record (HER) in US
[141]	ADR detection from EPR through temporal data analysis	Danish psychiatric hospital
[142]	ADR (hypersensitivity) signal detection of six anticancer agents	FDA released AERS reports (2004–2009), US
[139]	ADR caused by multiple drugs	FDA released AERS reports, US
[143]	ADR due to Statins used in Cardiovascular disease (CVD) and muscular and renal failure treatment	FDA released AERS reports, US
[144]	Creating a ranked list of Adverse Events (AEs)	EHR form European Union
[145]	Detecting ADR signals of Rosuvastatins compared to other statins users	Health Insurance Review and Assessment Service claims database (Seoul, Korea)
[146]	Unexpected and rare ADR detection technique	Medicare Benefits Scheme (MBS) and Queensland Linked Data Set (QLDS)

Researchers considered muscular and renal AEs caused by pravastatin, simvastatin, atorvastatin, and rosuvastatin by applying data mining techniques to the FDA's Adverse Event Reporting System (FAERS) database reports from 2004 to 2009 [143]. They found that all statins except simvastatin were associated with muscular AE; rosuvastatin had the strongest association. All statins, besides atorvastatin, were associated with acute renal failure. The criteria used to identify significant association were: proportional reporting ratio (PRR), reporting odds ratio (ROR), information component (IC), and empirical Bayes geometric mean (EBGM). In another study of AEs related to statin family, researchers used a Korean claims database [145] and showed that a relative risk-based data-mining approach successfully detected signals for rosuvastatin.

Three more studies used the FDA's AERS report database. In an examination of ADR "hypersensitivity" to six anticancer agents [142] data mining results showed that Paclitaxel is associated with mild to lethal reaction wherein Docetaxel is associated to lethal reaction, and the other four drugs were not associated to hypersensitivity [142]. Another researcher [139] argued that AEs can be caused not only by a single drug, but also by a combination of drugs [140]. They showed that that 84% of the AERs reports contain an association between at least one drug and two AEs or two drugs and one AE. Another group [138] increased precision in detecting ADRs by considering multiple data sources together. They achieved 31% (on average) improvement in identification by using publicly available EHRs in combination with the FDA's AERS reports.

Furthermore, dose-dependent ADRs have been identified by researchers using models developed from structured and unstructured EHR data [141]. Among the top five drugs associated with ADRs, four were found to be related to dose [141]. Pharmacovigilance activity has also been prioritized using unstructured text data in EHRs [144]. In traditional pharmacovigilance, ADRs are unknown. While looking for association between a drug and any possible ADR, it is possible to get false signals. Such false signals can be avoided if a list of possible ADRs is already known. Researchers [144] developed an ordered list of 23 ADRs which can be very helpful for future pharmacovigilance activities. To detect unexpected and rare ADRs in real-world healthcare administrative databases, another group of researchers [146] designed an algorithm—Unexpected Temporal Association Rules (UTARs)—that performs more effectively than existing techniques.

We identified one study that used data outside of adverse event reports or HER data. For early detection of ADR, one group of researchers used online forums [140]. They identified the side effect of a specific drug called "Erlotinib" used for lung cancer. Sentiment analysis—a technique of categorizing opinions—on data collected from different cancer discussion forums showed that 70% of users had a positive experience after using this drug. Users most frequently reported were acne and rash. Apart from pharmacovigilance, this type of analysis can be very helpful for the pharmaceutical companies to analyze customer feedback. Researchers can take advantage of the popularity of social media and online forums for identifying adverse events. These sources can provide signals of AEs quicker than FDA database as it takes time to update the database. By the time AE reports are available in the FDA database, there could already be significant damage to patient and society. Moreover, it can help to avoid the limitations of FDA AERS database like biased reporting and underreporting [141].

5. Theoretical Study

Twenty-five of the articles we reviewed focus on the theoretical aspects of the application of data mining in healthcare including designing the database framework, data collection, and management to algorithmic development. These intellectual contributions extend beyond the analytical perspective of data—descriptive, predictive or prescriptive analytics—to the sectors and problems highlighted in Table 11.

Table 11. Problem analyzed in theoretical studies.

Sector Highlight	Reference	Problem Analyzed
Disease Control, Current situation of different diseases (infection, epidemic, cancer, mental health)	[147]	Proposed an idea for dynamic clinical decision support
	[148]	Described current situation of infection control and predicted future challenges in this sector
	[149]	Described activities taken by national organization to control disease and provide better health care
	[150]	Reviewed efficient collection and aggregation of big data and proposed an intelligence based learning framework to help prevent cancer
Data quality, database framework and uncertainty quantification	[151]	Considered the management of uncertainty originating from data mining.
	[152]	Contemplated the quality of the data when collected from multimodal sources
	[150]	Provided the structure of the database of CancerLinQ that comprised of 4 key steps
	[153]	Described five major problems that need to be tackled in order to have an effective integration of big data analytics and VPH modeling in healthcare
	[152]	Discuss the issues of data quality in the context of big data health care analytics
	[154]	Discussed the necessity of proper management and confidentiality of healthcare data along with the benefit of big data analytics
Healthcare policy making	[155–157]	Addressed the challenges faced in implementing health care policies and considered the ethical and legal issues of performing predictive analysis on health care big data
	[150]	Focused on the US federal regulatory pathway by which CancerLinQ will have legislative authority to use the patients' records and the approach of ASCO toward the organizing and supervising the information
Patient Privacy	[158]	Focused on ensuring patient privacy while collecting data, storing them and using them for analysis aimed to eliminate discrimination in the health care provided to patients.
	[159]	Spotted light on ensuring Privacy and security while collecting Personal Health care Information (PHI)
	[160]	Highlighted those strategies appropriate for data mining from physicians' prescriptions while maintaining the patient's privacy
Personalized health care	[161]	Transforming big data into computational models to provide personalized health care
	[162]	Development of informed decision-making frameworks for person centered health care
	[163]	Looked into the availability of big data and the role of biomedical informatics on the personalized medicine. Also, emphasized on the ethical concerns related to personalized medicines
Others	[164]	Finding the aspects of big data that are most relevant to Health care
	[165]	Selecting dynamic simulation modeling approach based on the availability and type of big data
	[166]	Quantifying performance in the delivery of medical services
	[167]	Identifying high risk patients to ensure better care, and explored the analytics procedure, algorithms and challenges to implement analytics
	[168]	Addressed barriers for the exploitation of health data in Europe
	[169]	Analyzed the opportunity and obstacles in applying predictive analytics based on big data in case of evaluating emergency care
	[170]	Provided an overview of the uses of the Person-Event Data Environment to perform command surveillance and policy analysis for Army leadership
	[171]	Development of big data analytics in healthcare and future challenges

The existing theoretical literature on disease control highlighted the current state of epidemics, cancer and mental health. To help physicians make real-time decisions about patient care, one group of researchers [147] proposed a real-time EMR data mining based clinical decision support system. They emphasized the need to have an anonymized EMR database which can be explored by using a search engine similar to web search engine. In addition, they focused on designing a framework for next generation EMR-based database that can facilitate the clinical decision-making process, and is also capable of updating a central population database once patients' recent (new) clinical records are available. Another researcher [148] forecasted future challenges in infection control that entails the importance of having timely surveillance system and prevention programs in place. To that end, they necessitate the formation, control and utilization of fully computerized patient record and data-mining-derived epidemiology. Finally, they recommended performance feedback to caregivers, wide accessibility of infection prevention tools, and access to documents like lessons learned and evidence-based best practices to strengthen the infection control, surveillance, and prevention scheme. Authors in [150] addressed the activities executed by national Institute of Mental Health (NIMH) in collaboration with other state organizations (e.g., Substance Abuse and Mental Health Service Administration (SAMSHSA), Center for Mental Health Service (CMHS) to promote optimal collection, pooling/aggregation, and use of big data to support ongoing and future researches of mental health practices. The outcome summary showcased that effective pooling/aggregation of state-level data from different sources can be used as a dashboard to set priorities to improve service qualities, measure system performance and to gain specific context-based insights that are generalizable and scalable across other systems, leading to a successful learning-based mental health care system. Another group of researchers [150] outlined the barriers and potential benefits of using big data from CancerLinQ (a quality and measurement reporting system as an initiative of the American Society of Clinical Oncology (ASCO) that collects information from EHRs of cancer patients for oncologists to improve the outcome and quality of care they provide to their patients). However, the authors also mentioned that these benefits are contingent upon the confidence of the patients, encouraging them to share their data out of the belief that their health records would be used appropriately as a knowledge base to improve the quality of the health care of others, as it is for themselves. This motivated ASCO to ensure that proper policies and procedures are in place to deal with the data quality, data security and data access, and adopt a comprehensive regulatory framework to ensure patients' data privacy and security.

Another group of researchers [151] data quality and database management to quantify, and consequentially understand the inherent uncertainty originating from radiology reporting system. They discussed the necessity of having a structured reporting system and emphasized the use of standardize language, leading to Natural Language Processing (NLP). Furthermore, they also indicated the need for creating a Knowledge Discovery Database (KDD) which will be consistent to facilitate the data-driven and automated decision support technologies to help improving the care provided to patients based on enhanced diagnosis quality and clinical outcome. A group of authors in [152] pointed that the success derived from the current trend of big-data analytics largely depends on how better the quality of the data collected from variety of sources are ensured. Their findings imply that the data quality should be assessed across the entire lifecycle of health data by considering the errors and inaccuracies stemmed from multiple of sources, and should also quantify the impact that data collection purpose on the knowledge and insights derived from the big data analytics. For that to ensure, they recommend that enterprises who deal with healthcare big data should develop a systematic framework including custom software or data quality rule engines, leading to an effective management of specific data-quality related problems. Researchers in [155] uncovered the lack of connection between phenomenological and mechanistic models in computational biomedicines. They emphasized the importance of big data which, when successfully extracted and analyzed, followed by the combination with Virtual Physiological Human (VPH)—an initiative to encourage personalized healthcare—can afford with effective and robust medicine solutions. In order for that to happen, they mentioned some challenges (e.g., confidentiality, volume and complexity of big data; integration of bioinformatics, systems biology and phenomics data; efficient storage of partial or complete data within organization to maximize the performance of overall predictive analytics) and concluded that these need to be addressed for successful development of big data technologies in computational medicines, enabling their adoption in clinical settings. Even though big data can generate significant value in modern healthcare system, researchers in [154] stated that without a set of proper IT infrastructures, analytical and visualization tools, and interactive interfaces to represent the work flows, the insights generated from big data will not be able to reach its full potential. To overcome this, they recommended that health care organizations engaging in data sharing devise new policies to protect patients' data against potential data breaches.

Three papers [155–157] considered health care policies and ethical and legal issues. One [155] outlined a national action plan to incorporate sharable and comparable nursing data beyond documentation of care into quality reporting and translational research. The plan advocates for standardized nursing terminologies, common data models, and information structures within EHRs. Another paper [157] analyzed the major policy, ethical, and legal challenges of performing predictive analytics on health care big data. Their proposed recommendations for overcoming challenges raised in the four-phase life cycle of a predictive analytics model (i.e., data acquisition, model formulation and validation, testing in real-world setting and implementation and use in broader scale) included developing a governance structure at the earliest phase of model development to guide patients and participating stakeholders across the process (from data acquisition to model implementation). They also recommended that model developers strictly comply with the federal laws and regulations in concert with human subject research and patients information privacy when using patients' data. And another paper [156] explored four central questions regarding: (i) aspects of big-data most relevant to health care, (ii) policy implications, (iii) potential obstacles in achieving policy objectives, and (iv) availability of policy levers, particularly for policy makers to consider when developing public policy for using big data in healthcare. They discussed barriers (including ensuring transparency among patients and health care providers during data collection) to achieve policy objectives based on a recent UK policy experiment, and argued for providing real-life examples of ways in which data sharing can improve healthcare.

Three papers [158–160] offered examples of realistic ways such as establishing policy leadership and risk management framework combining commercial and health care entities to recognize existing privacy related problem and devise pragmatic and actionable strategies of maintaining patient privacy in big data analytics. One paper [158] provided a policy overview of health care and data analytics, outlined the utility of health care data from a policy perspective, reviewed a variety of methods for data collection from public and private sources, mobile devices and social media, examined laws and regulations that protect data and patients' privacy, and discussed a dynamic interplay among three aspects of today's big data driven personal health care—policy goals to tackle both cost, population health problem and eliminate disparity in patient care while maintaining their privacy. Another study [159] proposed a Secure and Privacy Preserving Opportunistic Computing (SPOC) framework to be used in healthcare emergencies focused on collecting intensive personal health information (through mobile devices like smart phone or wireless sensors) with minimal privacy disclosure. The premise of this framework is that when a user of this system (called medical user) faces any emergency, other users in the vicinity with similar disease or symptom (if available) can come to help that user before professional help arrives. It is assumed that two persons with similar disease are skilled enough to help each other and the threshold of similarity is controlled by the user. And in physician prescribing—another paper [160] identified strategies for data mining from physicians' prescriptions while maintaining patient privacy.

Theoretical research on personalized-health care services—treatment plans designed for someone based on the susceptibility of his/her genomic structure to a disease—also emerged from the literature review. One study [161] highlighted the potential of powerful analytical tools to open an avenue for predictive, preventive, participatory, and personalized (P4) medicine. They suggested a more nuanced understanding of the human systems to design an accurate computational model for P4 medicine. Reviewing the research paradgims of current person-centered approaches and traditions, another study [162] advocated a transdisciplinary and complex systems approach to improve the field. They synthesized the emerging aproaches and methodologies and highlighted the gaps between academic research and accessibility of evaluation, informatics, and big data from health information systems. Another paper [163] reviewed the availability of big data and the role of biomedical informatics in personalized medicine, emphasizing the ethical concerns related to personalized medicines and health equity. Personalized medicine has a potential to reduce healthcare cost, however, the researchers think it can create race, income, and educational disparity. Certain socioeconomic and demographic groups currently have less or no access to healthcare and data driven personalized medicine will exclude those groups, increasing disparities. They also highlighted the impact of EHRs and CDWs on the field of personalized medicine through acclerated research and decreased the delivery time of new technologies.

A myriad of extant theoretical points has also been identified in the literature. These topics range from exploiting big data to: study the paradigm shift in healthcare policy and management from prioritizing volume to value [164,167]; aid medical device consumers in their decision-making [166]; improve emergency departments [169]; perform command surveillance and policy analysis for Army leadership [170]; to comparing different simulation methods (i.e., systems dynamics, discrete event simulation and agent based modeling) for specific health care system problems like resource allocation, length of stay [165]; to the ethical challenges of security, management, and ownership [170]. Another researcher outlined the challenges the E.U. is facing in data mining given numerous historical, technical, legal, and political barriers [168].

6. Future Research and Challenges

Data mining has been applied in many fields including finance, marketing, and manufacturing [172]. Its application in healthcare is becoming increasingly popular [173]. A growing literature addresses the challenges of data mining including noisy data, heterogeneity, high dimensionality, dynamic nature, computational time. In this section, we focus on future research applications including personalized care, information loss in preprocessing, collecting healthcare data for research purposes, automation for non-experts, interdisciplinarity of study and domain expert knowledge, integration into the healthcare system, and prediction-specific to data mining application and integration in healthcare.

- Personalized care

The EMR is increasingly used to document demographic and clinician patient information [1]. EMR data can be utilized to develop personalized care plans, enhancing patient experience [162] and improving care quality.

- Loss of information in pre-processing

Pre-processing of data, including handling missing data, is the most time-consuming and costly part of data mining. The most common method used in the papers reviewed was deletion or elimination of missing data. In one study, approximately 46.5% of the data and 363 of 410 features were eliminated due to missing values [49]. In another, researchers [98] were only able to use 2064 of 4948 observations (42%) [98]. By eliminating missing value cases and outliers, we are losing a significant amount of information. Future research should focus on finding a better method of missing value estimation than elimination. Moreover, data collection techniques should be developed or modified to avoid this issue.

Similar to missing data, deletion or elimination is a common way to handle outliers [174]. However, as illustrated in one of the studies we reviewed [48], outliers can be used to gain information about rare forms of diseases. Instead of neglecting the outliers, future research should analyze them to gain insight.

- Collecting healthcare data for research purpose

Traditionally, the primary objective of data collection in healthcare is documentation of patient condition and care planning [109]. Including research objectives in the data collection process through structured fields could yield more structured data with fewer cases of error and missing values [64]. A successful example of data collection for research purpose is the Study of Health in Pomerania (SHIP) [175]. The objective of SHIP was to identify common diseases, population level risk factors, and overall health of people living in the north-east region of Germany. This study only suffered from one "mistake" for every 1000 data entries [175] which ensures a structured form of data with high reliability, less noise and fewer missing values. We can take advantage of current documentation processes (EMR or EHR) by modifying them to collect more reliable and structured data. Long-term vision and planning is required to introduce research purpose in healthcare data collection.

- Automation of data mining process for non-expert users

The end users of data mining in healthcare are doctors, nurses, and healthcare professionals with limited training in analytics. One solution for this problem is to develop an automated (i.e., without human supervision) system for the end users [134]. A cloud-based automated structure to prevent medical errors could also be developed [95]; but the task would be challenging as it involves different application areas and one algorithm will not have similar accuracy for all applications [134].

- Interdisciplinary nature of study and domain expert knowledge

Healthcare analytics is an interdisciplinary research field [134]. As a form of analytics, data mining should be used in combination with expert opinion from specific domains—healthcare and problem specific (i.e., oncologist for cancer study, cardiologist for CVD) [106]. Approximately 32% of the articles in analytics did not utilize expert opinion in any form. Future research should include members from different disciplines including healthcare.

- Integration in healthcare system

Very few articles reviewed made an effort to integrate the data mining process into the actual decision-making framework. The impact of knowledge discovery through data mining on healthcare professional's workload and time is unclear. Future studies should consider the integration of the developed system and explore the effect on work environments.

- Prediction error and "The Black Swan" effect

In healthcare, it is better not to predict than making an erroneous prediction [46]. A little under half of the literature we identified in analytics is dedicated to prediction but, none of the articles discussed the consequence of a prediction error. High prediction accuracy for cancer or any other disease does not ensure an accurate application to decision-making.

Moreover, prediction models may be better at predicting commonplace events than rare ones [176]. Researchers should develop more sophisticated models to address the unpredictable, "The Black Swan" [176]. One study [101] addressed a similar issue in evidence based recommendations for medical prescriptions. Their concern was, how much evidence should be sufficient to make a recommendation. Many of the studies in this review do not address these salient issues. Future research should address the implementation challenges of predictive models, especially how the decision-making process should adapt in case of errors and unpredictable incidents.

7. Conclusions

The development of an informed decision-making framework stems from the growing concern of ensuring a high value and patient-focused health care system. Concurrently, the availability of big data has created a promising research avenue for academicians and practitioners. As highlighted in our review, the increased number of publications in recent years corroborates the importance of health care analytics to build improved health care systems world-wide. The ultimate goal is to facilitate coordinated and well-informed health care systems capable of ensuring maximum patient satisfaction.

This paper adds to the literature on healthcare and data mining (Table 1) as it is the first, to our knowledge, to take a comprehensive review approach and offer a holistic picture of health care analytics and data mining. The comprehensive and methodologically rigorous approach we took covers the application and theoretical perspective of analytics and data mining in healthcare. Our systematic approach starting with the review process and categorizing the output as analytics or theoretical provides readers with a more widespread review with reference to specific fields.

We also shed light on some promising recommendations for future areas of research including integration of domain-expert knowledge, approaches to decrease prediction error, and integration of predictive models in actual work environments. Future research should recommend ways so that the analytic decision can effectively adapt with the predictive model subject to errors and unpredictable incidents. Regardless of these insightful outcomes, we are not constrained to mention some limitations of our proposed review approach. The sole consideration of academic journals and exclusion of conference papers, which may have some good coverage in this sector is the prime limitation of this review. In addition to this, the search span was narrowed to three databases for 12 years which may have ignored some prior works in this area, albeit the increasing trend since 2005 and less number of publications before 2008 can minimize this limitation. The omission of articles published in languages other than English can also restrict the scope of this review as related papers written in other languages might be evident in the literature. Moreover, we did not conduct forward (reviewing the papers which cited the selected paper) and backward (reviewing the references in the selected paper and authors' prior works) search as suggested by Levy and Ellis [31].

Despite these limitations, the systematic methodology followed in this review can be used in the universe of healthcare areas.

Author Contributions: Contribution of the authors can be summarized in following manner. Conceptualization: M.S.I., M.N.-E.-A.; Formal analysis: M.S.I., M.M.H., X.W.; Investigation: M.S.I., M.M.H., X.W.; Methodology: M.S.I.; Project administration: M.S.I., M.N.-E.-A.; Supervision: M.N.-E.-A.; Visualization: M.S.I., X.W.; Writing—draft: M.S.I., M.M.H., H.D.G.; Writing—review and editing: M.S.I., M.M.H., H.D.G., M.N.-E.-A.

Funding: Germack is supported by CTSA Grant Number TL1 TR001864 from the National Center for Advancing Translational Science (NCATS), a component of the National Institutes of Health (NIH). The content is solely the responsibility of the authors and does not necessarily represent the official views of this organization.

References

1. Yang, J.-J.; Li, J.; Mulder, J.; Wang, Y.; Chen, S.; Wu, H.; Wang, Q.; Pan, H. Emerging information technologies for enhanced healthcare. *Comput. Ind.* **2015**, *69*, 3–11. [CrossRef]

2. Cortada, J.W.; Gordon, D.; Lenihan, B. *The Value of Analytics in Healthcare*; Report No.: GBE03476-USEN-00; IBM Institute for Business Value: Armonk, NY, USA, 2012.

3. Center for Medicare and Medicaid Services. Available online: https://www.cms.gov/Research-Statistics-Data-and-Systems/Statistics-Trends-andReports/NationalHealthExpendData/NationalHealthAccountsHistorical.html (accessed on 1 August 2017).

4. Berwick, D.M.; Hackbarth, A.D. Eliminating waste in US health care. *J. Am. Med. Assoc.* **2012**, *307*, 1513–1516. [CrossRef]

5. Makary, M.A.; Daniel, M. Medical error-the third leading cause of death in the US. *Br. Med. J.* **2016**, *353*, i2139. [CrossRef] [PubMed]

6.   Prokosch, H.-U.; Ganslandt, T. Perspectives for medical informatics. *Methods Inf. Med.* **2009**, *48*, 38–44. [CrossRef] [PubMed]

7.   Simpao, A.F.; Ahumada, L.M.; Gálvez, J.A.; Rehman, M.A. A review of analytics and clinical informatics in health care. *J. Med. Syst.* **2014**, *38*, 45. [CrossRef] [PubMed]

8.   Ghassemi, M.; Celi, L.A.; Stone, D.J. State of the art review: The data revolution in critical care. *Crit. Care* **2015**, *19*, 118. [CrossRef] [PubMed]

9.   Tomar, D.; Agarwal, S. A survey on Data Mining approaches for Healthcare. *Int. J. Bio-Sci. Bio-Technol.* **2013**, *5*, 241–266. [CrossRef]

10. Herland, M.; Khoshgoftaar, T.M.; Wald, R. A review of data mining using big data in health informatics. *J. Big Data* **2014**, *1*, 2. [CrossRef]

11. Sigurdardottir, A.K.; Jonsdottir, H.; Benediktsson, R. Outcomes of educational interventions in type 2 diabetes: WEKA data-mining analysis. *Patient Educ. Couns.* **2007**, *67*, 21–31. [CrossRef] [PubMed]

12. Li, J.; Huang, K.-Y.; Jin, J.; Shi, J. A survey on statistical methods for health care fraud detection. *Health Care Manag. Sci.* **2008**, *11*, 275–287. [CrossRef] [PubMed]

13. Bellazzi, R.; Zupan, B. Predictive data mining in clinical medicine: Current issues and guidelines. *Int. J. Med. Inform.* **2008**, *77*, 81–97. [CrossRef] [PubMed]

14. Yoo, I.-H.; Song, M. Biomedical ontologies and text mining for biomedicine and healthcare: A survey. *J. Comput. Sci. Eng.* **2008**, *2*, 109–136. [CrossRef]

15. Ting, S.; Shum, C.; Kwok, S.K.; Tsang, A.H.; Lee, W. Data mining in biomedicine: Current applications and further directions for research. *J. Softw. Eng. Appl.* **2009**, *2*, 150–159. [CrossRef]

16. Iavindrasana, J.; Cohen, G.; Depeursinge, A.; Müller, H.; Meyer, R.; Geissbuhler, A. Clinical data mining: A review. *Yearb. Med. Inform.* **2009**, *2009*, 121–133.

17. Bellazzi, R.; Ferrazzi, F.; Sacchi, L. Predictive data mining in clinical medicine: A focus on selected methods and applications. *WIRE* **2011**, *1*, 416–430. [CrossRef]

18. Barati, E.; Saraee, M.; Mohammadi, A.; Adibi, N.; Ahmadzadeh, M. A survey on utilization of data mining approaches for dermatological (skin) diseases prediction. *J. Sel. Areas Health Inform.* **2011**, *2*, 1–11.

19. Jacob, S.G.; Ramani, R.G. Data mining in clinical data sets: A review. *Int. J. Appl. Inf. Syst.* **2012**, *4*, 15–26. [CrossRef]

20. Yoo, I.; Alafaireet, P.; Marinov, M.; Pena-Hernandez, K.; Gopidi, R.; Chang, J.-F.; Hua, L. Data mining in healthcare and biomedicine: A survey of the literature. *J. Med. Syst.* **2012**, *36*, 2431–2448. [CrossRef] [PubMed]

21. Shukla, D.; Patel, S.B.; Sen, A.K. A literature review in health informatics using data mining techniques. *Int. J. Softw. Hardw. Res. Eng.* **2014**, *2*, 123–129.

22. Mohammed, E.A.; Far, B.H.; Naugler, C. Applications of the MapReduce programming framework to clinical big data analysis: Current landscape and future trends. *BioData Min.* **2014**, *7*, 22. [CrossRef] [PubMed]

23. Raghupathi, W.; Raghupathi, V. Big data analytics in healthcare: Promise and potential. *Health Inf. Sci. Syst.* **2014**, *2*, 3. [CrossRef] [PubMed]

24. Belle, A.; Thiagarajan, R.; Soroushmehr, S.; Navidi, F.; Beard, D.A.; Najarian, K. Big data analytics in healthcare. *BioMed Res. Int.* **2015**, *2015*, 370194. [CrossRef] [PubMed]

25. Sarker, A.; Ginn, R.; Nikfarjam, A.; O'Connor, K.; Smith, K.; Jayaraman, S.; Upadhaya, T.; Gonzalez, G. Utilizing social media data for pharmacovigilance: A review. *J. Biomed. Inform.* **2015**, *54*, 202–212. [CrossRef] [PubMed]

26. Karimi, S.; Wang, C.; Metke-Jimenez, A.; Gaire, R.; Paris, C. Text and data mining techniques in adverse drug reaction detection. *ACM Comput. Surv.* **2015**, *47*, 56. [CrossRef]

27. Dinov, I.D. Methodological challenges and analytic opportunities for modeling and interpreting Big Healthcare Data. *Gigascience* **2016**, *5*, 12. [CrossRef] [PubMed]

28. Moher, D.; Liberati, A.; Tetzlaff, J.; Altman, D.G.; Group, P. Preferred reporting items for systematic reviews and meta-analyses: The PRISMA statement. *PLoS Med.* **2009**, *6*, e1000097. [CrossRef] [PubMed]

29. The Joanna Briggs Institute. Available online: http://joannabriggs.org/research/critical-appraisal-tools.html (accessed on 7 September 2017).

30. Critical Approsal Skills Programme. Available online: http://docs.wixstatic.com/ugd/dded87_25658615020e427da194a325e7773d42.pdf (accessed on 7 September 2017).

31. Levy, Y.; Ellis, T.J. A systems approach to conduct an effective literature review in support of information systems research. *Inf. Sci.* **2006**, *9*, 181–212. [CrossRef]

32. Webster, J.; Watson, R.T. Analyzing the past to prepare for the future: Writing a literature review. *Manag. Inf. Syst. Q.* **2002**, *22*, xiii–xxiii.

33. Russom, P. *Big Data Analytics*; TDWI Best Practices Report; Fourth Quarter; Report No.: 9.14.2011; TDWI: Renton, WV, USA, 2011.

34. Bastian, M.; Heymann, S.; Jacomy, M. Gephi: An open source software for exploring and manipulating networks. In Proceedings of the 3rd International AAAI Conference on Weblogs and Social Media, San Jose, CA, USA, 17–19 May 2009; pp. 361–362.

35. Issa, N.T.; Byers, S.W.; Dakshanamurthy, S. Big data: The next frontier for innovation in therapeutics and healthcare. *Expert Rev. Clin. Pharmacol.* **2014**, *7*, 293–298. [CrossRef] [PubMed]

36. Baldwin, T.; Cook, P.; Lui, M.; MacKinlay, A.; Wang, L. How noisy social media text, how diffrnt social media sources? In Proceedings of the Sixth International Joint Conference on Natural Language Processing, Nagoya, Japan, 14–19 October 2013; pp. 356–364.

37. Wang, C.; Guo, X.; Wang, Y.; Chen, Y.; Liu, B. Friend or foe?: Your wearable devices reveal your personal pin. In Proceedings of the 11th ACM on Asia Conference on Computer and Communications Security, Xi'an, China, 30 May–3 June 2016; pp. 189–200.

38. Yeh, W.-C.; Chang, W.-W.; Chung, Y.Y. A new hybrid approach for mining breast cancer pattern using discrete particle swarm optimization and statistical method. *Expert Syst. Appl.* **2009**, *36*, 8204–8211. [CrossRef]

39. jasondavies.com. Available online: https://www.jasondavies.com/wordcloud/ (accessed on 17 July 2017).

40. Karaolis, M.; Moutiris, J.A.; Hadjipanayi, D.; Pattichis, C.S. Assessment of the risk factors of coronary heart events based on data mining with decision trees. *IEEE Trans. Inf. Technol. Biomed.* **2010**, *14*, 559–566. [CrossRef] [PubMed]

41. Tsipouras, M.G.; Exarchos, T.P.; Fotiadis, D.I.; Kotsia, A.P.; Vakalis, K.V.; Naka, K.K.; Michalis, L.K. Automated diagnosis of coronary artery disease based on data mining and fuzzy modeling. *IEEE Trans. Inf. Technol. Biomed.* **2008**, *12*, 447–458. [CrossRef] [PubMed]

42. Nguyen, T.; Khosravi, A.; Creighton, D.; Nahavandi, S. Classification of healthcare data using genetic fuzzy logic system and wavelets. *Expert Syst. Appl.* **2015**, *42*, 2184–2197. [CrossRef]

43. Vock, D.M.; Wolfson, J.; Bandyopadhyay, S.; Adomavicius, G.; Johnson, P.E.; Vazquez-Benitez, G.; O'Connor, P.J. Adapting machine learning techniques to censored time-to-event health record data: A general-purpose approach using inverse probability of censoring weighting. *J. Biomed. Inform.* **2016**, *61*, 119–131. [CrossRef] [PubMed]

44. Bandyopadhyay, S.; Wolfson, J.; Vock, D.M.; Vazquez-Benitez, G.; Adomavicius, G.; Elidrisi, M.; Johnson, P.E.; O'Connor, P.J. Data mining for censored time-to-event data: A Bayesian network model for predicting cardiovascular risk from electronic health record data. *Data Min. Knowl. Discov.* **2015**, *29*, 1033–1069. [CrossRef]

45. Sufi, F.; Khalil, I. Diagnosis of cardiovascular abnormalities from compressed ECG: A data mining-based approach. *IEEE Trans. Inf. Technol. Biomed.* **2011**, *15*, 33–39. [CrossRef] [PubMed]

46. Kusiak, A.; Caldarone, C.A.; Kelleher, M.D.; Lamb, F.S.; Persoon, T.J.; Burns, A. Hypoplastic left heart syndrome: Knowledge discovery with a data mining approach. *Comput. Biol. Med.* **2006**, *36*, 21–40. [CrossRef] [PubMed]

47. Wang, F.; Lee, N.; Hu, J.; Sun, J.; Ebadollahi, S.; Laine, A.F. A framework for mining signatures from event sequences and its applications in healthcare data. *IEEE Trans. Pattern Anal. Mach. Intell.* **2013**, *35*, 272–285. [CrossRef] [PubMed]

48. Antonelli, D.; Baralis, E.; Bruno, G.; Cerquitelli, T.; Chiusano, S.; Mahoto, N. Analysis of diabetic patients through their examination history. *Expert Syst. Appl.* **2013**, *40*, 4672–4678. [CrossRef]

49. Huang, Y.; McCullagh, P.; Black, N.; Harper, R. Feature selection and classification model construction on type 2 diabetic patients' data. *Artif. Intell. Med.* **2007**, *41*, 251–262. [CrossRef] [PubMed]

50. Tapak, L.; Mahjub, H.; Hamidi, O.; Poorolajal, J. Real-data comparison of data mining methods in prediction of diabetes in Iran. *Healthc. Inform. Res.* **2013**, *19*, 177–185. [CrossRef] [PubMed]

51. Razavian, N.; Blecker, S.; Schmidt, A.M.; Smith-McLallen, A.; Nigam, S.; Sontag, D. Population-level prediction of type 2 diabetes from claims data and analysis of risk factors. *Big Data* **2015**, *3*, 277–287. [CrossRef] [PubMed]

52. Wei, W.-Q.; Leibson, C.L.; Ransom, J.E.; Kho, A.N.; Caraballo, P.J.; Chai, H.S.; Yawn, B.P.; Pacheco, J.A.; Chute, C.G. Impact of data fragmentation across healthcare centers on the accuracy of a high-throughput clinical phenotyping algorithm for specifying subjects with type 2 diabetes mellitus. *J. Am. Med. Assoc.* **2012**, *19*, 219–224. [CrossRef] [PubMed]

53. Barakat, N.; Bradley, A.P.; Barakat, M.N.H. Intelligible support vector machines for diagnosis of diabetes mellitus. *IEEE Trans. Inf. Technol. Biomed.* **2010**, *14*, 1114–1120. [CrossRef] [PubMed]

54. Delen, D. Analysis of cancer data: A data mining approach. *Expert Syst.* **2009**, *26*, 100–112. [CrossRef]

55. Iqbal, U.; Hsu, C.-K.; Nguyen, P.A.A.; Clinciu, D.L.; Lu, R.; Syed-Abdul, S.; Yang, H.C.; Wang, Y.C.; Huang, C.Y.; Huang, C.W.; et al. Cancer-disease associations: A visualization and animation through medical big data. *Comput. Methods Programs Biomed.* **2016**, *127*, 44–51. [CrossRef] [PubMed]

56. Agrawal, A.; Misra, S.; Narayanan, R.; Polepeddi, L.; Choudhary, A. Lung cancer survival prediction using ensemble data mining on SEER data. *Sci. Program* **2012**, *20*, 29–42. [CrossRef]

57. Ha, S.H.; Joo, S.H. A hybrid data mining method for the medical classification of chest pain. *Int. J. Comput. Eng.* **2010**, *4*, 33–38.

58. Ceglowski, R.; Churilov, L.; Wasserthiel, J. Combining data mining and discrete event simulation for a value-added view of a hospital emergency department. *J. Oper. Res. Soc.* **2007**, *58*, 246–254. [CrossRef]

59. Kim, S.; Kim, W.; Park, R.W. A comparison of intensive care unit mortality prediction models through the use of data mining techniques. *Healthc. Inform. Res.* **2011**, *17*, 232–243. [CrossRef] [PubMed]

60. Lee, J.; Maslove, D.M.; Dubin, J.A. Personalized mortality prediction driven by electronic medical data and a patient similarity metric. *PLoS ONE* **2015**, *10*, e0127428. [CrossRef] [PubMed]

61. Razali, A.M.; Ali, S. Generating treatment plan in medicine: A data mining approach. *Am. J. Appl. Sci.* **2009**, *6*, 345–351. [CrossRef]

62. Su, C.-T.; Wang, P.-C.; Chen, Y.-C.; Chen, L.-F. Data mining techniques for assisting the diagnosis of pressure ulcer development in surgical patients. *J. Med. Syst.* **2012**, *36*, 2387. [CrossRef] [PubMed]

63. Raju, D.; Su, X.; Patrician, P.A.; Loan, L.A.; McCarthy, M.S. Exploring factors associated with pressure ulcers: A data mining approach. *Int. J. Nurs. Stud.* **2015**, *52*, 102–111. [CrossRef] [PubMed]

64. Wright, A.; Chen, E.S.; Maloney, F.L. An automated technique for identifying associations between medications, laboratory results and problems. *J. Biomed. Inform.* **2010**, *43*, 891–901. [CrossRef] [PubMed]

65. Lee, C.-H.; Chen, J.C.-Y.; Tseng, V.S. A novel data mining mechanism considering bio-signal and environmental data with applications on asthma monitoring. *Comput. Methods Prog. Biomed.* **2011**, *101*, 44–61. [CrossRef] [PubMed]

66. Chawla, N.V.; Davis, D.A. Bringing big data to personalized healthcare: A patient-centered framework. *J. Gen. Intern. Med.* **2013**, *28*, S660–S665. [CrossRef] [PubMed]

67. Roque, F.S.; Jensen, P.B.; Schmock, H.; Dalgaard, M.; Andreatta, M.; Hansen, T.; Søeby, K.; Bredkjær, S.; Juul, A.; Werge, T.; et al. Using electronic patient records to discover disease correlations and stratify patient cohorts. *PLoS Comput. Biol.* **2011**, *7*, e1002141. [CrossRef] [PubMed]

68. Mookiah, M.R.K.; Acharya, U.R.; Lim, C.M.; Petznick, A.; Suri, J.S. Data mining technique for automated diagnosis of glaucoma using higher order spectra and wavelet energy features. *Knowl. Based Syst.* **2012**, *33*, 73–82. [CrossRef]

69. Murphy, D.R.; Meyer, A.N.; Bhise, V.; Russo, E.; Sittig, D.F.; Wei, L.; Wu, L.; Singh, H. Computerized triggers of big data to detect delays in follow-up of chest imaging results. *Chest* **2016**, *150*, 613–620. [CrossRef] [PubMed]

70. Khalilia, M.; Chakraborty, S.; Popescu, M. Predicting disease risks from highly imbalanced data using random forest. *BMC Med. Inform. Decis. Mak.* **2011**, *11*, 51. [CrossRef] [PubMed]

71. Kusiak, A.; Dixon, B.; Shah, S. Predicting survival time for kidney dialysis patients: A data mining approach. *Comput. Biol. Med.* **2005**, *35*, 311–327. [CrossRef] [PubMed]

72. Stamm, A.M.; Bettacchi, C.J. A comparison of 3 metrics to identify health care-associated infections. *Am. J. Infect. Control* **2012**, *40*, 688–691. [CrossRef] [PubMed]

73. Dinov, I.D.; Heavner, B.; Tang, M.; Glusman, G.; Chard, K.; Darcy, M.; Madduri, R.; Pa, J.; Spino, C.; Kesselman, C.; et al. Predictive big data analytics: A study of Parkinson's disease using large, complex, heterogeneous, incongruent, multi-source and incomplete observations. *PLoS ONE.* **2016**, *11*, e0157077. [CrossRef] [PubMed]

74. Yeh, J.-Y.; Wu, T.-H.; Tsao, C.-W. Using data mining techniques to predict hospitalization of hemodialysis patients. *Desic. Support Syst.* **2011**, *50*, 439–448. [CrossRef]

75. Mathias, J.S.; Agrawal, A.; Feinglass, J.; Cooper, A.J.; Baker, D.W.; Choudhary, A. Development of a 5 year life expectancy index in older adults using predictive mining of electronic health record data. *J. Am. Med. Inform. Assoc.* **2013**, *20*, e118–e124. [CrossRef] [PubMed]

76. Zhang, Y.; Fong, S.; Fiaidhi, J.; Mohammed, S. Real-time clinical decision support system with data stream mining. *BioMed Res. Int.* **2012**. Available online: https://www.hindawi.com/journals/bmri/2012/580186/cta/ (accessed on 11 July 2017). [CrossRef] [PubMed]

77. Mozaffarian, D.; Benjamin, E.J.; Go, A.S.; Arnett, D.K.; Blaha, M.J.; Cushman, M.; Das, S.R.; Ferranti, S.D.; Després, J.P.; Fullerton, H.J.; et al. Heart disease and stroke statistics—2016 update. *Circulation* **2016**, *133*, e38–e360. [CrossRef] [PubMed]

78. Sheridan, S.; Pignone, M.; Mulrow, C. Framingham-based tools to calculate the global risk of coronary heart disease. *J. Gen. Intern. Med.* **2003**, *18*, 1039–1052. [CrossRef] [PubMed]

79. Wang, Z.; Hoy, W.E. Is the Framingham coronary heart disease absolute risk function applicable to Aboriginal people? *Med. J. Aust.* **2005**, *182*, 66–69. [PubMed]

80. Rea, T.D.; Heckbert, S.R.; Kaplan, R.C.; Smith, N.L.; Lemaitre, R.N.; Psaty, B.M. Smoking status and risk for recurrent coronary events after myocardial infarction. *Ann. Intern. Med.* **2002**, *137*, 494–500. [CrossRef] [PubMed]

81. Karaolis, M.; Moutiris, J.A.; Papaconstantinou, L.; Pattichis, C.S. Association rule analysis for the assessment of the risk of coronary heart events. In Proceedings of the Annual International Conference of the IEEE Engineering in Medicine and Biology Society, Minneapolis, MN, USA, 3–6 September 2009; pp. 6238–6241.

82. Sturgeon, L.P.; Bragg-Underwood, D.; Tonya, M.; Blankenship, D. Practice matters: Prevention and care of individuals with type 2 diabetes. *Int. J. Faith Commun. Nurs.* **2016**, *2*, 32–40.

83. Siegel, R.L.; Miller, K.D.; Jemal, A. Cancer statistics, 2016. *CA* **2016**, *66*, 7–30. [CrossRef] [PubMed]

84. Chen, T.-C.; Hsu, T.-C. A GAs based approach for mining breast cancer pattern. *Expert Syst. Appl.* **2006**, *30*, 674–681. [CrossRef]

85. Sousa, T.; Silva, A.; Neves, A. Particle swarm based data mining algorithms for classification tasks. *Parallel Comput.* **2004**, *30*, 767–783. [CrossRef]

86. National Center for Health Statistics (US). *Health, United States, 2012: With Special Feature on Emergency Care*; Report No.: 2013-1232; National Center for Health Statistics (US): Hyattsville, MD, USA, 2013.

87. Angus, D.C.; Barnato, A.E.; Linde-Zwirble, W.T.; Weissfeld, L.A.; Watson, R.S.; Rickert, T.; Rubenfeld, G.D. Use of intensive care at the end of life in the United States: An epidemiologic study. *Crit. Care Med.* **2004**, *32*, 638–643. [CrossRef] [PubMed]

88. Saeed, M.; Villarroel, M.; Reisner, A.T.; Clifford, G.; Lehman, L.-W.; Moody, G.; Heldt, T.; Kyaw, T.H.; Moody, B.; Mark, R.G. Multiparameter Intelligent Monitoring in Intensive Care II (MIMIC-II): A public-access intensive care unit database. *Crit. Care Med.* **2011**, *39*, 952–960. [CrossRef] [PubMed]

89. Post, A.R.; Kurc, T.; Cholleti, S.; Gao, J.; Lin, X.; Bornstein, W.; Cantrell, D.; Levine, D.; Hohmann, S.; Saltz, J.H. The Analytic Information Warehouse (AIW): A platform for analytics using electronic health record data. *J. Biomed. Inform.* **2013**, *46*, 410–424. [CrossRef] [PubMed]

90. Zhou, X.; Chen, S.; Liu, B.; Zhang, R.; Wang, Y.; Li, P.; Guo, Y.; Zhang, H.; Gao, Z.; Yan, X. Development of traditional Chinese medicine clinical data warehouse for medical knowledge discovery and decision support. *Artif. Intell. Med.* **2010**, *48*, 139–152. [CrossRef] [PubMed]

91. Zhang, Y.; Qiu, M.; Tsai, C.-W.; Hassan, M.M.; Alamri, A. Health-CPS: Healthcare cyber-physical system assisted by cloud and big data. *IEEE Syst. J.* **2015**, *11*, 88–95. [CrossRef]

92. Erinjeri, J.P.; Picus, D.; Prior, F.W.; Rubin, D.A.; Koppel, P. Development of a Google-based search engine for data mining radiology reports. *J. Digit. Imaging* **2009**, *22*, 348–356. [CrossRef] [PubMed]

93. Mullins, I.M.; Siadaty, M.S.; Lyman, J.; Scully, K.; Garrett, C.T.; Miller, W.G.; Muller, R.; Robson, B.; Apte, C.; Weiss, S.; et al. Data mining and clinical data repositories: Insights from a 667,000 patient data set. *Comput. Biol. Med.* **2006**, *36*, 1351–1377. [CrossRef] [PubMed]

94. Praveenkumar, B.; Suresh, K.; Nikhil, A.; Rohan, M.; Nikhila, B.; Rohit, C.; Srinivas, A. Geospatial Technology in Disease Mapping, E-Surveillance and Health Care for Rural Population in South India. *Int. Arch. Photogr. Remote Sens. Spat. Inf. Sci.* **2014**, *40*, 221. [CrossRef]

95. Shen, C.-P.; Jigjidsuren, C.; Dorjgochoo, S.; Chen, C.-H.; Chen, W.-H.; Hsu, C.-K.; Muller, R.; Robson, B.; Apte, C.; Weiss, S.; et al. A data-mining framework for transnational healthcare system. *J. Med. Syst.* **2012**, *36*, 2565–2575. [CrossRef] [PubMed]

96. Bertsimas, D.; Bjarnadóttir, M.V.; Kane, M.A.; Kryder, J.C.; Pandey, R.; Vempala, S.; Wang, G. Algorithmic prediction of health-care costs. *Oper. Res.* **2008**, *56*, 1382–1392. [CrossRef]

97. Phillips-Wren, G.; Sharkey, P.; Dy, S.M. Mining lung cancer patient data to assess healthcare resource utilization. *Expert Syst. Appl.* **2008**, *35*, 1611–1619. [CrossRef]

98. Hachesu, P.R.; Ahmadi, M.; Alizadeh, S.; Sadoughi, F. Use of data mining techniques to determine and predict length of stay of cardiac patients. *Healthc. Inform. Res.* **2013**, *19*, 121–129. [CrossRef] [PubMed]

99. Pur, A.; Bohanec, M.; Lavrač, N.; Cestnik, B. Primary health-care network monitoring: A hierarchical resource allocation modeling approach. *Int. J. Health Plan. Manag.* **2010**, *25*, 119–135. [CrossRef] [PubMed]

100. Robinson, J.W. Regression tree boosting to adjust health care cost predictions for diagnostic mix. *Health Serv. Res.* **2008**, *43*, 755–772. [CrossRef] [PubMed]

101. Cercone, N.; An, X.; Li, J.; Gu, Z.; An, A. Finding best evidence for evidence-based best practice recommendations in health care: The initial decision support system design. *Knowl. Inf. Syst.* **2011**, *29*, 159–201. [CrossRef]

102. Zhuang, Z.Y.; Churilov, L.; Burstein, F.; Sikaris, K. Combining data mining and case-based reasoning for intelligent decision support for pathology ordering by general practitioners. *Eur. J. Oper. Res.* **2009**, *195*, 662–675. [CrossRef]

103. Delen, D.; Fuller, C.; McCann, C.; Ray, D. Analysis of healthcare coverage: A data mining approach. *Expert Syst. Appl.* **2009**, *36*, 995–1003. [CrossRef]

104. Greaves, F.; Ramirez-Cano, D.; Millett, C.; Darzi, A.; Donaldson, L. Use of sentiment analysis for capturing patient experience from free-text comments posted online. *J. Med. Internet Res.* **2013**, *15*, e239. [CrossRef] [PubMed]

105. Glowacka, K.J.; Henry, R.M.; May, J.H. A hybrid data mining/simulation approach for modelling outpatient no-shows in clinic scheduling. *J. Oper. Res. Soc.* **2009**, *60*, 1056–1068. [CrossRef]

106. Duan, L.; Street, W.N.; Xu, E. Healthcare information systems: Data mining methods in the creation of a clinical recommender system. *Enterp. Inf. Syst.* **2011**, *5*, 169–181. [CrossRef]

107. Koskela, T.-H.; Ryynanen, O.-P.; Soini, E.J. Risk factors for persistent frequent use of the primary health care services among frequent attenders: A Bayesian approach. *Scand. J. Prim. Health Care* **2010**, *28*, 55–61. [CrossRef] [PubMed]

108. Cubillas, J.J.; Ramos, M.I.; Feito, F.R.; Ureña, T. An Improvement in the Appointment Scheduling in Primary Health Care Centers Using Data Mining. *J. Med. Syst.* **2014**, *38*, 89. [CrossRef] [PubMed]

109. Lee, T.-T.; Liu, C.-Y.; Kuo, Y.-H.; Mills, M.E.; Fong, J.-G.; Hung, C. Application of data mining to the identification of critical factors in patient falls using a web-based reporting system. *Int. J. Med. Inf.* **2011**, *80*, 141–150. [CrossRef] [PubMed]

110. Tremblay, M.C.; Berndt, D.J.; Luther, S.L.; Foulis, P.R.; French, D.D. Identifying fall-related injuries: Text mining the electronic medical record. *Inf. Technol. Manag.* **2009**, *10*, 253–265. [CrossRef]

111. Feldman, K.; Chawla, N.V. Does Medical School Training Relate to Practice? Evidence from Big Data. *Big Data* **2015**, *3*, 103–113. [CrossRef] [PubMed]

112. Hao, H.; Zhang, K. The voice of chinese health consumers: A text mining approach to web-Based physician reviews. *J. Med. Internet Res.* **2016**, *18*. [CrossRef] [PubMed]

113. Christodoulakis, A.; Karanikas, H.; Billiris, A.; Thireos, E.; Pelekis, N. "Big data" in health care Assessment of the performance of Greek NHS hospitals using key performance and clinical workload indicators. *Arch. Hellenic Med.* **2016**, *33*, 489–497.

114. Torosyan, Y.; Hu, Y.; Hoffman, S.; Luo, Q.; Carleton, B.; Marinac-Dabic, D. An in silico framework for integrating epidemiologic and genetic evidence with health care applications: Ventilation-related pneumothorax as a case illustration. *J. Am. Med. Inform. Assoc.* **2016**, *23*, 711–720. [CrossRef] [PubMed]

115. Callahan, A.; Pernek, I.; Stiglic, G.; Leskovec, J.; Strasberg, H.R.; Shah, N.H. Analyzing information seeking and drug-safety alert response by health care professionals as new methods for surveillance. *J. Med. Internet Res.* **2015**, *17*, e204. [CrossRef] [PubMed]

116. Madigan, E.A.; Curet, O.L. A data mining approach in home healthcare: Outcomes and service use. *BMC Health Serv. Res.* **2006**, *6*, 18. [CrossRef] [PubMed]

117. Lin, C.-H.; Huang, L.-C.; Chou, S.-C.T.; Liu, C.-H.; Cheng, H.-F.; Chiang, I.-J. Temporal event tracing on big healthcare data analytics. *Big Data Appl. Use Cases* **2016**, 95–108. [CrossRef]

118. Liu, K.; Kargupta, H.; Ryan, J. Random projection-based multiplicative data perturbation for privacy preserving distributed data mining. *IEEE Trans. Knowl. Data Eng.* **2006**, *18*, 92–106.

119. Youssef, A.E. A framework for secure healthcare systems based on big data analytics in mobile cloud computing environments. *Int. J. Ambient Syst. Appl.* **2014**, *2*, 1–11. [CrossRef]

120. Li, F.; Zou, X.; Liu, P.; Chen, J.Y. New threats to health data privacy. *BMC BioInform.* **2011**, *12*, S7. [CrossRef] [PubMed]

121. Yang, W.-S.; Hwang, S.-Y. A process-mining framework for the detection of healthcare fraud and abuse. *Expert Syst. Appl.* **2006**, *31*, 56–68. [CrossRef]

122. Mohammed, N.; Fung, B.C.M.; Hung, P.C.K.; Lee, C.-K. Centralized and Distributed Anonymization for High-Dimensional Healthcare Data. *ACM Trans. Knowl. Discov. Data* **2010**, *4*, 1–33. [CrossRef]

123. Chong, S.A.; Abdin, E.; Vaingankar, J.A.; Heng, D.; Sherbourne, C.; Yap, M.; Lim, Y.W.; Wong, H.B.; Ghosh-Dastidar, B.; Kwok, K.W.; et al. A population-based survey of mental disorders in Singapore. *Ann. Acad. Med. Singap.* **2012**, *41*, 49–66. [PubMed]

124. Walker, E.R.; Druss, B.G. Cumulative burden of comorbid mental disorders, substance use disorders, chronic medical conditions, and poverty on health among adults in the USA. *Psychol. Health Med.* **2017**, *22*, 727–735. [CrossRef] [PubMed]

125. Panagiotakopoulos, T.C.; Lyras, D.P.; Livaditis, M.; Sgarbas, K.N.; Anastassopoulos, G.C.; Lymberopoulos, D.K. A contextual data mining approach toward assisting the treatment of anxiety disorders. *IEEE Trans. Inf. Technol. Biomed.* **2010**, *14*, 567–581. [CrossRef] [PubMed]

126. Chang, C.-L. A study of applying data mining to early intervention for developmentally-delayed children. *Expert Syst. Appl.* **2007**, *33*, 407–412. [CrossRef]

127. Candás, J.L.C.; Peláez, V.; López, G.; Fernández, M.Á.; Álvarez, E.; Díaz, G. An automatic data mining method to detect abnormal human behaviour using physical activity measurements. *Perv. Mob. Comput.* **2014**, *15*, 228–241. [CrossRef]

128. Diederich, J.; Al-Ajmi, A.; Yellowlees, P.E. X-ray: Data mining and mental health. *Appl. Softw. Comput.* **2007**, *7*, 923–928. [CrossRef]

129. Adomavicius, G.; Tuzhilin, A. Context-Aware Recommender Systems. In *Recommender Systems Handbook*; Springer: Boston, MA, USA, 2015; pp. 191–226.

130. Nimmagadda, S.L.; Dreher, H.V. On robust methodologies for managing public health care systems. *Int. J. Environ. Res. Public Health* **2014**, *11*, 1106–1140. [CrossRef] [PubMed]

131. Buczak, A.L.; Baugher, B.; Guven, E.; Moniz, L.; Babin, S.M.; Chretien, J.-P. Prediction of Peaks of Seasonal Influenza in Military Health-Care Data. *Biomed. Eng. Copmut. Biol.* **2016**, *7*, 15–26. [CrossRef] [PubMed]

132. Hosseini, Z.Z.; Mohammadzadeh, M. Knowledge discovery from patients' behavior via clustering-classification algorithms based on weighted eRFM and CLV model: An empirical study in public health care services. *Iran. J. Pharm. Res.* **2016**, *15*, 355–367.

133. Kostkova, P.; Fowler, D.; Wiseman, S.; Weinberg, J.R. Major infection events over 5 years: How is media coverage influencing online information needs of health care professionals and the public? *J. Med. Internet Res.* **2013**, *15*, e107. [CrossRef] [PubMed]

134. Santos, R.S.; Malheiros, S.M.; Cavalheiro, S.; De Oliveira, J.P. A data mining system for providing analytical information on brain tumors to public health decision makers. *Comput. Methods Prog. Biomed.* **2013**, *109*, 269–282. [CrossRef] [PubMed]

135. Lavrač, N.; Bohanec, M.; Pur, A.; Cestnik, B.; Debeljak, M.; Kobler, A. Data mining and visualization for decision support and modeling of public health-care resources. *J. Biomed. Inform.* **2007**, *40*, 438–447. [CrossRef] [PubMed]

136. Rathore, M.M.; Ahmad, A.; Paul, A.; Wan, J.; Zhang, D. Real-time Medical Emergency Response System: Exploiting IoT and Big Data for Public Health. *J. Med. Syst.* **2016**, *40*, 283. [CrossRef] [PubMed]

137. Ma, B.L.W.H.Y.; Liu, B. Integrating classification and association rule mining. In Proceedings of the Fourth International Conference on Knowledge Discovery and Data Mining, New York, NY, USA, 27–31 August 1998.

138. Harpaz, R.; Vilar, S.; DuMouchel, W.; Salmasian, H.; Haerian, K.; Shah, N.H.; Chase, H.S.; Friedman, C. Combing signals from spontaneous reports and electronic health records for detection of adverse drug reactions. *J. Am. Med. Inform. Assoc.* **2012**, *20*, 413–419. [CrossRef] [PubMed]

139. Harpaz, R.; Chase, H.S.; Friedman, C. Mining multi-item drug adverse effect associations in spontaneous reporting systems. *BMC BioInform.* **2010**, *11*, S7. [CrossRef] [PubMed]

140. Akay, A.; Dragomir, A.; Erlandsson, B.-E. Network-based modeling and intelligent data mining of social media for improving care. *IEEE J. Biomed. Health Inform.* **2015**, *19*, 210–218. [CrossRef] [PubMed]

141. Eriksson, R.; Werge, T.; Jensen, L.J.; Brunak, S. Dose-specific adverse drug reaction identification in electronic patient records: Temporal data mining in an inpatient psychiatric population. *Drug Saf.* **2014**, *37*, 237–247. [CrossRef] [PubMed]

142. Kadoyama, K.; Kuwahara, A.; Yamamori, M.; Brown, J.; Sakaeda, T.; Okuno, Y. Hypersensitivity reactions to anticancer agents: Data mining of the public version of the FDA adverse event reporting system, AERS. *J. Exp. Clin. Cancer Res.* **2011**, *5*, 93. [CrossRef] [PubMed]

143. Sakaeda, T.; Kadoyama, K.; Okuno, Y. Statin-associated muscular and renal adverse events: Data mining of the public version of the FDA adverse event reporting system. *PLoS ONE* **2011**, *6*, e28124. [CrossRef] [PubMed]

144. Trifirò, G.; Pariente, A.; Coloma, P.M.; Kors, J.A.; Polimeni, G.; Miremont-Salamé, G.; Catania, M.A.; Salvo, F.; David, A.; Moore, N.; et al. Data mining on electronic health record databases for signal detection in pharmacovigilance: Which events to monitor? *Pharmacoepidemiol. Drug Saf.* **2009**, *18*, 1176–1184. [CrossRef] [PubMed]

145. Choi, N.K.; Chang, Y.; Choi, Y.K.; Hahn, S.; Park, B.J. Signal detection of rosuvastatin compared to other statins: Data-mining study using national health insurance claims database. *Pharmacoepidemiol. Drug Saf.* **2010**, *19*, 238–246. [CrossRef] [PubMed]

146. Jin, H.; Chen, J.; He, H.; Williams, G.J.; Kelman, C.; O'Keefe, C.M. Mining unexpected temporal associations: Applications in detecting adverse drug reactions. *IEEE Trans. Inf. Technol. Biomed.* **2008**, *12*, 488–500. [PubMed]

147. Celi, L.A.; Zimolzak, A.J.; Stone, D.J. Dynamic clinical data mining: Search engine-based decision support. *JMIR Med. Inform.* **2014**, *2*, e13. [CrossRef] [PubMed]

148. Pittet, D. Infection control and quality health care in the new millenium. *Am. J. Infect. Control* **2005**, *33*, 258–267. [CrossRef] [PubMed]

149. Chambers, D.A.; Rupp, A. Sharing state mental health data for research: Building toward ongoing learning in mental health care systems. *Adm. Policy Ment. Health Serv. Res.* **2015**, *42*, 586–587. [CrossRef] [PubMed]

150. Schilsky, R.L.; Michels, D.L.; Kearbey, A.H.; Yu, P.P.; Hudis, C.A. Building a rapid learning health care system for oncology: The regulatory framework of CancerLinQ. *J. Clin. Oncol.* **2014**, *32*, 2373–2379. [CrossRef] [PubMed]

151. Reiner, B. Uncovering and improving upon the inherent deficiencies of radiology reporting through data mining. *J. Digit. Imaging* **2010**, *23*, 109–118. [CrossRef] [PubMed]

152. Sukumar, S.R.; Natarajan, R.; Ferrell, R.K. Quality of Big Data in health care. *Int. J. Qual. Health Care* **2015**, *28*, 621–634. [CrossRef] [PubMed]

153. Viceconti, M.; Hunter, P.; Hose, R. Big data, big knowledge: Big data for personalized healthcare. *IEEE J. Biomed. Health Inform.* **2015**, *19*, 1209–1215. [CrossRef] [PubMed]

154. Roski, J.; Bo-Linn, G.W.; Andrews, T.A. Creating value in health care through big data: Opportunities and policy implications. *Health Aff.* **2014**, *33*, 1115–1122. [CrossRef] [PubMed]

155. Westra, B.L.; Latimer, G.E.; Matney, S.A.; Park, J.I.; Sensmeier, J.; Simpson, R.L.; Swanson, M.J.; Warren, J.J.; Delaney, C.W. A national action plan for sharable and comparable nursing data to support practice and translational research for transforming health care. *J. Am. Med. Inform. Assoc.* **2015**, *22*, 600–607. [CrossRef] [PubMed]

156. Heitmueller, A.; Henderson, S.; Warburton, W.; Elmagarmid, A.; Darzi, A. Developing public policy to advance the use of big data in health care. *Health Aff.* **2014**, *33*, 1523–1530. [CrossRef] [PubMed]

157. Cohen, I.G.; Amarasingham, R.; Shah, A.; Xie, B.; Lo, B. The legal and ethical concerns that arise from using complex predictive analytics in health care. *Health Aff.* **2014**, *33*, 1139–1147. [CrossRef] [PubMed]

158. Hiller, J.S. Healthy Predictions? Questions for Data Analytics in Health Care. *Am. Bus. Law J.* **2016**, *53*, 251–314. [CrossRef]

159. Lu, R.; Lin, X.; Shen, X. SPOC: A secure and privacy-preserving opportunistic computing framework for mobile-healthcare emergency. *IEEE Trans. Parallel Distrib. Syst.* **2013**, *24*, 614–624. [CrossRef]

160. Orentlicher, D. Prescription data mining and the protection of patients' interests. *J. Law Med. Ethics* **2010**, *38*, 74–84. [CrossRef] [PubMed]

161. Soroushmehr, S.R.; Najarian, K. Transforming big data into computational models for personalized medicine and health care. *Dialogues Clin. Neurosci.* **2016**, *18*, 339–343.

162. Martin, C.M.; Félix-Bortolotti, M. Person-centred health care: A critical assessment of current and emerging research approaches. *J. Eval. Clin. Pract.* **2014**, *20*, 1056–1064. [CrossRef] [PubMed]

163. Estape, E.S.; Mays, M.H.; Sternke, E.A. Translation in Data Mining to Advance Personalized Medicine for Health Equity. *Intell. Inf. Manag.* **2016**, *8*, 9–16. [CrossRef] [PubMed]

164. Kimberly, J.; Cronk, I. Making value a priority: How this paradigm shift is changing the landscape in health care. *Ann. N. Y. Acad. Sci.* **2016**, *1381*, 162–167. [CrossRef] [PubMed]

165. Marshall, D.A.; Burgos-Liz, L.; IJzerman, M.J.; Crown, W.; Padula, W.V.; Wong, P.K.; Pasupathy, K.S.; Higashi, M.K.; Osgood, N.D. Selecting a dynamic simulation modeling method for health care delivery research—Part 2: Report of the ISPOR Dynamic Simulation Modeling Emerging Good Practices Task Force. *Value Health* **2015**, *18*, 147–160. [CrossRef] [PubMed]

166. Reiner, B.I. Transforming health care service delivery and provider selection. *J. Digit. Imaging* **2011**, *24*, 373–377. [CrossRef] [PubMed]

167. Bates, D.W.; Saria, S.; Ohno-Machado, L.; Shah, A.; Escobar, G. Big data in health care: Using analytics to identify and manage high-risk and high-cost patients. *Health Aff.* **2014**, *33*, 1123–1131. [CrossRef] [PubMed]

168. Auffray, C.; Balling, R.; Barroso, I.; Bencze, L.; Benson, M.; Bergeron, J.; Bergeron, J.; Bernal-Delgado, E.; Blomberg, N.; Bock, C.; et al. Making sense of big data in health research: Towards an EU action plan. *Genome Med.* **2016**, *8*, 71–83. [CrossRef] [PubMed]

169. Janke, A.T.; Overbeek, D.L.; Kocher, K.E.; Levy, P.D. Exploring the potential of predictive analytics and big data in emergency care. *Ann. Emerg. Med.* **2016**, *67*, 227–236. [CrossRef] [PubMed]

170. Vie, L.L.; Griffith, K.N.; Scheier, L.M.; Lester, P.B.; Seligman, M.E. The Person-Event Data Environment: Leveraging big data for studies of psychological strengths in soldiers. *Front. Psychol.* **2013**, *4*, 934. [CrossRef] [PubMed]

171. Andreu-Perez, J.; Poon, C.C.; Merrifield, R.D.; Wong, S.T.; Yang, G.-Z. Big data for health. *IEEE J. Biomed. Health Inform.* **2015**, *19*, 1193–1208. [CrossRef] [PubMed]

172. Fayyad, U.; Piatetsky-Shapiro, G.; Smyth, P. From data mining to knowledge discovery in databases. *AI Mag.* **1996**, *17*, 37–55.

173. Koh, H.C.; Tan, G. Data mining applications in healthcare. *J. Healthc. Inform. Manag.* **2011**, *19*, 65–73.

174. Aguinis, H.; Gottfredson, R.K.; Joo, H. Best-practice recommendations for defining, identifying, and handling outliers. *Organ. Res. Meth.* **2013**, *16*, 270–301. [CrossRef]

175. John, U.; Hensel, E.; Lüdemann, J.; Piek, M.; Sauer, S.; Adam, C.; Adam, C.; Born, G.; Alte, D.; Greiser, E.; et al. Study of Health In Pomerania (SHIP): A health examination survey in an east German region: Objectives and design. *Sozial-und Präventivmedizin* **2001**, *46*, 186–194. [CrossRef] [PubMed]

176. Nicholas, T.N. *The Black Swan: The Impact of the Highly Improbable*; Random: New York, NY, USA, 2007.

4

Impact of Veteran Status and Timing of PTSD Diagnosis on Criminal Justice Outcomes

Brandt A. Smith

Department of Psychology, Columbus State University, Columbus, GA 31907, USA;
smith_brandt@columbusstate.edu

Abstract: Previous research has demonstrated that jurors show a bias towards treatment for veterans with post-traumatic stress disorder (PTSD). The present research examines this bias when jurors are faced with cases of potential malingering, in which the defendant's claim of PTSD is a perceived attempt to escape legal punishments. Trial vignettes, in which veteran status and PTSD diagnosis timing were manipulated, were used to explore this phenomenon. It was found that veterans who received their diagnosis after being arrested were found guilty more often, and were diverted to treatment less often, than those who were diagnosed before an arrest. This has critical implications for mental healthcare in that it is crucial to properly diagnose and treat people before they find themselves in court. Further, the negative outcomes in court demonstrate one of the severe social impacts of untreated or late-diagnosed PTSD.

Keywords: PTSD; veterans; court; malingering

1. Introduction

Post-traumatic stress disorder (PTSD) has received attention because of the prevalence of the condition in veterans from Operation Iraqi Freedom (OIF), Operation Enduring Freedom (OEF), and Operation New Dawn (OND). Associated with this is the supposed connection between some symptoms of PTSD and criminal behavior [1], for example, hypervigilance. The scientific evidence linking PTSD and criminal behavior is inconclusive [2], though still believed by some to resolved. Though in many cases defense attorneys avoid the so-called insanity-defense [3,4] PTSD has been shown to be a mitigating factor in criminal proceedings [5]. Unfortunately, there is a stigma associated with PTSD (real or perceived is immaterial) that could discourage people from seeking assistance and mental healthcare [6]. This stigma can lead to people not seeking help until they reach a negative social position and find themselves involved in the criminal justice system. A defense attorney may attempt to use PTSD as a defense for their client, which would require an evaluation by mental health professionals after the person has been arrested. This post-arrest diagnosis may be perceived as malingering by jurors and not serve to help a person who is suffering. This is the reason that defense attorneys often avoid the insanity defense, as it is often seen by juries to be an attempt to avoid responsibility [3,4]. For this reason, it is hypothesized that a post-arrest diagnosis is mistrusted and could be viewed as self-serving.

This phenomenon illustrates why it is necessary to diagnose and help those in need, before their lives are disrupted by criminal court proceedings. The present research examines one facet of this problem, PTSD diagnosis before or after an arrest. Previous research has shown a bias towards treatment for veterans with PTSD when verdict options beyond "guilty" and "not guilty" were available [7]. That research did not examine the influence of perceived malingering on juror verdicts. The present research was designed to remedy this. Examining the impact of said issues in a criminal court setting allows us to see the impact of perceived malingering of PTSD. This approach details, in a practical setting, the importance of early diagnosis and intervention to avoid future criminal justice issues and quality of life problems.

Jurors may view a post-arrest diagnosis of PTSD as an attempt to escape punishment, and some may note the ease by which PTSD can be malingered [8]. Some people may not seek treatment because of perceived stigma [9], which could leave them in a situation where their PTSD diagnosis is given after an arrest. This can lead to perceptions of malingering, which, in turn, would remove the bias towards treatment seen in previous research [7].

1.1. Malingering

Malingering and/or symptom exaggeration is fairly common in some instances, though, in criminal cases, researchers show a 19% prevalence [10]. Nearly one-fifth of criminal cases were found to have some evidence of malingering. This is problematic because a person could benefit from receiving a PTSD diagnosis if it helped them escape punishment. Whether or not the person truly has PTSD is immaterial to the purposes of the present research, as the examination is about juror responses to what could be malingered PTSD. The present research does not differentiate between exaggerated symptoms and malingering.

Research has shown that PTSD diagnoses are susceptible to malingering because the diagnosis relies heavily on a person's self-report of symptoms [11]. There are several reasons why a person may malinger PTSD. Financial gains are obvious in that a person can receive money from their government in the form of disability payments. These payments can be substantial and result in other gains, money for school, and other considerations. Personal gain is particularly highlighted in the case of escaping criminal liability, where a PTSD diagnosis can alleviate personal responsibility. When there is a real or perceived gain from the diagnosis, it is more likely that a juror perceives the PTSD claim as malingered. No previous research has empirically examined the effects of perceived malingering in relation to juror verdicts.

1.2. Untreated PTSD

Taking into account the desire to avoid stigma associated with PTSD [6] and the notion that certain symptoms of PTSD can contribute to criminal behavior, a person can find themselves in court because of, at least in part, untreated PTSD. This reluctance to seek mental healthcare has been related to several other negative health outcomes. Untreated PTSD is persistent [12] and has been associated with damaging stress on family and social relationships [13]. Further, PTSD has been associated with general physical health symptoms [14,15], and it has a known comorbidity with alcoholism and other substance abuse disorders that carry their own health and social risks [16,17].

Veterans are disproportionately represented in the criminal justice system in the United States [18], in which veterans comprise approximately 9% of the prison population while comprising 7% of the overall population. This disproportionate representation of veterans in the criminal justice system is not accounted for by any social characteristics associated with veterans. The present research examined the impact of a post-arrest diagnosis on juror decision making. This was done to add to a small but growing corpus of knowledge related to the issue of PTSD and the criminal justice system.

2. Materials and Methods

The present study was a 2 (veteran status: veteran vs. non-veteran) by 3 (diagnosis timing: no diagnosis vs. post-arrest diagnosis vs. pre-arrest diagnosis) between-subjects design. The research protocol was approved by the university IRB (17-071). Two-hundred and twenty-eight people participated in this study. Two participants did not render a verdict, so they were excluded from analysis (final $N = 226$). The average age of the participants was 20.85 years ($SD = 4.123$; range 18–43 years old). The sample was predominately female ($n = 166$). The sample was comprised of college students in a small southeastern United States university.

Participants were randomly assigned to read a trial vignette that showed a defendant who was either a veteran or a non-veteran and revealed information about PTSD diagnosis. The trial vignette detailed a violent encounter in which a person suffered personal injury that was not life threatening. For the non-veteran condition, military service, or the lack thereof, was not mentioned. In the no diagnosis condition, there was no mention of PTSD. The no diagnosis condition was included in this study to serve as a control condition. After participants had read the trial vignette, they were asked to render a verdict of guilty, not guilty, or diverted to treatment. The participants that rendered a guilty verdict were presented with a short survey consisting of three items that measured the severity of the recommended punishment ("how long should the defendant spend in prison"). Participants who rendered a diverted to treatment verdict were shown a list of prohibitions and required activities that they could endorse for the defendant, and they were questioned as to how long the defendant should be under court supervision. All participants were given a short survey that assessed their trust of the criminal justice system. This was assessed to test for a potential moderator of verdict.

3. Results

Veteran status (non-veteran vs. veteran), timing of the diagnosis (no diagnosis vs. post-arrest diagnosis vs. pre-arrest diagnosis), and the interaction between the two variables were entered into a logistic regression analysis. The primary outcome—verdict—was given as guilty, not guilty, or diverted to treatment. Assumptions of linearity for independent variables and log odds were met. The model was significant, χ^2 (10, $N = 229$) = 56.55, $p < 0.0001$, $R^2 = 0.12$. Veteran status did not predict verdict, χ^2 (2, $N = 229$) = 0.995, $p = 0.61$. The timing of diagnosis predicted verdict, χ^2 (4, $N = 229$) = 44.23, $p < 0.0001$, which shows that defendants who were diagnosed with PTSD after arrest are given guilty verdicts more often than defendants who were diagnosed before arrest. Both pre- and post-arrest diagnosis conditions were given fewer guilty verdicts than the no diagnosis condition (Table 1).

Table 1. Verdict by diagnosis condition.

Diagnosis	Guilty	Not Guilty	Diverted
No Diagnosis	51	9	17
Pre-Arrest	17	16	43
Post-Arrest	36	21	16

The interaction between veteran status and timing of diagnosis was a significant predictor of verdict, χ^2 (4, $N = 226$) = 16.03, $p = 0.003$ (Table 2). Examining this interaction revealed that veteran status in the no diagnosis condition did not predict verdict, χ^2 (2, $N = 78$) = 1.24, $p = 0.54$. Veteran status in the post-arrest diagnosis condition predicted verdict, χ^2 (2, $N = 77$) = 6.41, $p = 0.04$, $r^2 = 0.04$. This shows that veterans with a pre-arrest diagnosis were found guilty less often than their non-veteran counterparts and were diverted to treatment more often. Veteran status in the pre-arrest diagnosis condition did predict verdict, χ^2 (2, $N = 74$) = 8.93, $p = 0.01$, $r^2 = 0.06$, showing that non-veterans with a pre-arrest diagnosis of PTSD were given more guilty verdicts and less diversion to treatment. Unexpectedly, participant trust in the justice system did not affect verdict, all p-values > 0.28.

Table 2. Verdict by interaction between diagnosis and veteran status.

Diagnosis	Veteran Status	Guilty	Not Guilty	Diverted
No Diagnosis	Non-Veteran	24	6	9
Post-Arrest	Non-Veteran	15	8	13
Pre-Arrest	Non-Veteran	13	7	18
No Diagnosis	Veteran	27	3	8
Post-Arrest	Veteran	21	13	3
Pre-Arrest	Veteran	4	9	25

3.1. Guilty

Examining those participants that rendered a guilty verdict (n = 98) showed that veteran status did not predict severity of sentence, $F(1, 97)$ = 0.884, p = 0.35. The timing of the diagnosis did, however, predict severity of the sentence, $F(1, 97)$ = 6.319, p = 0.003, r^2 = 0.111. This shows that the non-diagnosis condition (M = 1.502, SE = 0.213) and the pre-arrest diagnosis condition (M = 1.738, SE = 0.262) did not differ, $t(97)$ = −1.713, p = 0.76. Sentence severity for the pre-arrest diagnosis and the post-arrest diagnosis (M = 3.215, SE = 0.434) conditions, $t(97)$ = 2.912, p = 0.013, differed. This shows the importance of early detection and diagnosis of PTSD, as it may serve to lessen sentences for people who become involved in the criminal justice system. The interaction between veteran status and timing of diagnosis was not predictive of sentence severity, $F(2, 97)$ = 1.588, p = 0.21.

3.2. Diverted to Treatment

Examining those participants who rendered a diverted to treatment verdict (n = 71) did not differ on the amount of time that a person should be in supervised treatment regardless of veteran status, $F(1, 70)$ = 0.071, p = 0.791, the timing of diagnosis, $F(1, 70)$ = 0.814, p = 0.447, or the interaction between the two independent variables, $F(2, 70)$ = 1.516, p = 0.227. However, there were differences for the restrictions of treatment by the experimental conditions (Table 3). To a great extent, veterans with a pre-arrest diagnosis of PTSD were held to a higher standard when diverted to treatment.

Table 3. Treatment restrictions by condition.

Restriction	Non-Veteran/ No PTSD	Non-Veteran/ Post Arrest	Non-Veteran/ Pre-Arrest	Veteran/ No PTSD	Veteran/ Post-Arrest	Veteran/ Pre-Arrest
Alcohol Testing	8	10	12	8	2	16
Drug Testing	5	8	10	4	2	14
Anger Management	8	11	12	7	2	19
Therapy	5	10	18	5	3	20
Group Therapy	5	8	11	3	1	13
Prison: Failure to Complete	4	6	6	6	0	7

4. Discussion

The present research illustrated the need for early diagnosis of PTSD because of the manner in which diagnoses after the fact (post-arrest) could be viewed as malingering. Veterans who had been diagnosed with PTSD before they had been arrested were diverted to treatment more often than those who received a diagnosis after their arrest. Previous research has shown that jurors have a preference for diverting a veteran to treatment instead of finding them guilty [7]. The present research has built on those findings by including a condition in which a PTSD diagnosis could be perceived as a malingering or as an attempt to avoid responsibility in a criminal case.

Veterans may, because of the "hero" status that they have, be held to a higher standard than non-veterans. While sometimes good for the veteran—discounts with certain companies and other social benefits—the status can result in an expectation of better behavior. According to a study commissioned by the Chairman of the Joint Chiefs of Staff, veterans can deal with any challenges that they face [19]. This could explain why veterans appear to be held to a higher standard than non-veterans when diverted to treatment.

The impact of being diagnosed after there are criminal or social problems can be problematic for a defendant, in that PTSD, which could be seen as a mitigating factor, would not be considered such in a post-arrest diagnosis. Receiving a diagnosis of PTSD after an arrest could be seen as self-serving on the part of the defendant when that diagnosis is presented as a mitigating factor in the criminal case. This hypothesis was supported in the present research, which showed that pre-arrest diagnoses resulted in higher rates of being diverted to treatment.

People who are suffering may be less likely to receive proper treatment for their condition. Though the present research examined this problem for veterans, there is no reason to presume that the impact would not be the same for non-veterans. There are several barriers to treatment that minority groups face, such as finances or family/cultural inhibitions [20]. Another reason that there is a barrier to care is self-stigma. Self-stigma has been shown to be a barrier to care for US [21] and UK [22] armed forces veterans. This stigmatization of PTSD could create the situation in which a person would not be diagnosed until after an arrest. This post-arrest diagnosis could then be seen as self-serving.

In short, addressing PTSD early will provide more avenues for remedy. Late diagnoses, as seen in the present research, can result in negative consequences for people who are already suffering. Prison is far from an environment that would lend itself to proper mental healthcare [23]. Overcoming stigma, including self-stigma, and taking a proactive approach to diagnosing and caring for people who are suffering would lead to better outcomes for the individual and for society as a whole.

Limitations and Future Directions

The present research is limited in that it used trial vignettes and a convenience sample of college students to test the hypotheses. This does call into question, to some degree, the generalizability of the findings. Previous research used similar methods [7]. Research comparing college samples and community samples have produced mixed results in that a community sample was more punitive than a college sample in some research [24], while other research has detected no differences between college and community samples [25]. Additional research is needed to determine if there is a difference for college and community samples when it comes to questions of PTSD and the criminal justice system.

Future research, using a community sample, should include information such as mock juror occupation, income, and other potential moderators. This information could useful for attorneys in the voir dire procedure. As the present research did not differentiate between exaggerated symptoms and malingering, future research should examine the impact of how juries understand this difference and integrate that understanding into their verdicts.

Funding: This research received no external funding.

References

1. Wilson, J.P.; Zigelbaum, S.D. The Vietnam veteran on trial: The relation of post-traumatic stress disorder to criminal behavior. *Behav. Sci. Law* **1983**, *1*, 69–83. [CrossRef]
2. Elbogen, E.B.; Johnson, S.C.; Newton, V.M.; Straits-Troster, K.; Vasterling, J.J.; Wagner, H.R.; Beckham, J.C. Criminal justice involvement, trauma, and negative affect in Iraq and Afghanistan war era veterans. *J. Consult. Clin. Psychol.* **2012**, *80*, 1097–1102. [CrossRef] [PubMed]
3. Aprilakis, C. The warrior returns: Struggling to address criminal behavior by veterans with PTSD. *Georget. J. Law Public Policy* **2005**, *3*, 541–566.
4. Valdes, S.G. Frequency and success: An empirical study of criminal law defenses, federal constitutional evidentiary claims, and plea negotiations. *Univ. Pa. Law Rev.* **2005**, *153*, 1709–1814. [CrossRef]
5. Berger, O.; McNiel, D.E.; Binder, R.L. PTSD as a criminal defense: A review of case law. *J. Am. Acad. Psychiatry Law* **2012**, *40*, 509–521. [PubMed]
6. Blais, R.K.; Renshaw, K.D. Self-stigma fully mediates the association of anticipated enacted stigma and help-seeking intentions in National Guard service members. *Mil. Psychol.* **2014**, *26*, 114–119. [CrossRef]
7. Smith, B.A. Juror preference for curative alternative verdicts for veterans with PTSD. *Mil. Psychol.* **2016**, *28*, 174–184. [CrossRef]
8. Burges, C.; McMillan, T.M. The ability of naïve participants to report symptoms of post-traumatic stress disorder. *Br. J. Soc. Clin. Psychol.* **2010**, *40*, 209–214. [CrossRef]
9. Pietrzak, R.H.; Johnson, D.C.; Goldstein, M.B.; Malley, J.C.; Southwick, S.M. Perceived stigma and barriers to mental health care utilization among OEF-OIF veterans. *Psychiatr. Serv.* **2009**, *60*, 1118–1122. [CrossRef] [PubMed]
10. Mittenberg, W.; Patton, C.; Canyock, E.M.; Condit, D.C. Base rates of malingering and symptom exaggeration. *J. Clin. Exp. Neuropsychol.* **2002**, *24*, 1094–1102. [CrossRef] [PubMed]

11. Ali, S.; Jabeen, S.; Alam, F. Multimodal approach to identifying malingered posttraumatic stress disorder: A review. *Innov. Clin. Neurosci.* **2015**, *12*, 12–20. [PubMed]
12. Priebe, S.; Matanov, A.; Jankovic, J.; McCrone, P.; Ljubotina, D.; Knezevic, G.; Kucukalic, A.; Franciskovic, T.; Schutzwohl, M. Consequences of untreated posttraumatic stress disorder following war in former Yugoslavia: Morbidity, subjective quality of life, and care costs. *Clin. Sci.* **2009**, 465–475. [CrossRef]
13. Dekel, R.; Monson, C.M. Military-related post-traumatic stress disorder and family relations: Current knowledge and future directions. *Aggress. Violent Behav.* **2010**, *15*, 303–309. [CrossRef]
14. Pacella, M.L.; Hruska, B.; Delahanty, D.L. The physical health consequences of PTSD and PTSD symptoms: A meta-analytic review. *J. Anxiety Disord.* **2013**, *27*, 33–46. [CrossRef] [PubMed]
15. Asnaani, A.; Reddy, M.K.; Shea, M.T. The impact of PTSD symptoms on physical and mental health functioning in returning veterans. *J. Anxiety Disord.* **2014**, *28*, 310–317. [CrossRef] [PubMed]
16. Stewart, S.H.; Pihl, R.O.; Conrod, P.J.; Dongier, M. Functional associations among trauma, PTSD, and substance-related disorders. *Addict. Behav.* **1998**, *23*, 797–812. [CrossRef]
17. Keane, T.M.; Wolfe, J. Comorbidity in post-traumatic stress disorder: An analysis of community and clinical studies. *J. Appl. Soc. Psychol.* **1990**, *20*, 1776–1788. [CrossRef]
18. Bronson, J.; Carson, A.; Noonan, M.; Berzofsky, M. *Veterans in Prison and Jail, 2011–2012*; U.S. Department of Justice Special Report: Washington, DC, USA, 2015.
19. Office of the Chairman of the Joint Chiefs of Staff. *Veteran Stereotypes: A Closer Look*; White Paper; Office of the Chairman of the Joint Chiefs of Staff: Arlington County, VA, USA, 2014.
20. Davis, R.G.; Ressler, K.J.; Schwartz, A.C.; Stephens, K.J.; Bradley, R.G. Treatment barriers for low-income, urban African Americans with undiagnosed posttraumatic stress disorder. *J. Trauma. Stress* **2008**, *21*, 218–222. [CrossRef] [PubMed]
21. Gould, M.; Greenberg, N.; Hetherton, J. Stigma and the military: Evaluation of a PTSD psychoeducational program. *J. Trauma. Stress* **2007**, *20*, 505–515. [CrossRef] [PubMed]
22. Murphy, D.; Busuttil, W. PTSD, stigma and barriers to help-seeking within the UK armed forces. *J. R. Army Med. Corps* **2014**, 1–5. [CrossRef] [PubMed]
23. Daniel, A.E. Care of the mentally ill in prisons: Challenges and solutions. *J. Am. Acad. Psychiatry Law* **2007**, *35*, 406–410. [PubMed]
24. McCabe, J.G.; Krauss, D.A.; Lieberman, J.D. Reality check: A comparison of college students and community sample of mock jurors in a simulated sexual violent predator civil commitment. *Behav. Sci. Law* **2010**, *28*, 730–750. [CrossRef] [PubMed]
25. Hosch, H.M.; Culhane, S.E.; Tubb, V.A.; Granillo, E.A. Town v. gown: A direct comparison of community residents and student mock jurors. *Behav. Sci. Law* **2011**, *29*, 452–466. [CrossRef] [PubMed]

5

The "Centrality of Sepsis": A Review on Incidence, Mortality, and Cost of Care

Jihane Hajj [1,*], Natalie Blaine [2] (ID), Jola Salavaci [2] and Douglas Jacoby [3]

[1] Department of Nursing, Widener University, One University Pl, Chester, PA 19013, USA
[2] Department of Pharmacy, Penn Presbyterian Medical Center, 51 N 39th St, Philadelphia, PA 19104, USA; Natalie.blaine@uphs.upenn.edu (N.B.); jola.salavaci@uphs.upenn.edu (J.S.)
[3] Department of Cardiology, Penn Presbyterian Medical Center, 51 N 39th St, Philadelphia, PA 19104, USA; Douglas.jacoby@uphs.upenn.edu
* Correspondence: jihane.hajj@uphs.upenn.edu

Abstract: Sepsis is a serious and fatal medical condition that has overburdened the US healthcare system. The purpose of this paper is to provide a review of published literature on severe sepsis with a distinct focus on incidence, mortality, cost of hospital care, and postdischarge care. A review of the nature of postsepsis syndrome and its impact on septic patients is also included. The literature review was conducted utilizing the PubMed database, identifying 34 studies for inclusion. From the evaluation of these studies, it was determined that the incidence of sepsis continues to be on the rise according to three decades of epidemiological data. Readmissions, mortality, and length of stay were all higher among septic patients when compared to patients treated for other conditions. The cost of treating sepsis is remarkably high and exceeds the cost of treating patients with congestive heart failure and acute myocardial infarction. The overall cost of sepsis is reflective of not only the cost of initial hospitalization but also the postdischarge care costs, including postsepsis syndrome and cognitive and functional disabilities that require a significant amount of healthcare resources long term. Sepsis and its impact on patients and the US healthcare system is a current quality-of-life and cost-burden issue that needs to be addressed with a greater focus on preventative strategies.

Keywords: severe sepsis; incidence; mortality; cost; postsepsis syndrome

1. Introduction

Sepsis is a serious medical condition that has historically overburdened the US healthcare system. It is important to note the evolution of definitions used for sepsis in the latest guidelines. Sepsis, formerly "severe sepsis", is defined as life-threatening organ dysfunction caused by a dysregulation of the host response following infection. Septic shock is a subset of sepsis which includes circulatory and metabolic dysfunction associated with higher mortality risk [1]. Hereinafter, "sepsis" and "severe sepsis" are used interchangeably, as the literature evaluated includes both terms. The burden of sepsis has been reported worldwide [1–6]. According to the most recent Center for Disease Control (CDC) report, it is estimated that sepsis affects around 1.5 million individuals in the United States annually, causing the death of 250,000 individuals and being responsible for 1 out of every 3 hospital deaths [7]. The treatment of sepsis can include fluid resuscitation, antimicrobial therapy, source control interventions, vasoactive medications, corticosteroids, blood products, and mechanical ventilation when necessary. The cost of each individual case of sepsis varies based on the presence or absence of septic shock as well as patient comorbidities and other patient-specific considerations. Sepsis is generally remarkably expensive to treat and has been associated with high readmission rates.

Despite its overwhelming severity, cost, and mortality, sepsis has not significantly attracted the public's attention.

Since its inception in 2002, the Surviving Sepsis Campaign (SSC) has achieved several milestones. These include establishing standards of care through the development of treatment guidelines, increasing sepsis awareness, and improving diagnosis, treatment, and post-intensive care unit (ICU) care. Despite these advances, sepsis care remains quite expensive. While significant savings could be achieved, this has not been attained due to the economic dynamic of healthcare reimbursement that does not currently reward avoided costs but rather the potential for new revenues. For example, Medicare has reimbursed around $40,000 per case of severe sepsis that required mechanical ventilation compared to $12,000 for nonmechanically ventilated severe sepsis cases [8]. The objective of this paper is to provide a review of the literature that has addressed sepsis in regards to incidence and mortality, with a distinct focus on cost of care during and post hospitalization, as well as to provide a review of postsepsis syndrome and its burden on septic patients.

2. Materials and Methods

This was a comprehensive review of the literature that aimed to evaluate severe sepsis in the United States and internationally. The databases utilized for the purpose of this review were PubMed and Google Scholar. Web pages pertaining to the CDC and sepsis organizations were also examined for the purpose of this review. A wide and comprehensive list of subject headings were utilized, and these were: (1) severe sepsis; (2) incidence; (3) mortality; (4) cost; (5) readmissions; and (6) postsepsis syndrome. The search of manuscripts was restricted to original studies published in English and conducted in the United States and internationally which addressed the main topics pertaining to the purpose of this review. A detailed description of the literature search approach is summarized in Figure 1. A total of 34 studies were utilized for the purpose of this review. While a statistical assay was not used by these authors, the statistical findings of those studies reviewed are summarized and reported within the results section as a reference to assays performed externally.

The results of the literature review led to the emergence of various themes that highlighted the nature of severe sepsis incidence, mortality, cost, and postsepsis syndrome. A summary of the result findings is highlighted in Table 1.

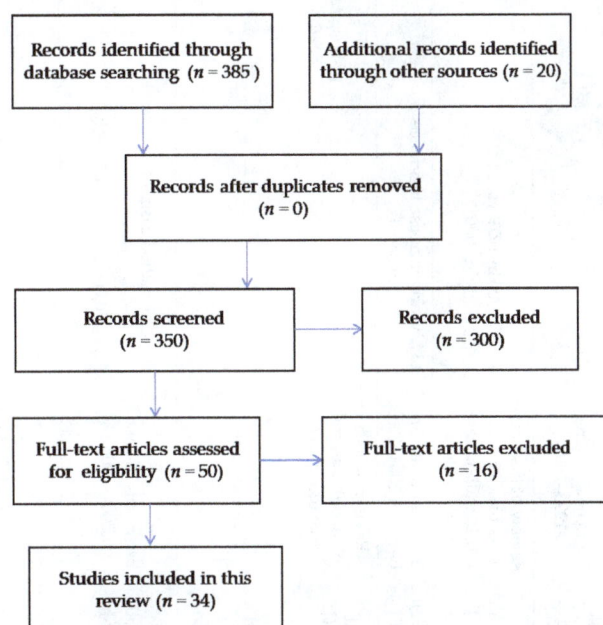

Figure 1. Literature search using the Preferred Reporting Items for systematic Reviews and Meta Analyses (PRISMA) flow diagram approach.

Table 1. Review table of literature review findings.

Studies	Designs/Setting	Incidence			Mortality			Cost		Readmissions	Comments
		Not Specified	60–64	>65	In-Hospital	At 1 Year	At 2/5 Year	Hospital	Post Hospital		
Angus et al. (2001) [14]	Observational/50 nonfederal hospitals in US		5/1000	26/1000	Hospital mortality rate estimated at 28%			○ Surgical patients: 30K ○ Medical patients: 19 K (p < 0.0001)			1.5% increase in the cases of sepsis per annum
Dombrovskiy et al. (2007) [15]	Trend analysis from 1993–2003										Percentage of cases of severe sepsis increased from 25% to 44%
Martin et al. (2003) [17]	Review of discharge data over 22 years and 10 million cases of sepsis	82/100,000 in 1979 vs. 240,000 in 2000									8% annual increase in the incidence of sepsis
Gaieski et al. (2013) [18]	Four national data between 2004-2009	13% yearly increase incidence of sepsis									
Hall et al. (2011) [21]	Review of 2008 National Hospital Discharge Survey				17% in-hospital deaths						Compared to 2% of deaths from conditions other than sepsis
Pfuntner et al., 2013 [31]	Data analysis of hospital costs in 2011							Highest aggregate cost of hospital among adults with septicemia estimated around $ 20 billion in 2011 or $ 55 million daily			This represents an 11% increase yearly since 1997
Wang et al. (2007) [16]	Analysis of data 2001–2004	○ 2.3 million cases of severe sepsis ○ 570,000 cases annually									
Lee et al. (2004) [34]	Analysis of data on 800 severe sepsis patients					12% death			Mean cost for year 1 was 14K–35K		○ Risk of death increased with age ○ PPPM outpatient and pharmacy cost was $ 1300
Weycker et al. (2003) [25]	Retrospective study. Data from US insurance claims 1991–2000				Estimate mortality: 21%	Doubled at 51%	Estimate mortality: 74%	Admission cost 45 K	○ At 1 year: 78K ○ At 5 year: 119K		○ 50% discharge home ○ 30% discharged to outside facility

Table 1. *Cont.*

Studies	Designs/Setting	Incidence			Mortality			Cost		Readmissions	Comments
		Not Specified	60–64	>65	In-Hospital	At 1 Year	At 2/5 Year	Hospital	Post Hospital		
Jagodic et al., (2006) [26]	Observational: long term survival of sepsis vs. trauma patients				○ Mortality 58 % vs. 38% ($p = 0.002$) ○ Post hospital mortality 22% vs. 8% ($p = 0.049$) ○ 2 years mortality 67% vs. 43% ($p = 0.0002$)						
Goodwin et al. (2015) [28]	Observational/data analysis/HCUP									○ Average cost: $ 25K ○ Cumulative cost at 180 days: $ 1.1 billions	○ 26% readmissions at 30 days ○ 48% readmissions at 180 days
Prescott et al. (2014) [27]	Observational 1998–2005 Health Retirement Survey						44% was the 1 year mortality				Significantly different than matched nonspesis cohort, 31% vs. 15% ($p < 0.01$)
Braun et al. (2004) [29]	Retrospective data analysis 1995–1999	○ <50 years old: 1 per 1000 ○ >50 years old: 4 per 1000			20% deaths. The odds of death were 9 for ages 80 and older				Average cost of $ 26K		
Karlsson et al. (2007) [24]	Prospective Study /24 ICUs and 21 hospitals					One year mortality: 40%	2 years mortality: 42%				2 fold increase in mortality for adults >65 years of age (40% vs. 20%)

3. Results

3.1. Incidence of Sepsis

There were several reports that addressed the epidemiology of sepsis over the past three decades. Most trials continue to report on the increase in the incidence of sepsis [9–12]. Most recently, Stoller and colleagues examined 4-year epidemiological trends on severe sepsis utilizing data from the 2010 US Census [13]. Severe sepsis incidence increased annually ($p < 0.05$). The incidence of sepsis was remarkably higher among the oldest old (>85 years), with around a 30-fold higher incidence reported from a 10-year data evaluation of Taiwanese health insurance claims [12]. Additionally, Angus and colleagues conducted an observational cohort study and analyzed data retrieved from 850 nonfederal hospitals in seven US states [14]. There were 750,000 cases of sepsis per annum nationally, which is equivalent to a national incidence rate of 3 in 1000 individuals. The incidence rate per 1000 based on age ranged between 5/1000 for 60–64 years of age and 26/1000 for persons greater than 85 years of age. The results of this data analysis suggest that the overall number of cases of sepsis has increased faster than the anticipated population growth. Angus and colleagues commented on a 1.5% increase in the cases of sepsis per annum, which is equivalent to 900,000 in 2010 and 1.10 million in 2020 [14]. Recent data estimate around 1.5 million cases of sepsis in the United States. Dombrovskiy and colleagues conducted a trend analysis of severe sepsis data from 1993 to 2003 and commented on a rapid increase in the rate of hospitalization annually [15]. The percentage of cases of severe sepsis continuously increased throughout the years, ranging from 25% in 1993 to 44% in 2003 ($p < 0.01$). The age-adjusted rate of hospitalization with severe sepsis also steadily increased annually by 9% ($p < 0.001$). Wang and colleagues analyzed data from the National Hospital Ambulatory Medical Care Survey between 2001 and 2004 [16]. There were around 2.3 million cases of suspected severe sepsis, accounting for 570,000 annually. Martin and colleagues also commented on the annual increase in the incidence of sepsis [17]. This was a review of discharge data over a 22-year period which included data on 10 million cases of sepsis. There was an 8% annual increase in the incidence of sepsis, which accounted for 82/100,000 in 1979 and 240/100,000 in 2000 (160,000 cases vs. 660,000 cases). In subsequent data from the 2010 US Census that accounted for around 310 individuals and estimated the epidemiological trends between the years 2008 and 2012, the incidence of sepsis continued to increase from 346/100,000 to 436/100,000 ($p < 0.05$) [13]. Lastly, Gaieski and colleagues evaluated four nationally representative samples of data that were previously published on severe sepsis between 2004 and 2009 [18]. This study reinforces the reality surrounding the continuous increase of incidence of sepsis in the United States. There was an average increase in incidence of sepsis by 13% yearly. In summary, the incidence of sepsis significantly varies by age group and has been steadily increasing throughout the years.

3.2. Hospital Length of Stay, Readmissions, and Mortality

Sepsis was one of the major risk factors identified that led to in-hospital death, discharge to hospice facilities, or 30-day readmissions [19]. Mortality related to sepsis was up to 140% higher compared to annual estimates of mortality from other causes [20]. Hall and colleagues reported on the results of their review of data from the National Hospital Discharge Survey, 2008 [21]. The average length of stay (LOS) for septic patients was 75% longer compared to those hospitalized for other conditions, and septic patients were eight times more likely to die during hospitalization. There were 17% in-hospital deaths among patients treated for septicemia compared to 2% of those treated for other conditions. This was similar to the 4-year epidemiological trends from the 2010 US census, which described a decrease in the overall mortality estimate from 22% to 17% over 4 years [13]. This was similar to the 2011 Nationwide Inpatient Sample, which estimated an all-cause mortality rate of around 15% and an average length of stay of 7 days [22]. A retrospective analysis of 12-year data on severe septic patients in Australia and New Zealand demonstrated a significant decrease in absolute mortality, estimated at 18% ($p < 0.001$) [2]. The account on readmission rates was also remarkable. Among Medicare patients, septicemia ranked second (after heart failure) as a condition with the highest 30-day readmission rates, accounting for 93,000 readmissions. These were substantial findings that have attracted the attention of stakeholders to devise strategies that aim at improving care coordination with the goal of decreasing the number of readmissions and achieving cost savings [23]. The in-hospital mortality data among septic patients remains remarkably high and worse mortality data are reported at 1 and 5 years posthospitalization with septic patients. The odds of death varied by age. In a retrospective analysis of data involving managed care organization enrollees between 1995 and 1999, the odds of death within the first year since hospital admission increased dramatically for the older group, reaching as high as 9 ($p < 0.0001$). Angus and colleagues reported on an overall hospital mortality rate of 28%, which is a number that is identical to septic ICU patients from the Finnsepsis study [14,24]. In this study, age was found to be an independent risk factor for sepsis mortality, where adults greater than 65 years had a two-fold increase in mortality compared to younger patients (40% vs. 20%). The 1-year mortality in this cohort was estimated around 40%, and mortality at 2 years was 1.5 times higher when compared to hospital mortality of 28%. The 1-, 2-, and 5-year mortality data continued to be remarkably high in several studies. In a retrospective study that examined the long-term mortality of severely septic patients, in-hospital mortality accounted for 21%, while 1-year hospital mortality doubled at 51%, and 5-year hospital mortality was estimated at 74% [25]. When comparing trauma and septic patients with similar Acute Physiology and Chronic Healthy Evaluation III (APACHEII) scores, in-hospital mortality was higher among ICU septic patients compared to trauma patients (58% vs. 38%, $p = 0.002$). Posthospital mortality of septic patients was also higher than trauma patients (22% vs. 8%, $p = 0.049$), as well as the 2-year mortality (67% vs. 43%, $p = 0.002$) [26]. When matched to a nonsepsis cohort, the 90-day and 1-year mortality was also significantly higher, accounting for 27% and 44% vs. 15% and 31%, respectively ($p < 0.01$). An observational cohort study that examined participants from the Health and Retirement Survey showed a remarkable use of healthcare resources after severe sepsis. The percentage of readmissions to the hospital at any point in time in the first year reached 63%. Also remarkable to note, patients spent a mean of 25% of their days alive in the first year following severe sepsis being admitted to an inpatient facility such as Long Term Acute Care (LTAC) or Skilled Nursing Facility (SNF) [27]. Finally, a more recent study conducted by Goodwin and colleagues highlighted the very high rate of readmissions among severe sepsis survivors [28]. In an observational cohort study that examined data from the Healthcare Cost and Utilization Project (HCUP), there were 26% and 48% readmissions after 30-day and 180-day postdischarge from severe sepsis respectively. The length of stay was comparable, with an average of 16–20 days [14,29].

3.3. The Cost Burden of Sepsis

The cost of sepsis and postsepsis care continues to be a serious healthcare burden. Based on the 2013 HCUP statistical brief, sepsis costs accounted for $23 billion and was the most expensive condition treated in US hospitals [30]. A recent report evaluated by the CDC commented on the healthcare resources used, and it is estimated that 7 out of 10 patients who were once treated for sepsis will continue to utilize a variety of healthcare services or will have chronic illnesses that require frequent medical care. In 2011, sepsis was estimated to cost $20 billion annually or $55 million daily. This is considered the highest aggregate hospital cost and represents a quadrupled increase in cost or an increase of around 11% compared to data from 1997 [31]. The median hospital cost of sepsis was estimated at around $16,000 [22]. The cost of sepsis may also vary based on the etiology of sepsis (healthcare, community, or hospital sepsis), where the highest cost has been attributed to hospital-acquired severe sepsis. The cost of hospital-acquired severe sepsis was remarkably higher and estimated at $38,000 compared to the community-acquired cost of $7000 [32]. Sepsis care is a challenge to both patients and hospitals. A significant portion of healthcare costs stem not only from inpatient hospital costs but also from postsepsis care costs. The percentage of patients discharged to long-term care institutions is more than double when compared to patients hospitalized with conditions other than sepsis (36% vs. 14%) [31].

The increase in the cost of sepsis is indirectly related to the major increase in survivorship of severe sepsis. In a retrospective analysis of data pertaining to Medicare beneficiaries between 1996 and 2008, there was around a 120% increase in 3-year survivorship of severe sepsis, 16% of which had a moderate-to-severe cognitive impairment, and 75% or 500,000 patients had a functional disability. This is clearly an added cost that is indirectly related to sepsis survivorship. When compared to acute myocardial infarction (AMI), severe sepsis data are much more dramatic in regards to cost. While there was a small decrease in the cost of treatment over a decade for AMI patients, the cost of severe sepsis has more than doubled ($6 billion vs. $15 billion in 2008) [33]. These data are a clear representation of the population burden posthospitalization with severe sepsis and also aligns with other studies that demonstrated the threefold increase in the odds of developing cognitive impairment and the addition of functional limitations [33].

Comorbidities and acuity of illness played a substantial role in determining the cost of care for sepsis survivors. For example, the cost of care of patients with known diabetes and associated complications was more than double the cost of care of those without diabetes ($32,000 vs. $13,000). This is notably different when compared with the cost of care for patients with diabetes in the general population, which is estimated at $2300. When examined in terms of APACHE II score, patients with greater than or equal to a score of 25 incurred an average cost of $84,500. The cost of care also differed by the year postsepsis survival. The costliest care was accrued during the first year, which not only accounted for $14,000 but also reflected the cost of readmissions. This was much greater than the second and third year postsepsis, which accounted for $5000 [34].

As noted earlier, the cost of sepsis is not restricted to hospital care but is a reflection of the healthcare services received postdischarge as well as the cost of readmissions. In a retrospective analysis of data that involved managed care organization enrollees, the average cost of hospital care was $26,000 for a mean LOS of 16 days; however, these numbers differed drastically between medicine and surgery patients, with an estimated cost of $6000 and $35,000 respectively. In regards to posthospitalization costs, per patient per month (PPPM) outpatient and pharmacy costs were estimated to be around $1300 for sepsis survivors. Emergency room (ER) costs and inpatient visit costs certainly contributed to the overall costs, further complicating the healthcare burden imposed by sepsis survivors [29]. Data from US insurance claims between 1991 and 2000 also addressed the cost of severe sepsis, which was once again substantial. The admission cost of severe sepsis was estimated at $45,000, and the cumulative cost of care at 1 year and 5 years was estimated at $78,000 and $119,000, respectively. More recently, Goodwin and colleagues examined HCUP data and found that the average cost of readmission was $25,000 and the cumulative cost of readmissions amounted to $1.1 billion for those admissions at 180-days postdischarge, which accounted for 43,000 total admissions [28]. Finally, a record of hospitalizations between 2009 and 2011 were retrieved from HCUP and the State Inpatient Database (SID). This was a retrospective cohort analysis that examined the cost of 30-day readmissions. Sepsis was the costliest condition, with an estimated annual cost of $500 million, which is not nearly comparable to Congestive Heart Failure (CHF) and Acute Myocardial Infarction (AMI) costs of $229 million and $149 million, respectively. This discrepancy delineates the "centrality of sepsis" in regard to the readmission problem.

Severe sepsis remains a burden on the US healthcare system and worldwide despite the available advances in technology and treatment [34–40]. This condition remains the costliest to treat, as its cost dramatically exceeds that of CHF and AMI. There is a notable difference between the cost of hospitalization of severe sepsis compared to all-cause admissions, and this reflects in many instances the burden imposed by the younger population on the healthcare system [29]. The overall cost of sepsis is not only a reflection of the hospitalization cost but also of other attributions such as readmissions and the chronic use of healthcare resources afterward. Additionally, survivorship of sepsis has played an important role in driving the increase in cost, as a great percentage of sepsis survivors have some sort of cognitive and functional disability.

3.4. Postsepsis Syndrome

Postsepsis syndrome, as evidenced by cognitive and functional disabilities, is another major burden that is assumed by a great percentage of sepsis survivors. In a prospective cohort study that examined cognitive and physical functioning among severe septic patients as compared to nonsepsis hospitalized patients, there were significant differences found. Among severe sepsis survivors, the odds ratio of developing moderate-to-severe cognitive impairment was 3.3 as compared to no change in cognitive impairment among nonsepsis hospitalized patients ($p = 0.01$) [39]. Similarly, severe sepsis survivors developed more functional limitations compared to nonsepsis hospitalized patients ($p = 0.001$). The extent of limitations and the experienced decline in both cognitive and functional abilities persisted for 8 years postsepsis hospitalization [33]. In another study that evaluated around 800 critically ill patients, including septic shock patients, approximately 70% of patients had a decline in cognitive functioning and had global cognition scores that were similar to those patients with traumatic brain injury and mild Alzheimer's disease condition [35]. This type of cognitive impairment is not only chronic but overburdening to patients and their families, and it is associated with high healthcare costs that are estimated in one study to be around $34,000 and $15,000 per year for patients and families, respectively [36]. Benros and colleagues (2015) evaluated around 160,000 men from the Danish Nationwide Register and concluded that men who were previously exposed to infection had a significantly lower cognitive ability ($p < 0.001$) [37]. This finding, while not addressing severe sepsis specifically, is highly relevant as it addresses the association of infection and change in immune system responses with significant decline in cognitive functioning. Finally, a systematic review of the literature that evaluated 12 studies also concluded that cognitive impairment is a major sequela that is observed among postsepsis survivors [38]. This is clearly a serious quality of life and cost burden issue that needs to be addressed, and measures to address prevention of cognitive decline should be established. This surely calls for several initiatives such as further research in the area of cognitive neurology, establishment of guidelines that address specifically the issue of postsepsis cognitive impairment (perhaps via instituting preventive management strategies in the early stages of sepsis), as well as further research that is much needed in regard to exploring variables or risk factors contributing to cognitive decline following critical illness. Considering the high cost of therapy of this overburdening condition, an increase in federal funding may be warranted. Such funding would involve the recruitment of specialists in the fields of occupational therapy and neurology as well as other scientists to pursue further research.

4. Conclusions

The burden of sepsis on our population has been reviewed and is clearly multifactorial. The incidence of sepsis has been steadily increasing over the past three decades and varies significantly by age group, with the most elderly patients carrying the greatest burden. Readmissions, length of stay, and mortality rates are all much higher in patients with sepsis when compared to patients admitted with nonsepsis diagnoses. This disparity in outcomes correlates to a substantially higher financial burden associated with this disease state. The cost of sepsis is both a reflection of the cost of initial hospitalization of these patients as well as care required postdischarge. Survivorship of sepsis has played an important role in driving the increase in cost, as a great percentage of sepsis survivors endure postsepsis syndrome and as such have cognitive and functional disabilities requiring significant healthcare resources long term.

The impact on patient outcomes and the increasing incidence of sepsis is a serious quality-of-life and cost-burden issue that needs to be addressed. Measures to address prevention of cognitive decline have not been and should be established. Initiatives that may aid in the development of these preventative strategies include: further research in cognitive neurology, establishment of guidelines that address the issue of postsepsis cognitive impairment via institution of preventive management strategies in the early stages of sepsis, and further research exploring contributory variables associated with cognitive decline following critical illness.

Funding: This research received no external funding.

References

1. Adrie, C.; Alberti, C.; Chaix-Couturier, C.; Azoulay, E.; De Lassence, A.; Cohen, Y.; Meshaka, P.; Cheval, C.; Thuong, M.; Troche, G.; et al. Epidemiology and economic evaluation of severe sepsis in France: Age, severity, infection site, and place of acquisition as determinants of workload and cost. *J. Crit. Care* **2005**, *20*, 46–58. [CrossRef] [PubMed]

2. Kaukonen, K.M.; Bailey, M.; Suzuki, S.; Pilcher, D.; Bellomo, R. Mortality related to severe sepsis and septic shock among critically ill patients in Australia and New Zeland, 2000–2012. *JAMA* **2014**, *311*, 1308–1316. [CrossRef] [PubMed]

3. Dellinger, R.P.; Levy, M.M.; Rhodes, A.; Annane, D.; Gerlach, H.; Opal, S.M.; Sevransky, J.E.; Sprung, C.L.; Douglas, I.S.; Jaeschke, R.; et al. Surviving Sepsis Campaign: International guidelines for management of severe sepsis and septic shock: 2012. *Crit. Care Med.* **2013**, *41*, 580–637. [CrossRef] [PubMed]

4. Schmid, A.; Burchardi, H.; Clouth, J.; Schneider, H. Burden of illness imposed by severe sepsis in Germany. *Eur. J. Health Econ.* **2002**, *3*, 77–82. [CrossRef] [PubMed]

5. Sogayar, A.M.; Machado, F.R.; Rea-Neto, A.; Dornas, A.; Grion, C.M.; Lobo, S.M.; Tura, B.R.; Silva, C.L.; Cal, R.G.; Beer, L.; et al. A multicenter, prospective study to evaluate costs of septic patients in Brazilian intensive care units. *Pharmacoeconomics* **2008**, *26*, 425–434. [CrossRef] [PubMed]

6. Vincent, J.L.; Marshall, J.C.; Namendys-Silva, S.A.; Francois, B.; Martin-Loeches, I.; Lipman, J. Assessment of the Worldwide Burden of Critical Illness: The Intensive Care Over Nations (ICON) Audit. 2014. Volume 2. Available online: www.Thelancet.com/respiratory (accessed on 2 February 2018).

7. Center for Disease Control and Prevention (CDC). Making Health Care Safer: Think Sepsis. 2017. Available online: https://www.cdc.gov/vitalsigns/pdf/2016-08-vitalsigns.pdf (accessed on 2 February 2018).

8. O'Brien, J. The Cost of Sepsis. 2015. Available online: https://blogs.cdc.gov/safehealthcare/the-cost-of-sepsis/ (accessed on 2 February 2018).

9. Alvaro-Meca, A.; Jimenez-sousa, M.A.; Micheloud, D.; Sanchez-Lopez, A.; Heredia-Rodrigez, M.; Tamayo, E.; Resino, S. Epidemiological trends of sepsis in the twenty first century (2000–2013): An analysis of incidence, mortality, and associated costs in Spain. *Popul. Health Metr.* **2018**, *16*, 4. [CrossRef] [PubMed]

10. Lagu, T.; Rothberg, M.B.; Shieh, M.S.; Pekow, P.S.; Steingrub, J.S.; Lindenauer, P.K. Hospitalizations, costs, and outcomes of severe sepsis in the United States 2003–2007. *Crit. Care Med.* **2012**, *40*, 754–761. [CrossRef] [PubMed]

11. Meyer, N.; Harhay, M.O.; Small, D.S.; Prescott, H.C.; Bowles, K.H.; Gaieski, D.F.; Mikkelsen, M.F. Temporal trends in incidence, sepsis-related mortality, and hospital-based acute care after sepsis. *Crit. Care Med.* **2018**, *46*, 354–360. [CrossRef] [PubMed]

12. Wu, M.C.; Chen, S.C.; Hsu, W.T.; Chen, S.T.; Su, K.Y. Nationwide trend of sepsis: A comparison among octogeneranians, elderly, and young adults. *Crit. Care Med.* **2018**, *46*, 926–934. [CrossRef]

13. Stoller, J.; Halpin, L.; Weis, M.; Aplin, B.; Qu, W.; Georgescu, C.; Nazzal, M. Epidemiology of severe sepsis: 2008-2012. *J. Crit. Care* **2016**, *31*, 58–62. [CrossRef] [PubMed]

14. Angus, D.C.; Linde-Zwible, W.T.; Lidicker, J.; Clermont, G.; Carcillo, J.; Pinsky, M.R. Epidemiology of severe sepsis in the Unites States: Analysis of incidence, outcome, and associated costs of care. *Crit. Care Med.* **2001**, *29*, 1303–1310. [CrossRef] [PubMed]

15. Dombrovskiy, V.Y.; Martin, A.A.; Sunderram, J.; Paz, H. Rapid increase in hospitalization and mortality rates for severe sepsis in the United States: A trend analysis from 1993 to 2003. *Crit. Care Med.* **2007**, *35*, 1244–1250. [CrossRef] [PubMed]

16. Wang, H.E.; Shapiro, N.I.; Angus, D.C.; Yealy, D.M. National estimates of severe sepsis in United States emergency departments. *Crit. Care Med.* **2007**, *35*, 1928–1936. [CrossRef] [PubMed]

17. Martin, G.S.; Mannino, D.M.; Eaton, S.; Moss, M. The epidemiology of sepsis in the United States from 1979 through 2000. *N. Engl. J. Med.* **2003**, *348*, 1546–1554. [CrossRef] [PubMed]

18. Gaieski, D.F.; Edwards, M.; Kallan, M.J.; Carr, B.G. Benchmarking the incidence and mortality of severe sepsis in the United States. *Crit. Care Med.* **2013**, *41*, 1167–1174. [CrossRef] [PubMed]

19.   Dietz, B.W.; Jones, T.K.; Small, D.S.; Gaieski, D.F.; Mikkelson, M.E. The relationship between index hospitalizations, sepsis, and death or transition to hospice care during 30-day hospital readmissions. *Med. Care* **2017**, *55*, 362–370. [CrossRef] [PubMed]

20.   Epstein, L.; Dantes, R.; Magill, S.; Fiore, A. Varying estimates of sepsis mortality using death certificates and administrative codes–Unites States, 1999–2014. *MMWR Morb. Mortal. Wkly. Rep.* **2016**, *65*, 342–345. [CrossRef] [PubMed]

21.   Hall, M.J.; Williams, S.N.; DeFrances, C.J.; Golosinskiy, A. Inpatient Care for Septicemia or Sepsis: A Challenge for Patients and Hospitals. 2011. Available online: https://www.cdc.gov/nchs/data/databriefs/db62.pdf (accessed on 5 March 2018).

22.   Nguyen, A.T.; Tsai, C.L.; Hwang, L.Y.; Lai, D.; Markjam, C.; Patel, B. Obesity and mortality, length of stay and hospital cost among patients with sepsis: A nationwide inpatient retrospective cohort study. *PLoS ONE* **2016**, *11*. [CrossRef] [PubMed]

23.   Hines, A.L.; Barrett, M.L.; Jiang, H.J.; Steiner, C.A. Conditions with the Largest Number of Adult Hospital Readmissions by Payer. 2011. Available online: https://www.hcup-us.ahrq.gov/reports/statbriefs/sb172-Conditions-Readmissions-Payer.jsp (accessed on 12 March 2018).

24.   Karlsson, S.; Varpula, M.; Ruokonen, E.; Pettila, V.; Parviainen, I.; Ala-Kokko, T.I.; Kolho, E.; Rintala, E.M. Incidence, treatment, and outcome of severe sepsis in ICU-treated adults in Finland: The Finnsepsis Study. *Intens. Care Med.* **2007**, *33*, 435–443. [CrossRef] [PubMed]

25.   Weycker, D.; Akhras, K.S.; Edelsberg, J.; Angus, D.C.; Oster, G. Long-term mortality and medical care charges in patients with severe sepsis. *Crit. Care Med.* **2003**, *31*, 2316–2323. [CrossRef] [PubMed]

26.   Jagodic, H.K.; Jagodic, K.; Podbregar, M. Long-term outcome and quality of life of patients treated in surgical intensive care: A comparison between sepsis and trauma. *Crit. Care* **2006**, *10*, P423. [CrossRef]

27.   Prescott, H.C.; Langa, K.M.; Liu, V.; Escobar, G.J.; Lwashyna, T.J. Increased 1-year healthcare use in survivors of severe sepsis. *Am. J. Respir. Crit. Care Med.* **2014**, *190*, 62–69. [CrossRef] [PubMed]

28.   Goodwin, A.J.; Rice, D.A.; Simpson, K.N.; Ford, D.W. Frequency, Cost, and Risk Factors of readmissions among severe sepsis survivors. *Crit. Care Med.* **2015**, *43*, 738–746. [CrossRef] [PubMed]

29.   Braun, L.; Riedel, A.A.; Cooper, M. Severe sepsis in managed care: Analysis of incidence, one-year mortality, and associated costs of care. *J. Manag. Care Pharm.* **2004**, *10*, 521–530. [CrossRef] [PubMed]

30.   Torio, V.M.; Moore, B.J. National Inpatient Hospital Costs: The Most Expensive Conditions by Payer. 2013. Available online: https://hcup-us.ahrq.gov/reports/statbriefs/sb204-Most-Expensive-Hospital-Conditions.jsp (accessed on 2 February 2018).

31.   Pfuntner, A.; Wier, L.M.; Stocks, C. Most Frequent Conditions in U.S. Hospitals, 2010. Available online: https://www.hcup-us.ahrq.gov/reports/statbriefs/sb148.jsp (accessed on 16 February 2018).

32.   Page, D.B.; Donnelly, J.P.; Wang, H.E. Community-, healthcare-, and hospital-acquired severe sepsis hospitalizations in the university healthsystem consortium. *Crit. Care Med.* **2015**, *43*, 1945–1951. [CrossRef] [PubMed]

33.   Lwashyna, T.J.; Cooke, C.R.; Wunsch, H.; Kahn, J.M. Population burden of long-term survivorship after severe sepsis in older Americans. *J. Am. Geriat. Soc.* **2012**, *60*, 1070–1077. [CrossRef] [PubMed]

34.   Lee, H.; Doig, J.D.; Ghali, W.; Donaldson, C.; Johnson, D.; Manns, B. Detailed cost analysis of care for survivors of severe sepsis. *Crit. Care Med.* **2004**, *32*, 981–985. [CrossRef] [PubMed]

35.   Pandharipande, P.P.; Girard, T.D.; Morandi, J.A.; Thompson, J.L.; Pun, B.T.; Brummel, N.E.; Hughes, C.G.; Vasilevskis, E.E.; Sintani, A.K.; Moons, K.G.; et al. Long-term cognitive impairment after critical Illness. *NEJM* **2013**, *14*, 1306–1316. [CrossRef] [PubMed]

36.   Handels, R.L.; Wolfs, C.A.; Aalten, P.; Verhey, F.R.; Severens, J.L. Determinants of care costs of patients with dementia or cognitive impairment. *Alzheimer Dis. Assoc. Disdord* **2013**, *27*, 30–36. [CrossRef] [PubMed]

37.   Benros, M.E.; Sorensen, H.J.; Nielsen, P.R.; Nordentoft, M.; Mortensen, P.B.; Petersen, L. The association between infections and general cognitive ability in young men—A nationwide study. *PLoS ONE* **2015**, *10*, e0124005. [CrossRef] [PubMed]

38.   Calsavara, A.J.C.; Nobre, V.; Barichello, T.; Teixeira, A.L. Post-sepsis cognitive impairment and associated risk factors: A systematic review. *Aust. Crit. Care* **2016**, *31*, 242–253. [CrossRef] [PubMed]

39. Iwashyna, J.T.; Wesley Ely, E.; Smith, D.M.; Langa, K.M. Long-term Cognitive Impairment and Functional Disability among Survivors of Severe Sepsis. *JAMA* **2010**, *304*, 1787–1794. [CrossRef] [PubMed]
40. Schmid, A.; Pugin, J.; Chevrolet, J.C.; Marsch, S.; Ludwig, S.; Stocker, R.; Finnern, H. Burden of illness imposed by severe sepsis in Switzerland. *Swiss Med. Wkly.* **2004**, *134*, 97–102. [PubMed]

6

A Rationale for Music Training to Enhance Executive Functions in Parkinson's Disease: An Overview of the Problem

Teresa Lesiuk [1],*, Jennifer A. Bugos [2] and Brea Murakami [3]

[1]   Music Therapy, University of Miami, Frost School of Music 5499 San Amaro Dr., N306, Coral Gables, FL 33146, USA

[2]   Music Education, University of South Florida, School of Music, 4202 E. Fowler Ave., MUS 101, Tampa, FL 33620, USA; bugosj@usf.edu

[3]   Department of Music, Pacific University, Forest Grove, OR 97116, USA; brea@ymail.com

*   Correspondence: tlesiuk@miami.edu

Abstract: Music listening interventions such as Rhythmic Auditory Stimulation can improve mobility, balance, and gait in Parkinson's Disease (PD). Yet, the impact of music training on executive functions is not yet known. Deficits in executive functions (e.g., attention, processing speed) in patients with PD result in gait interference, deficits in emotional processing, loss of functional capacity (e.g., intellectual activity, social participation), and reduced quality of life. The model of temporal prediction and timing suggests two networks collectively contribute to movement generation and execution: the basal ganglia-thalamocortical network (BGTC) and the cerebellar-thalamocortical network (CTC). Due to decreases in dopamine responsible for the disruption of the BGTC network in adults with PD, it is hypothesized that rhythmic auditory cues assist patients through recruiting an alternate network, the CTC, which extends to the supplementary motor areas (SMA) and the frontal cortices. In piano training, fine motor finger movements activate the cerebellum and SMA, thereby exercising the CTC network. We hypothesize that exercising the CTC network through music training will contribute to enhanced executive functions. Previous research suggested that music training enhances cognitive performance (i.e., working memory and processing speed) in healthy adults and adults with cognitive impairments. This review and rationale provides support for the use of music training to enhance cognitive outcomes in patients with Parkinson's Disease (PD).

Keywords: Parkinson's Disease; executive functions; music training; fine motor; cerebellar-thalamocortical network (CTC)

---

1. A Rationale for Music Training to Enhance Executive Function in Parkinson's Disease: An Overview of the Problem

Parkinson's Disease (PD), a neurodegenerative disorder that affects more than five million adults in the U.S. alone, is often accompanied by deficits in executive functions in addition to motor symptoms such as bradykinesia, tremors, rigidity, and gait and postural difficulties [1]. Deficits in executive functions (e.g., attention, processing speed) in patients with PD result in gait interference, deficits in emotional processing, loss of functional capacity (e.g., intellectual activity, social participation), and reduced quality of life [2,3]. While research supports the effectiveness of music listening interventions (e.g., Rhythmic Auditory Stimulation) on mobility, balance, and gait [4–7], the impact of more enactive music experiences (i.e., music training) on deficits in executive functions in PD is not yet known. The use of music training to enhance cognitive outcomes in adults with PD is supported in this rationale.

2. Deficits in Executive Functions in PD

In a meta-analysis of executive function ability in adults with PD, Kudlicka, Clare, and Hindle [8] found significant deficits in all tested skills including cognitive flexibility, set switching, inhibition, selection attention, working memory, and concept formation. These deficits may be compounded by typical age-related cognitive decline and may be the precursor to mild cognitive impairment (PD-MCI) and dementia (PDD) [9]. Yet, despite these cognitive deficits, most interventions focus upon implementing movement for patients with PD and fail to discriminate between differential cognitive profiles.

Discrepancies in whole-brain functional connectivity may be explained by the different levels of cognitive ability found in patients with PD. Lopes et al. [10] examined four categories of cognitive profiles from 119 patient participants: cognitively intact, those with only slight mental slowing, those with mild to moderate deficits predominantly in executive functions, and those with severe deficits in all cognitive domains. Age and education accounted for, there were significant group neural connectivity differences in each category. Essentially, the main neural areas involved the ventral prefrontal, parietal, temporal, and occipital cortices as well as the basal ganglia. As cognitive levels decrease, the network organization is progressively disrupted, with increased numbers of altered connections between the above-mentioned brain regions. Mak et al. [11] examined structural magnetic resonance imaging of 105 patients with PD and 37 controls at baseline and at 18 months. Those patients with PD without dementia at baseline developed significant frontal cortical thinning over 18 months. The researchers concluded that the increased frontal thinning is associated with concurrent dopaminergic, serotonergic, cholinergic, or noradrenergic frontal–striatal circuit disruptions.

Deficits in executive functions can lead to mild cognitive impairment, and eventually progress to dementia [12]. Specifically, the longitudinal status of cognitive ability in adults with PD was examined by Pedersen et al. [12] at baseline ($n = 178$), and then at 1 ($n = 175$), 3 ($n = 163$), and 5 ($n = 150$) years. One observed trend was a progression of cognitive decline, regardless of baseline cognitive status. For those with normal cognition at baseline ($n = 142$), the incidence of mild cognitive impairment (MCI) was 9.9%, 23.2%, and 28.9% by year 1, 3, and 5, respectively. While 39.1% of those with baseline or incident MCI progressed to dementia by year 5, a greater percent of those with persistent MCI, 59.1%, progressed to dementia by the fifth year. Of patients with normal cognition at baseline, 7.2% converted to dementia by the fifth year. Still, progressive decline was not definite; the remainder of those with normal cognition at baseline retained their ability. Moreover, 24% of those with incident MCI reverted to normal cognition by year 5. However, the researchers stated that those who reverted to normal cognition within the first three years are at a continued risk for developing dementia. Given these findings, those patients with MCI who revert to normal cognition may be excellent candidates for cognitive interventions to prevent progressive cognitive decline.

3. A Theory for Improving Cognition in Adults with PD

Aging is associated with decreases in white matter tracts, resulting in a reduced supply of motor resources when compared to young adults [13]. Consequently, aging adults demonstrate structural and functional reductions in motor-based performance and cognitive resources. As the long white matter tracts degenerate, the neuronal assemblies which link sensory awareness, cognitive drive, emotional efficacy, and motor action de-differentiate. The capacity for differentiated adaptive action is consequently reduced. To optimally re-differentiate remaining resources, compensation can engage the mechanisms of neuronal plasticity.

The cerebellum, an area associated with fine motor movements, may hold the key to improving cognition in aging as explained in part by the Supply and Demand Framework [13]. According to this framework, older adults rely upon cognitive brain processes for motor control, resulting in increased cognitive demand. Specifically, the dopaminergic degeneration observed in aging adults (and especially in patients with PD) leads to increased dependence on prefrontal regions to consciously control motor and cognitive tasks. Thus, rehabilitation interventions targeting motor skills, cognitive skills, or the dopaminergic system may have a shared benefit to other behavioral or neural systems. Successful regulation and maintenance of cognition in aging depends upon coordination and integration between brain areas dominated by a critical neurochemical modulatory system.

The frontal, dopaminergic system is concerned fundamentally with motivated behavior and the capacity to plan and control a course of action and to successfully evaluate, in real time, the consequences of actions. Seidler's [13] Supply and Demand Framework asserts that the dopaminergic system acts on the cortico-cerebellar neural pathways that project from the cerebellum to the frontal cortices—areas associated with higher-level cognitive processing. Thus, if the cortico-cerebellar pathway is strengthened through fine motor skills in music training, this may result in enhanced cognitive performance or mitigate potential cognitive deficits.

4. Neuroplasticity and Cognitive Improvements

Improvements in cognitive functioning may be explained by structural and functional neural plasticity. Neural plasticity is defined as, "the ability of the nervous system to respond to intrinsic and extrinsic stimuli by reorganizing its structure, function, and connections" [14]). An extensive review by Sweatt [15] explains how these neural and biochemical mechanisms have been understood in recent decades. First, behavior may be influenced by synaptic plasticity via long-term potentiation (LTP)—a strengthening of the synapses between neurons. LTP is directly implicated in cognitive functions such as learning and memory as related to neural structures including the amygdala, cerebral cortex, and hippocampus. In contrast to structural plasticity, functional plasticity is associated with Hebbian synaptic plasticity, a theory suggesting that the strength of a neural connection may be dependent upon repeated and persistent shared activity between neurons [16].

Neurogenesis, or the development of new and functional neurons, within behavioral circuits is a third mechanism underlying behavioral changes. Finally, experiences can drive the production and regulation of epigenetic molecular mechanisms and impact gene transcription within the CNS. This process impacting the expression of epigenetic marks in adults may underlie enduring changes in behaviors associated with cognition function including memory formation and attention. These cognitive functions contribute to executive functions.

Current understanding of how cognitive training programs protect older adults from cognitive decline is sparse. Kim et al. [17] point to neuroplasticity as an essential mechanism behind cognitive rehabilitation in several clinical populations and in older adults. However, they point out that many studies implicated in neuroplasticity and learning are limited to simple forms of learning, while the relationship between higher-order cognitive functions and neuroplasticity is not fully understood. The authors provide a theoretical framework for understanding the mechanisms underlying cognitive rehabilitation in older adults. Neural changes induced by cognitive rehabilitation can be generally divided into two categories: (1) stimulation, which induces functional brain reorganization via interaction with external stimuli; and (2) compensation, which involves an adaptive reorganization in response to internal damage or degeneration. Cognitive training may mediate these neural mechanisms. Stimulation-based training may restore functional connectivity across diverse brain regions as targeted by specific cognitive exercises (e.g., attention, working memory, and language). Meanwhile, compensation-based training targeting attention or executive functions may be supported by frontal-mediated adjustments. Thus, mechanisms for neuroplasticity observed in response to cognitive rehabilitation may be explained by multiple neural adaptations.

4.1. Neuroplasticity and Music Training

Many researchers suggest that musicians' brains may serve as models for neuroplasticity [18–23]. Neurological data confirm transferability from specific musical skills to a broad range of neural correlates not limited to the motor cortices, superior temporal gyrus, basal ganglia, and cerebellum. For instance, research suggests that fine motor skills implicated in piano training result in increased gray matter density in pianists compared with in nonmusicians [24]. Similarly, results of another study implicating piano training showed an increased positive connectivity in the left primary motor cortical area to the right cerebellum post-training in youth with neurodevelopmental disorders [25]. Data in both of these studies showed enhanced activations in the left primary sensorimotor cortex and right cerebellum.

In music training, structural and functional neural plasticity have been associated with specific musical instruments [26]. Imaging data confirm that musical experiences in terms of instrument training and the level of practice strengthened connections between auditory and motor regions. The strengthened neurological connections, evident in musicians with long-term music training, show enhanced sensorimotor and cognitive performance.

4.2. Music, Temporal Entrainment, and Cognition

Temporal entrainment to music via the auditory–motor system is well understood, but less so with cognition. Short-term interventions with temporal elements may improve executive functions in patients with PD [5,27,28]. For instance, rhythmic complexity in tango dancing (18 h over 12 weeks) enhanced spatial cognition compared to education training [29]. The model of temporal prediction and timing suggests that two networks collectively contribute to movement generation and execution: the basal ganglia-thalamocortical network (BGTC) and the cerebellar-thalamocortical network (CTC) [30, 31]. Due to decreases in dopamine responsible for the disruption of the BGTC network in PD, it is hypothesized that rhythmic auditory cues, like those used in piano training, assist patients through recruiting an alternate CTC network which extends to the supplementary motor areas (SMA) and the frontal cortices [31,32]. In piano training, fine rhythmic motor finger movements that activate the cerebellum and SMA essentially exercise the CTC network [31,33].

Additionally, evidence from temporal entrainment in music mnemonic training of learning and recall of word lists has shown changes in brain plasticity of oscillatory neural networks [34]. The music-induced plasticity, indicated by higher electroencephalography synchrony in learning-related networks, was concomitant with significantly better recall during music (sung) versus spoken recall. The improved word recall performance was found in both healthy adults and those with multiple sclerosis, a condition known for deficits in executive functions, similar to those seen in adults with PD.

4.3. Music Training and Healthy Adults with Age-Related Cognitive Decline

Music training includes complex fine motor skills that rely upon sensorimotor processing. Music training can transfer to a broad range of cognitive and learning domains and may serve as an effective cognitive training intervention for older adults. The *Model of Successful Aging and Music Participation* suggests that musical performance modulates psychological, physiological, and emotional health in older adults through necessary components critical for cognitive training programs: task novelty, progressive difficulty, sensorimotor integration, practice requirements, and social components [35]. This model has many implications for the benefits of music training in patients with Parkinson's disease. For instance, learning a new musical skill necessitates the facilitation of increased attention and concentration, believed to exercise areas of executive functions [36]. Task novelty contributes to attentional demands. Sustained attention and selective attention have been shown to contribute to enhanced performance in child musicians when compared with nonmusicians on measures of executive functions [37]. These attentional benefits may be extended into adulthood for those engaging in the highly novel experience of learning a musical instrument.

Age-related cognitive deficits of 60–85-year-old naïve musicians, namely, abilities found in working memory and planning, were significantly improved with piano instruction [38]. The individualized piano instruction required high levels of temporal and spatial processing, requiring the participant to plan, organize, and sequence a cohesive musical event [38]. Increased reliance upon sustained attention was attributed to enhancements in working memory and processing speed in older adults who received piano training compared to those who did not receive piano trainng. This study is important for the present rationale in that it shows evidence of general executive function enhancement, in contrast to solely music executive function skill. These benefits are particularly important to extend to and investigate in the PD population. A recent systematic review [39] of the efficacy of controlled and noncontrolled studies of cognitive rehabilitation, physical rehabilitation, exercise, and brain stimulation techniques for patients with PD found that interventions should target those with no significant cognitive impairment, those with MCI, or those with dementia.

In patients with PD, it is even more critical to receive opportunities to exercise executive functions to mitigate further decline. Patients with PD exhibit differentiating levels of deficits in executive functions. Compensation for such deficits is evident in patients in the moderate stages of the disease [40]. Compensation strategies include planning for cognitive tasks to account for limitations in psychomotor speed. Interventions such as music training can facilitate increases in motor and cognitive processing speed through practice of progressively difficult passages requiring neurological processing of rhythmic and sequential musical structures. Further, music therapy for adults with PD enhances their ability to perceive rhythm in rhythmic auditory cuing, a rhythm-based treatment that improves gait in PD [41]. Fine motor training may facilitate a different layer of complexity in music education programs with progressive difficulty. As such, these programs have the potential to activate cerebellar structures contributing to neuroplasticity.

4.4. Music and Adults with Deficits in Executive Functions

Cognitive flexibility, a higher-order executive function, was significantly improved in adults with executive function deficits (e.g., stroke, traumatic brain injury) following one neurologic music therapy session [42]. While not a music training session per se, the adults participated in instrument playing and made decisions about their group improvisation. Exercising decision-making, planning, and problem-solving through facilitated music experiences constitutes the neurologic music therapy technique referred to as music executive function training (MEFT) [43]. Music training that emphasizes these executive functions as goal areas may also be referred to as MEFT. Indeed, feasibility and intervention criteria for MEFT successfully employed to address task-shifting in adults with acquired brain injury are outlined by Lynch and LaGasee [44]. Music training that involves attainable incremental challenges, novelty, emotional arousal, and exercises task-shifting, sequencing, and so forth may also be of benefit to the executive function needs of adults with PD.

Therapeutic music activities have successfully targeted and improved executive functioning in adult clinical populations. "Chemo-brain," a frequent side effect of chemotherapy treatments, often produces attention and memory problems. Fifteen women receiving adjuvant chemotherapy for breast cancer received individualized once-weekly mindfulness-based music therapy, along with daily homework, for four weeks. While not music training per se, the women learned to play simple patterns on percussion and harmonic instruments (e.g., xylophone, piano) as part of the mindfulness-based music therapy four-week program. Information processing speed, as measured through a standardized computer test, was significantly improved, and, as well, symptom distress was significantly decreased [45]. The resulting cognitive improvement may be explained by the stimulation of the music program as opposed to a compensatory mechanism as mentioned by Kim et al. [17].

5. Conclusions and Recommendations

Together, this evidence presents a compelling case for music training to improve executive functioning for adults with PD. First, music training activates the cerebellar-thalamocortical network (CTC) network providing a rerouting to activate executive functions through fine motor activity [33]. We hypothesize that exercising the CTC network through music training will contribute to enhanced cognitive performance. The Movement Disorder Society (MDS) values the identification and intervention of cognitive impairment in adults with PD, and sees it as part of essential care—a need yet to be met [46]. Cognitive interventions that include repeated practice exercising the CTC network through sensorimotor integration may assist patients with PD. While research has shown that music training enhances cognitive performance (i.e., working memory and processing speed) in healthy older adults [38,47,48], there is a need to extend the benefits of music training to patients with PD. It will be necessary to fully ascertain the benefits of music training through large-scale randomized controlled trials. Researchers, patients, and caregivers would greatly benefit from published protocols that provide clear descriptions and manuals for musical interventions. Music training, as a type of cognitive rehabilitation, should also adhere to these guidelines and provide an evidence base for its use for adults with PD.

Acknowledgments: This review is supported by the GRAMMY FOUNDATION and the University of Miami Provost Research Award.

References

1.   Miura, K.; Matsui, M.; Takashima, S.; Tanaka, K. Neuropsychological characteristics and their association with higher-level functional capacity in Parkinson's Disease. *Dement. Geriatr. Cogn. Disord.* **2015**, *5*, 271–284. [CrossRef] [PubMed]

2.   Halpern, A.; Golden, H.L.; Magdalinou, N.; Witoonpanich, P.; Warren, J.D. Musical tasks targeting preserved and impaired functions in two dementias. *Ann. N. Y. Acad. Sci.* **2015**, *1337*, 241–248. [CrossRef] [PubMed]

3.   Lord, S.; Rochester, L.; Hetherington, V.; Allcock, A.L.; Burn, D. Executive dysfunction and attention contribute to gait interference in 'off' state Parkinson's Disease. *Gait Posture* **2010**, *31*, 169–174. [CrossRef] [PubMed]

4.   De Dreu, M.J.; van der Wilk, A.S.D.; Poppe, E.; Kwakkel, G.; van Wegen, E.E.H. Rehabilitation, exercise therapy and music in patients with Parkinson's disease: A meta-analysis of the effects of music-based movement therapy on walking ability, balance, and quality of life. *Parkinsonism Relat. Disord.* **2012**, *18*, S114–S119. [CrossRef]

5.   Nombela, C.; Hughes, L.E.; Owen, A.M.; Grahn, J.A. Into the groove: Can rhythm influence Parkinson's disease? *Neurosci. Biobehav. Rev.* **2013**, *37*, 2564–2570. [CrossRef] [PubMed]

6.   Thaut, M.H.; McIntosh, G.C.; Rice, R.R.; Miller, R.A.; Rathbun, J.; Brault, J.M. Rhythmic auditory stimulation in gait training for Parkinson's disease patients. *Mov. Disord.* **1996**, *11*, 193–200. [CrossRef] [PubMed]

7.   Thaut, M.H. *Rhythm, Music, and the Brain: Scientific Foundation and Clinical Applications*; Taylor and Francis Group: New York, NY, USA, 2005.

8.   Kudlicka, M.A.; Clare, L.; Hindle, J.V. Executive functions in Parkinson's Disease: Systematic review and meta-analysis. *Mov. Disord.* **2015**, *26*, 2306–2315. [CrossRef] [PubMed]

9.   Biundo, R.; Weis, L.; Antonini, A. Cognitive decline in Parkinson's disease: The complex picture. *NPJ Parkinsons Dis.* **2016**, *2*, 16018. [CrossRef] [PubMed]

10.   Lopes, R.; Delmaire, C.; Defebvre, L.; Moonen, A.J.; Duits, A.A.; Hofman, P.; Leentjens, A.F.; Dujardin, K. Cognitive phenotypes in Parkinson's Disease differ in terms of brain-network organization and connectivity. *Hum. Brain Mapp.* **2017**, *38*, 1604–1621. [CrossRef] [PubMed]

11.   Mak, E.; Su, L.; Williams, G.B.; Firbank, M.J.; Lawson, M.J.; Yarnall, R.A.; Owen, A.M.; Khoo, T.K.; Brooks, D.J.; Rowe, J.B.; et al. Baseline and longitudinal grey matter changes in newly diagnosed Parkinson's disease: ICICLE-PD study. *Brain* **2015**, *138*, 2974–2986. [CrossRef] [PubMed]

12.   Pederson, K.F.; Larsen, J.P.; Tysnes, O.B.; Alves, G. Natural course of mild cognitive impairment in Parkinson disease: A 5-year population-based study. *Neurology* **2017**, *88*, 767–774. [CrossRef] [PubMed]

13.   Seidler, R.D.; Bernard, J.A.; Burutolu, T.B.; Fling, B.W.; Gordon, M.T.; Kwak, Y.; Lipps, D.B. Motor control and aging: Links to age-related brain structural, functional and biochemical effects. *Neurosci. Biobehav. Rev.* **2010**, *34*, 721–733. [CrossRef] [PubMed]

14.   Cramer, S.C.; Sur, M.; Dobkin, B.H.; O'Brien, C.; Sanger, T.D.; Trojanowski, J.W.; Rumsey, J.M.; Hicks, R.; Cameron, J.; Chen, D.; et al. Harnessing neuroplasticity for clinical applications. *Brain* **2011**, *134*, 1591–1609. [CrossRef] [PubMed]

15.   Sweatt, J.D. Neural plasticity and behavior—Sixty years of conceptual advances. *J. Neurochem.* **2016**, *139*, 179–199. [CrossRef] [PubMed]

16. Hebb, D.O. *The Organization of Behavior*; Wiley: New York, NY, USA, 1949.

17. Kim, E.Y.; Kim, K.W. A theoretical framework for cognitive and non-cognitive interventions for older adults: Stimulation versus compensation. *Aging Ment. Health* **2014**, *18*, 304–315. [CrossRef] [PubMed]

18. Alain, C.; Zendel, B.R.; Hutka, S.; Bidelman, G.M. Turning down the noise: The benefit of musical training on the aging auditory brain. *Hear. Res.* **2014**, *308*, 162–173. [CrossRef] [PubMed]

19. Chang, X.; Wang, P.; Zhang, Q.; Feng, X.; Zhang, C.; Zhou, P. The effect of music training on unimanual and bimanual responses. *Music. Sci.* **2014**, *18*, 464–472. [CrossRef]

20. Herholz, S.C.; Zatorre, R.J. Musical training as a framework for brain plasticity: Behavior, function, and structure. *Neuron* **2012**, *76*, 486–502. [CrossRef] [PubMed]

21. Moreno, S.; Bidelman, G.M. Examining neural plasticity and cognitive benefit through the unique lens of musical training. *Hear. Res.* **2014**, *308*, 84–97. [CrossRef] [PubMed]

22. Pantev, C.; Herholz, S.C. Plasticity of the human auditory cortex related to musical training. *Neurosci. Biobehav. Rev.* **2011**, *35*, 2140–2154. [CrossRef] [PubMed]

23. Wan, C.Y.; Schlaug, G. Music making as a tool for promoting brain plasticity across the life span. *Neuroscientist* **2010**, *16*, 566–577. [CrossRef] [PubMed]

24. Huang, Y.; Zhen, Z.; Song, Y.; Zhu, Q.; Wang, S.; Liu, J. Motor training increases the stability of activation patterns in the primary motor cortex. *PLoS ONE* **2013**, *8*, e53555. [CrossRef] [PubMed]

25. Alves-Pinto, A.; Turova, V.; Blumenstein, T.; Thienel, A.; Wohlschlager, A.; Lampe, R. fMRI assessment of neuroplasticity in youths with neurodevelopmental-associated motor disorders after piano training. *Eur. J. Paediatr. Neurol.* **2015**, *19*, 15–28. [CrossRef] [PubMed]

26. Münte, T.F.; Altenmüller, E.; Jäncke, L. The musician's brain as a model of neuroplasticity. *Nat. Rev. Neurosci.* **2002**, *3*, 473–478. [CrossRef] [PubMed]

27. Bloem, B.R.; de Vries, N.M.; Eberbach, G. Nonpharmacological treatments for patients with Parkinson's Disease. *Mov. Disord.* **2015**, *30*, 1504–1520. [CrossRef] [PubMed]

28. Leung, I.H.K.; Walton, C.C.; Hallock, H.; Lewis, S.J.G.; Valenzuela, M.; Lampit, A. Cognitive training in Parkinson's Disease: A systematic review and meta-analysis. *Neurology* **2015**, *85*, 1843–1850. [CrossRef] [PubMed]

29. McKee, K.E.; Hackney, M.E. The effects of adapted tango on spatial cognition and disease severity in Parkinson's disease. *J. Motor Behav.* **2013**, *45*, 519–529. [CrossRef] [PubMed]

30. Bologna, M.; di Biasio, F.; Conte, A.; Iezzi, E.; Modugno, N.; Berardelli, A. Effects of cerebellar continuous theta bursts stimulation on resting tremor in Parkinson's disease. *Parkinsonism Relat. Disord.* **2015**, *21*, 1061–1066. [CrossRef] [PubMed]

31. Hasslinger, B.; Erhard, P.; Altenmuller, E.; Hennenlotter, A.; Schwaiger, M.; Einsiedel, H.G.C. Reduced recruitment of motor association areas during bimanual coordination in concert pianists. *Hum. Brain Mapp.* **2004**, *22*, 206–215. [CrossRef] [PubMed]

32. Bella, S.D.; Benoit, C.E.; Farrugia, N.; Schwartze, M.; Kotz, S.A. Effects of musically cued gait training in Parkinson's disease: Beyond a motor benefit. *Ann. N. Y. Acad. Sci.* **2015**, *1337*, 77–85. [CrossRef] [PubMed]

33. Zuk, J.; Benjamin, C.; Kenyon, A.; Gaab, N. Behavioral and neural correlates of executive functioning in musicians and non-musicians. *PLos ONE* **2014**, *9*, e99868. [CrossRef] [PubMed]

34. Thaut, M.H.; Peterson, D.A.; McIntosh, G.C. Temporal entrainment of cognitive functions: Musical mnemonics induce brain plasticity and oscillatory synchrony in neural networks underlying memory. *Ann. N. Y. Acad. Sci.* **2005**, *1060*, 243–254. [CrossRef] [PubMed]

35. Bugos, J.A. Community music as a cognitive training programme for successful ageing. *Int. J. Community Music* **2014**, *7*, 339–341. [CrossRef]

36. Posner, M.I.; Patoine, B. How arts training improves attention and cognition. *Cerebrum* **2009**, *2009*, 2–4.

37. Degé, F.; Kubicek, C.; Schwarzer, G. Music lessons and intelligence: A relation mediated by executive functions. *Music Percept.* **2011**, *29*, 195–201. [CrossRef]

38. Bugos, J.A.; Perlstein, W.M.; McCrae, C.S.; Brophy, T.S.; Bedenbaugh, P.H. Individualized piano instruction enhances executive functioning and working memory in older adults. *Aging Ment. Health* **2007**, *11*, 464–471. [CrossRef] [PubMed]

39. Hindle, J.V.; Petrelli, A.; Claire, L.; Kalbe, E. Nonpharmacological enhancement of cognitive function in Parkinson's Disease: A systematic review. *Mov. Disord.* **2013**, *28*, 1034–1049. [CrossRef] [PubMed]

40. Koerts, J.; van Beilen, M.; Tucha, O.; Leenders, K.L.; Brouwer, W.H. Executive functioning in daily life in Parkinson's Disease: Initiative, planning and multi-task performance. *PLoS ONE* **2011**, *6*, e29254. [CrossRef] [PubMed]

41. De Cock, V.C.; Dotov, D.G.; Ihalainen, P.; Bégel, V.; Galtier, F.; Lebrun, C.; Bella, S.D. Rhythmic abilities and musical training in Parkinson's disease: Do they help? *Nat. Partn. J. Parkinsons Dis.* **2018**, *4*, 8. [CrossRef] [PubMed]

42. Thaut, M.H.; Gardiner, J.C.; Holmberg, D.; Horwitz, J.; Kent, L.; Andrews, G.; Donelan, B.; McIntosh, G.R. Neurologic music therapy improves executive function and emotional adjustment in traumatic brain injury rehabilitation. *Ann. N. Y. Acad. Sci.* **2009**, *1169*, 406–416. [CrossRef] [PubMed]

43. Gardiner, J.C.; Thaut, M.H. Musical executive function training. In *Handbook of Neurologic Music Therapy*; Thaut, M.H., Hoemberg, V., Eds.; Oxford University Press: New York, NY, USA, 2014; pp. 279–293.

44. Lynch, C.; LaGasse, B. Training endogenous task shifting using music therapy: A feasibility study. *J. Music Ther.* **2016**, *53*, 279–307. [CrossRef] [PubMed]

45. Lesiuk, T. The effect of a mindfulness-based music therapy program (MBMT) on attention and mood in women receiving adjuvant chemotherapy for breast cancer: A pilot study. *Oncol. Nurs. Forum* **2015**, *42*, 276–282. [CrossRef] [PubMed]

46. Litvan, I.; Goldman, J.G.; Troster, A.I.; Schmand, B.A.; Weintraub, B.A.; Peterson, R.C.; Mollenhauer, B.; Adler, C.H.; Marder, K.; Williams-Gray, C.H.; et al. Diagnostic criteria for mild cognitive impairment in Parkinson's disease; Movement Disorder Society task force guidelines. *Mov. Disord.* **2012**, *27*, 349–356. [CrossRef] [PubMed]

47. Bugos, J.A.; Maxfield, N.; Kochar, S. Intense piano training on self-efficacy and physiological stress in aging. *Psychol. Music* **2016**, *44*, 611–624. [CrossRef] [PubMed]

48. Bugos, J.A. Intense piano training enhances verbal fluency in older adults. Presented at Meeting of the Society for Music Perception and Cognition (SMPC) Nashville, TN, USA, 1–5 August 2015.

7

What People Want to Know About Their Genes: A Critical Review of the Literature on Large-Scale Genome Sequencing Studies

Courtney L. Scherr [1,*], Sharon Aufox [2], Amy A. Ross [1], Sanjana Ramesh [1], Catherine A. Wicklund [2] and Maureen Smith [2]

[1] Center for Communication and Health, Department of Communication Studies, Northwestern University, 710 North Lake Shore Drive, 15th Floor, Chicago, IL 60611; USA; amyross2019@u.northwestern.edu (A.A.R.); sanjanaramesh2022@u.northwestern.edu (S.R.)

[2] Center for Genetic Medicine, Feinberg School of Medicine, Northwestern University, 645 N Michigan Ave, Suite 630, Chicago, IL 60611, USA; s-aufox@northwestern.edu (S.A.); c-wicklund@northwestern.edu (C.A.W.); m-smith6@northwestern.edu (M.S.)

* Correspondence: courtney.scherr@northwestern.edu

Abstract: From a public health perspective, the "All of Us" study provides an opportunity to isolate targeted and cost-effective prevention and early-detection strategies. Identifying motivations for participation in large-scale genomic sequencing (LSGS) studies, and motivations and preferences to receive results will help determine effective strategies for "All of Us" study implementation. This paper offers a critical review of the literature regarding LSGS for adult onset hereditary conditions where results could indicate an increased risk to develop disease. The purpose of this review is to synthesize studies which explored peoples' motivations for participating in LSGS studies, and their desire to receive different types of genetic results. Participants were primarily motivated by altruism, desire to know more about their health, and curiosity. When asked about hypothetically receiving results, most participants in hypothetical studies wanted all results except those which were uncertain (i.e., a variant of uncertain significance (VUS)). However, participants in studies where results were returned preferred to receive only results for which an intervention was available, but also wanted VUS. Concerns about peoples' understanding of results and possible psychosocial implications are noted. Most studies examined populations classified as "early adopters," therefore, additional research on motivations and expectations among the general public, minority, and underserved populations is needed.

Keywords: all of us; genetic studies; participant expectations; precision medicine; public health; results return

---

1. Introduction

Over three years ago, President Obama announced the Precision Medicine Initiative (PMI), a research effort to personalize medicine based on an individual's genes, environment, and lifestyle [1]. Since the PMI announcement, research has intensified to improve the understanding of disease mechanisms, diagnosis, and treatment outcomes using genomic sequencing projects [2]. From a public health perspective, the promise of the PMI is the identification of personalized interventions that not only include treatment, but also more targeted and cost-effective prevention and early-detection strategies [3–5]. Furthermore, hope exists that providing people with individualized genetic risk information will inform prevention and early-detection behaviors [6]. Yet, these outcomes will not be achieved without efforts to identify effective strategies for study implementation that ensure generalizability and motivate prevention behaviors.

Prior to the PMI, several federally funded research consortia were established to ascertain best practices in genomic sequencing research and practice. These consortia examined practical challenges related to recruitment and informed consent, data management, big data analysis, information and data sharing, and the dissemination and use of genetic results [7]. The PMI aims to use knowledge gained from these consortia to create a nationally-representative database with one million individual genetic profiles, called the "All of Us Research Program", led by the National Institutes of Health (NIH). Recruitment is underway, and plans to return genetic results are in development (see: https://allofus.nih.gov/), which makes the present an ideal time to consider how efforts from consortia studies can inform practices and future research efforts surrounding the PMI to ensure the advancement of public health goals.

This paper offers a critical review of existing literature related to participation in hypothetical and actual genomic research in the United States. The purpose of a critical review is not to aggregate all existing literature on the topic under review, but rather to extract what is valuable to inform conceptual development [8]. As such, we reviewed existing literature to identify, analyze, and synthesize studies exploring expectations and motivations for participating in LSGS studies, and participants' desires to receive different types of genetic results. The purpose of this methodology is to organize competing attitudes towards reasons for participation in LSGS studies, and preferences towards receiving results [8]. In doing so, we hope to synthesize what is currently known to inform recruitment processes and guideline development for the return of results. We conclude by highlighting gaps in existing literature and provide suggestions for future investigation.

2. Methodology

Given our emphasis on population health, we explored studies focused on large-scale genomic sequencing (LSGS) for adult onset hereditary conditions where results could indicate an increased risk to develop disease, and excluded LSGS testing for clinical purposes, for conditions in which disease onset is certain (e.g., Huntington's), or for pediatric conditions. We use the acronym LSGS to refer to testing where many genes are being analyzed at once, including genome-wide association studies (GWAS), whole exome and/or whole-genome sequencing (WES/WGS), and/or targeted sequencing of a large panel of genes. In addition, because guidelines, cultural, and social norms vary by country with respect to genetic testing, and genetics in general, we focused on studies carried out in the United States.

We conducted an initial search between 2015 and 2016 by examining the websites of existing LGSG studies which had a listing of publications. For example, Clinical Sequencing Evidence-Generating Research (CSER): https://cser-consortium.org/publications, Electronic Medical Records and Genomics (eMERGE): https://emerge.mc.vanderbilt.edu/publications/, and CLINSEQ: https://www.genome.gov/25521307/clinseq-study-news--updates/. A study team member reviewed the listing of publications for those which described participation in LSGS studies. In addition to selecting relevant manuscripts from the publication list, we entered manuscript titles into the Web of Science to identify additional relevant papers cited by or citing the paper from the publication listing. We also used Web of Science, Google Scholar, and our institution's library using search terms including patient and "experiences", or "expectations", or "motivations" plus "genetic testing", "GWAS", or "WGS", or "WES". At the beginning of 2018, two study team members updated the list of publications by entering in each earlier identified manuscript to the Web of Science search to determine any literature that had cited the previous studies since 2015. Likewise, the websites and publication listings of relevant LSGS studies were reviewed from 2015 to the present for any additional relevant publications (see Table 1 for the list of included publications).

Table 1. Included Studies.

In Text Citation	Article	LSGS	Methods	Purpose	Population	Disease	Return of Results
[9]	Facio, F.M., Brooks, S., Loewenstein, J., Green, S., Biesecker, L.G., & Biesecker, B.B. (2011). Motivators for participation in a whole-genome sequencing study: Implications for translational genomics research.	ClinSeq	Quantitative-participants completed surveys	To understand motivations and expectations of individuals who are choosing to have their whole genome or exome sequenced, and have the opportunity to learn about their results in the future	Individuals age 45-65 with a risk of developing coronary artery disease, including asymptomatic and symptomatic individuals	Individuals age 45-65 with a risk of developing coronary artery disease, including asymptomatic and symptomatic individuals	Yes; Selected, but not all- results are returned; a subset of data considered high-throughput results was determined as appropriate to return
[10]	Sanderson, S.C., Linderman, M.D., Suckiel, S.A., Diaz, G.A., Zinberg, R.E., Ferryman, K., Wasserstein, M., Kasarskis, A., & Schadt, E.E. (2016). Motivations, concerns and preferences of personal genome sequencing research participants: Baseline findings from the HealthSeq project.	HealthSeq	Mixed methods-participants completed questionnaires and in-depth interviews at multiple points during study	To assess motivations and concerns that participants have about genome sequencing; to understand preferences around return of results and informed consent	Unselected healthy adult population	Various diseases	Yes; A range of results including Alzheimer's, type 3 diabetes, rare disease-associated variants, ancestry, and pharmacogenomics; participants also offered raw data
[11]	Gollust, S.E., Gordon, E.S., Zayac, C., Griffin, G., Christman, M.F., Pyeritz, R.E., Wawak, L., & Bernhardt, B.A. (2012). Motivations and perceptions of early adopters of personalized genomics: Perspectives from research participants.	Coriell Personalized Medicine Collaborative	Quantitative-participants completed surveys	To ascertain motivation for enrolling, perceptions around risks and benefits, and intention to share results	Selected healthy adult populations	Various diseases	Yes; Actionable genetic variant results, non-genetic risk factors, and drug responses; participants decide whether they wish to view each actionable result
[12]	Kauffman, T.L., Irving, S.A., Leo, M.C., Gilmore, M.J., Himes, P., McMullen, C.K., Morris, E., Schneider, J., Wilfond, B.S., & Goddard, K.A.B. (2017). The NextGen study: Patient motivation for participation in genome sequencing for carrier status.	NextGen	Qualitative-participants were asked two open-ended questions about motivation to participate during an informed consent and education session with genetic counselor	To explore motivations in healthy pre-conception women to participate in genome sequencing research	Pre-conception women who were planning for pregnancy, and had undergone carrier screening	Various diseases	Yes; Medically actionable secondary findings, carrier findings
[13]	Bollinger, J.M., Joan, S., Dvoskin, R., & Kaufman, D. (2012). Public preferences regarding the return of individual genetic research results: Findings from a qualitative focus group study.	N/A-hypothetical	Qualitative-participants were divided into 10 focus groups	To explore preferences around the return of individual research results in genetic research	Unselected healthy adult population	N/A-hypothetical	N/A-hypothetical
[14]	Murphy, J., Scott, J., Kaufman, D., Geller, G., Leroy, L., & Hudson, K. (2008). Public expectations for return of results from large-cohort genetic research.	N/A	Qualitative-participants were divided into 6 focus groups	To learn values and perspectives about the return of individual research results in genetic studies	Unselected adults	Various diseases	Yes; Individual research results

Table 1. *Cont.*

In Text Citation	Article	LSGS	Methods	Purpose	Population	Disease	Return of Results
[15]	Allen, N.L. Karlson, E.W., Malspeis, S., Lu, B., Seidman, C.E., & Lehmann, L.S. (2014). Biobank participants' preferences for disclosure of genetic research results: Perspectives from the OurGenes, OurHealth, OurCommunity project.	Our Genes, Our Health, Our Community	Quantitative-participants completed a survey	To understand biobank participants preferences in the disclosure of results	Selected healthy adult patients	Various diseases	Yes; Hypothetically all results including results indicating high penetrance and risk for serious conditions
[16]	Facio, F.M., Eidem, H., Fisher, T., Brooks, S., Linn, A., Kaphingst, K.A., Biesecker, L.G., & Biesecker, B.B. (2013). Intentions to receive individual results from whole-genome sequencing among participants in the ClinSeq study.	ClinSeq	Mixed methods-participants completed surveys with open-ended questions	To learn general preferences and attitudes towards learning different types of genetic test results	Individuals age 45-65 with a risk of developing coronary artery disease, including asymptomatic and symptomatic individuals	Coronary artery disease	All results ranging from medically actionable to unknown significance
[17]	Wright, M.F., Lewis, K.L., Fisher, T.C., Hooker, G.W. Emanuel, T.E., Biesecker, L.G., & Biesecker, B.B. (2014). Preferences for results delivery from exome sequencing/genome sequencing.	ClinSeq	Qualitative-participants were divided into 6 focus groups	To understand enthusiasm towards and implications for returning genetic test results	Individuals age 45-65 with a risk of developing coronary artery disease, including asymptomatic and symptomatic individuals	Coronary artery disease	All results ranging from medically actionable to unknown significance
[18]	Hitch, K., Joseph, G., Guiltinan, J., Kianmahd, J., Youngbolm, J., & Blanco, A. (2014). Lynch Syndrome Patients' Views of and Preferences for Return of Results Following Whole Exome Sequencing.	N/A	Qualitative-participants completed individual interviews	To explore preferences of cancer patients about return of results from WES	Patients previously diagnosed with Lynch syndrome but received uninformative negative Lynch syndrome genetic results through traditional genetic testing	Lynch Syndrome	Yes; They only would receive cancer-related results generated from WES
[19]	Lupo, P.J., Robinson, J.O., Diamond, P.M., Jamal, L, Danysh, H.E., Blumenthal-Barby, J., Lehmann, L.S., Vassy, J.L., Christensen, K.D., & Green, R.C. (2016). Patients' perceived utility of whole-genome sequencing for their healthcare: Findings from the MedSeq project.	MedSeq	Quantitative-participants completed surveys	To understand participants' perceived utility, and how attitudes, behaviors, and demographic factors predict perceived utility	Healthy primary care participants 40–70 years old; Cardiology patients >18 years old	Various diseases in healthy participants; cardiovascular disease (hypertrophic and dilated cardiomyopathy) in cardiology patients	Yes; All results, including results in which clinical significance is uncertain

Note: LSGS: Large-scale genomic sequencing study; N/A: Not applicable.

3. Motivations for Participation in LSGS Studies

The success of the "All of Us Research Program" and other similar studies examining links between genetics and health outcomes depend on the enrollment of large numbers of people willing to longitudinally share their data with researchers [20,21]. Some studies examined hypothetical participation on LSGS studies. Other studies are "proof-of-principle" studies, designed to accumulate evidence about the impact of introducing new genomic sequencing technologies in defined populations [9,22]. These studies have evolved over time, some began by only recruiting populations with disease, or those who were at risk of developing disease, and later included healthy individuals (e.g., ClinSeq). We first discuss motivations for participating in LSGS studies and then explore preferences for the return of results from LSGS studies.

3.1. Intrinsic Motivations for Participating in LSGS Studies

Exploring peoples' motivations to enroll in LSGS studies is an important aspect of federally funded LSGS research consortia efforts. Most studies found participants held multiple motivations for participating in LSGS studies, but three motivations were consistent across studies: altruism, personal/family benefit, and curiosity.

3.2. Altruism

Debates regarding the definition of altruism are beyond the scope of this paper see: [23–25]. Given existing debates, it is unsurprising that studies used the term altruism inconsistently, if at all. When the term altruism was used, slight variations in operational definitions emerged. For the purposes of this review, and consistent with prior definitions of altruism in research studies, we define altruism as a prosocial behavior including either or both aspects: (1) the desire to help others; and (2) the desire to advance research or science. When authors did not use the term altruism, we still categorized it as such, based on the aforementioned definition.

Interviews conducted with a subsample of unselected members of the general population in the longitudinal HealthSeq study identified altruism as a motivator, which was framed as either "an altruistic desire to help others and the field of medicine", or "to contribute to the advancement of science" [10]. Altruism in the ClinSeq study was operationalized as a desire to help someone who may be at risk of specific disorders, such as coronary artery disease (CAD), to "help others in the future", and advance research in genetics or health [9]. However, the survey conducted with unselected volunteers in the Coriell Personalized Medicine Collaborative (CPMC) only included the response option, "participating in research to help others", and did not include a response option regarding the opportunity to advance science [11]. Of note, the authors did not describe this as altruism. In contrast, responses from the NextGen study focused on the advancement of research, but not on helping others, and again, the authors did not refer to this type of response as altruism [12].

Altruism was identified across studies as motivating participation in LSGS, but the number of people who reported altruism as a motivating factor varied. In qualitative interviews conducted prior to genetic results disclosure in the ClinSeq study of affected or at-risk participants, altruism was found to be a motivator for approximately half of participants. For example, approximately 44% of participants with or at risk of CAD reported altruism as a primary motivation for taking part [9]. Similarly, altruism was a motivating factor for unselected (i.e., healthy) participants. The CPMC, a study in which unselected volunteer participants receive 'medically actionable' genetic test results, found 56.2% of participants indicated "participating in research to help others" was a "very important" reason for taking part in the study [11].

The most divergent finding was in the NextGen study, which explored motivation to participate in LSGS research among healthy women and couples actively planning a pregnancy [12]. Participants were asked an open-ended question after enrollment about "what they hoped to learn from being in the study." Compared with the aforementioned studies, support of research was the least reported motivation (11%); however, the lower rate could be influenced by the way the question was asked.

3.3. Personal and Family Benefits

Interestingly, responses from the ClinSeq cohort, indicated motivation for participation was either driven by altruism or seeking personal health information, with little overlap [9]. Those who reported seeking personal health information wanted to learn about their risk for CAD, while others wanted information about genetic risk and predispositions to disease more generally, especially in the case of a family history of disease [9]. Most other studies found motivations for participation often included both altruism and a desire for personal information, among other motivators. In contrast with LSGS studies of affected or at-risk populations, studies of unselected or healthy participants more often cited personal benefit as the primary motivator for participation [10–12]. For example, in qualitative interviews conducted with unselected individuals, Sanderson, Linderman, Suckiel, Diaz, Zinberg, Ferryman, Wasserstein, Kasarskis and Schadt [10] found most participants reported the potential benefit for themselves and their family, some of whom also indicated altruism. Related to personal benefit, participants were hopeful that information from genetic testing could help them avoid or reduce their risk of disease, or help them to prepare or plan for the future. In some cases, they did not expect information from genetic testing would be immediately available or beneficial, but hoped additional research and investigation would provide more information in the future.

Among unselected healthy participants in the CPMC, approximately 78% indicated finding out about diseases for which they were at risk, and finding out what they can do to improve their health as very important motivators for participation [11]. Half of participants were interested in risk information related specifically to either heart disease, diabetes, or cancer. Of note, a minority (3.3%) wanted to know their risk of Alzheimer's disease, even though they were told at enrollment this information would not be available. A smaller proportion (47%) reported obtaining information about risk of health conditions for children and grandchildren as a motivating their participation. Consistently, the NextGen study of healthy women and couples actively planning a pregnancy with an indication for offering sequencing for carrier status and medically actionable secondary findings (SF) found knowledge about a particular health condition in their family (69%) as the most motivating factor for participation, tied with curiosity, and followed by reproductive planning (52%) [12].

3.4. Curiosity

In addition to altruism and personal benefit, curiosity was another motivator for participation in these studies. Interestingly, the majority of participants in the in the CPMC study (81%), the HealthSeq study (71%), and the NextGen (69%) study, all of which were conducted with unselected participants, were motivated to participate due to curiosity or general health information seeking [10–12]. The ClinSeq study also identified curiosity as a motivating factor, but at a much lower rate (19%) [9]. Although less often noted, or less common across studies, other motivating factors similar to curiosity included: having an interest in personal ancestry [10,11], and being adopted and wanting information about genetics [11].

4. Results Disclosure

In the United States, guidelines continue to recommend that disclosing genetic results in research studies, and returning SF findings be deliberated on a "protocol-by-protocol" basis [26,27]. Prior to determining whether results will be returned, serious considerations should be given to the steps that will be taken to confirm the appropriate infrastructure, support, and approval of relevant institutions (i.e., institutional review board), maintain quality in the conduct of the analysis (e.g., CLIA-certified laboratory), and incorporate participants' preferences (for detailed guidance, see: [27]).

Analytic and clinical validity, clinical or reproductive significance, and whether a result is clinically actionable are recommended considerations for determining results disclosure. Variations in the definition of "actionable" are debated, but most often, actionable means a genetic risk can be managed through "established interventions aimed at preventing or significantly reducing morbidity and mortality" [28,29]. From a public health perspective, the advantage of providing results to participants is the anticipation that such information can be used by the person to guide individual prevention and treatment decisions. Indeed, studies indicate participants' preference to receive results for such reasons.

Focus group studies conducted across the United States with members of the general public (i.e., not currently participating in an LSGS study) believed results could serve as compensation for study participation, and many felt researchers had an obligation to at least offer to disclose the results, particularly in the case of treatable and preventable conditions [13,14]. Similarly, a study of a subsample of biobank participants in the OurGenes, OurHealth, OurCommunity examined preferences for hypothetical results disclosure and found most (90%) believed it was very or somewhat important to receive their results [15]. Although there was a preference to receive results, there was divergence in the type of results people wanted to receive.

4.1. The Type of Results People Want

Studies with members of the general public found most participants wanted to receive all possible results, including conditions for which treatment is not currently available, but most did not want to receive variant of uncertain significance (VUS) results [13,14]. Consistent with views of the general public, the vast majority of a sample of mostly healthy participants in ClinSeq ($n = 311$), who will receive results as a condition of their participation, indicated they wanted to learn all of their results (95%) including those for which no intervention is available [16]. A focus group study of healthy participants and those at risk of CAD in the ClinSeq study confirmed the preference to receive all positive results, including those not medically actionable (i.e., diseases for which there is no known treatment) [17].

In contrast with perceptions of the general public and those in the ClinSeq study, healthy biobank participants, who would not receive results, were more favorable about receiving results for which an intervention or treatment was available [15]. Similarly, an LSGS study of cancer patients who would receive only cancer-related results found participants were less interested in receiving all results, only 63% indicated a preference to receive all possible results, and 6% wanted only those relevant to their medical care [18].

Studies of the general public, and of LSGS participants who would not receive results, found less favorable attitudes towards receiving uncertain results (i.e., VUS) [13–15]. In contrast, participants in LSGS studies who would receive results were interested in receiving VUS. Most (84%) cancer patients who would receive cancer-related results preferred to receive VUS; all wanted to receive updates in the case of VUS reclassification [18], and a significant majority of participants in the ClinSeq study wanted to receive VUS [16].

One study of the general public found result accuracy and conclusiveness were not critical to participants, they understood and expected that information from research could change over time [13]. However, another study of participants in the general public and one with healthy individuals found result accuracy was important [10,14]. Specifically, participants believed the lab should be reliable, and results should be conclusive and have a known correlation with health and disease prior to being shared with the participant.

4.2. What People Plan to Do with Their Results

Consistent with arguments for providing participants with results, that it may help promote preventive behavior, studies found participants planned to use results to engage in preventive health behaviors, and would share information with their family members. In addition, participants shared that genetic test results could be useful to them for other reasons, for example, to plan for the future.

Members of the general public reported a desire to receive all SF because they believed it could improve their health by directing treatment or disease prevention and through changing their health-related behaviors [13]. Similarly, other qualitative studies uncovered participants' perceptions of perceived benefits from learning genetic results. Cancer patients who consented to participate in an LSGS study and who would receive results wanted this information because they believed the knowledge would help with medical decision-making and prevention decisions, including altering their lifestyle [18]. Participants who would receive results as part of ClinSeq wanted to know their results for preventive reasons, including improving diet and exercise [16].

4.3. Participant Perspectives on Actionability

In addition to assisting with their own medical and preventive health decisions, participants viewed actionability to be important, as in, being able to "do" something with the information. Among the general population, such actions included: informing family members of risk, making reproductive decisions, working for environmental action or remediation, life and financial planning, and participating in future research [13,14]. Such views about actionability were also found among participants in LSGS studies who were asked about hypothetical results disclosure. Cancer patients believed results could help them prepare financially and psychologically for their future [18]. A third of a cohort of healthy participants in ClinSeq wanted to know their results to inform their children and family members [16]. Participants in the ClinSeq focus group believed results would allow for "peace of mind" and "more control" in the future [17]. When considering the development of guidelines for results return, it is important to recognize the general public may hold a broader definition of "actionable," and view results as personally useful, even in the absence of clinical intervention.

Of note, a study which explored perceived utility as a motivation for participation in the MedSeq study identified trust as a driving factor [19]. Participants generally fell into one of three groups: enthusiasts, health conscious, and skeptics (i.e., lowest perceived utility). Enthusiasts believed results had utility beyond medical purposes, including family and end-of-life planning. Health conscious believed results only had utility for medical purposes, and skeptics did not believe results would have personal utility. Trust in result interpretation and dissemination was the only predictor of utility, skeptics reported the least trust [19]. Additional studies that identify other predictors of participant preference may be useful for determining what information participants want to receive, and in some cases, anticipating how they may use results.

4.4. Concerns about Receiving Results

The preponderance of respondents across studies were favorable about receiving results, but some studies identified concerns. For example, cancer patients raised the possibility to experience negative psychosocial outcomes in response to learning about a serious untreatable disease, but they noted that their experience with a cancer diagnosis helped them to feel better able to cope with such genetic test results [18]. Often, participants' concerns about potential negative consequences of learning results emerged after additional discussion. Focus group participants in the ClinSeq study indicated a preference to receive all results, yet upon further discussion about possible results, participants experienced hesitations, and some reported not wanting to learn about untreatable progressive disease risk [17]. By providing an extended discussion about the possible outcomes from learning about specific types of disease, participants changed their minds, raising concerns about how informed their initial preferences were.

Collectively, study results indicate people desire to receive all genetic results for value beyond clinical prevention or treatment. The general public was not interested in results which were uncertain, but participants enrolled in studies which included result disclosure as a condition of enrollment wanted all results, including VUS. Similarly, additional discussions about what each result means in a focus group led to some participants changing their preference, which suggests participants must be provided with clear informed consent which describes possible results and the implications of those results (i.e., psychosocial implications) in detail prior to making decisions about participating and potentially receiving results. Such results highlight the importance of providing anticipatory guidance, encouraging participants to consider possible thoughts and emotions they may experience with the possible range of outcomes [30].

5. Discussion and Conclusions

The increased focus on precision medicine and the use of LSGS in research studies and clinical practice has implications for public health. White papers, perspectives and opinions of those in public health have identified the PMI's potential and the pitfalls from recruitment to the return of results. Beginning with recruitment, we identified altruism, personal and family benefit, and general curiosity among the most common motivators for participating in LSGS studies. In all but one study [9], participants identified more than one motivating factor for participating. Those affected or at risk were slightly more likely to identify altruism as a motivating factor compared with the general population, who were most motivated by personal benefit and curiosity. Given the vast majority of participants in LSGS studies are likely to receive negative results, additional research should examine how to balance participants' excitement about the prospect of receiving personal health information with the reality that most results will be negative.

There is considerable debate in the research community over whether LSGS studies should return results to participants [31]. Concerns have been raised by researchers about providing participants with genetic test results due to the potential for a participant to conflate research and clinical care. Questions about appropriateness, training, and boundary blurring are raised when a researcher provides SF results to a participant [7,26,32]. How to manage the logistics of delivering the information, and what to tell participants whose phenotypes are not indicative of the condition needs to be considered [33,34]. Conversely, others feel a sense of responsibility due to the potential for the participant or patient to undergo disease prevention or early-detection behaviors [35–37]. The recent Consensus Study Report from the National Academy of Sciences committee on Return of Individual-Specific Research Results Generated in Research Laboratories is moving away from strict recommendations against returning results to research participants [27]. This move appears to recognize the interest of research participants in learning about their genetic health as well as a move towards better laboratory testing in research.

In this review, we found members of the general population and participants in ClinSeq wanted to receive all genetic results, except VUS. The most common reasons for wanting results were consistent with motivations for participating and included a sense of rights or ownership, believing the information can inform future decision-making and health behavior, and the desire to share information with their family members. In contrast, studies of LSGS participants found the majority was favorable towards receiving results, but preferred results for which an intervention was available, and wanted VUS results. Given preference variability, particularly related to SF and even more so VUS, suggestions have been made to allow participants the option to make ongoing choices and modify their preferences for the type of results they receive [14].

A focus group study, which probed more deeply into the potential consequences of learning of certain results [17], found participants hesitated in their initial desire to receive all results. Additional research should examine participants' understanding of genetic results, including possible implications to their psychosocial well-being, and how their understanding (or lack thereof) informs their preferences. Determining key information and identifying appropriate levels of understanding could be useful to guiding informed consent processes for research and clinical practice. Allowing participants to select which results they will receive in absence of complete understanding of the consequences could cause negative psychosocial outcomes and impact future recruitment efforts.

Studies in this review examined hypothetical preferences, or were conducted on participants who agreed to participate in a study where genomic sequencing information will be returned to them in the future. Those not enrolled in an LSGS study and those unaffected individuals in the process of enrolling in a study where results will be returned were more likely to be favorable towards receiving results compared with those who were affected or who enrolled in a study where results would not be returned. Given these differences, research which allows participants a choice about receiving results could improve participant heterogeneity. Additionally, studies where participants were told they would not receive results at enrollment (e.g., some biobank studies), but are now considering returning results, should do so with caution. Research conducted on the process of actually returning results in such cases could inform our understanding of actual preferences.

Most studies in this review included participants who could be classified as "early adopters of new technologies", specifically those who are white, of higher socioeconomic status, higher education, and more interested in taking risks [9]. As such, extrapolating their intentions and experiences with LSGS to the general population is not reasonable. Although this information provides a foundation for understanding public perceptions, it is unlikely that it will be consistent with the general population [38]. A conclusion reached by nearly every study was the need for additional research on diverse populations in terms of location (urban vs. rural), accessibility, ethnicity, race, education, socioeconomic status and drawing participants who have varied experience with disease, illness, and knowledge or experience with genetics [18].

Strategies to engage minority and underserved communities include making initial contact by phone, using community-based strategies such as engaging community leaders, and involving community members with research-based activities throughout the duration of the study [39]. Continued efforts to identify best practices for recruitment of minority and underserved populations is urgent for behavioral and biomedical reasons. Genetic heterogeneity exists between population groups, which impacts disease risk (e.g., some diseases are more common than others in certain populations), and treatment responses [40]. Failing to include minority racial and ethnic populations in LSGS studies will increase knowledge of disease risk in majority populations only, thereby perpetuating health disparities [41]. Continued research to determine methods for improving trust of racial/ethnic minority populations and improving recruitment to LSGS studies is a priority.

LSGS studies are beginning to return results to their participants, and data soon will be available about the type of actions participants take in response to learning about their genetic risk. Despite the desire to receive results to inform choices about health protective behaviors, little is known about how participants will use this information. A revised and updated Cochrane review published in 2016 found the disclosure of genetic risk has little or no effect on health-related behavior [42]. These results are not surprising. For decades, health behaviorists have known information alone does not change behavior. The development of health behavior theories for communicating risk information such as the Health Belief Model [43], the Extended Parallel Process Model [44], the Transtheoretical Model [45] were the direct result of this acknowledgement. Information delivered in absence of a theoretical framework is unlikely to be motivating. Furthermore, behavior change is difficult. Even among patients who experienced life-changing health events such as a heart attack or cancer often fail to sustain behavior change over time.

In addition to asking about motivations to participate in the aforementioned CPMC study, Gollust, Gordon, Zayac, Griffin, Christman, Pyeritz, Wawak and Bernhardt [11] also asked about participants' intentions to share their results with their healthcare providers. Perhaps consistent with the desire for genetic information to improve their health, the vast majority (91.7%) stated they were likely or very likely to share their results with their physicians. In part, the researchers noted that participants in the CPMC study were encouraged to share their results with their healthcare providers when they enrolled in the study, which may have skewed these results. Identifying pathways between genetics professionals (who disclose the result) and healthcare providers who have ongoing contact and can monitor and encourage patients' prevention behavior, may have advantages for adherence. Although actual follow-up with physicians was low in the CPMC study, the authors indicated that primary care physicians may not have the training required to assist patients in interpreting and managing their healthcare based on genetic test results. They suggested additional research which follows early adopter's use of primary care services after receiving genetic test results to evaluate whether regulatory guidance is needed on a public health level [11].

The ability for LSGS studies and the "All of Us" study to positively impact public health will largely be determined by several important factors that will require additional investigation. First, continued efforts are needed to identify effective methods for recruiting a diverse cohort of participants. Second, additional research is needed to determine which results will be most likely to improve prevention behaviors and the least likely to cause negative psychosocial consequences. Preferences related to race/ethnicity, gender, age, and other socioeconomic factors should continue to be explored. Finally, determining communication strategies to disclose results which have the greatest potential to motivate prevention behaviors, and identifying pathways to improve adherence will be critical. The inclusion of a diverse cohort, development of guidelines for results disclosure, and messages and systems to support prevention behavior will lay the groundwork to achieve the promise of precision public health.

Author Contributions: C.L.S. conceived of and developed the overview with conceptual contributions from M.S., S.A. and C.W. A preliminary review of the literature was conducted by A.R. and C.L.S., with a supplemental review provided by C.L.S. and S.R. The original manuscript was written by C.L.S., A.R. and S.R., and significant editorial suggestions and reviews were provided by M.S., S.A. and C.W.

Funding: This research received no external funding.

References

1. The White House. Fact Sheet: President Obama's Precision Medicine Initiative. Available online: http://www.whitehouse.gov/the-press-office/2015/01/30/fact-sheet-president-obama-s-precision-medicine-initiative (accessed on 14 May 2018).

2. Auffray, C.; Caulfield, T.; Griffin, J.L.; Khoury, M.J.; Lupski, J.R.; Schwab, M. From genomic medicine to precision medicine: Highlights of 2015. *Genet. Med.* **2016**, *8*, 1–5. [CrossRef] [PubMed]

3. Khoury, M.J.; Iademarco, M.F.; Riley, W.T. Precision public health for the era of precision medicine. *Am. J. Prev. Med.* **2016**, *50*, 398–401. [CrossRef] [PubMed]

4. Khoury, M.J.; Galea, S. Will precision medicine improve population health? *JAMA* **2016**, *316*, 1357–1358. [CrossRef] [PubMed]

5. Ashley, E.A. The precision medicine initiative: A new national effort. *JAMA* **2015**, *313*, 2119–2120. [CrossRef] [PubMed]

6. Ramaswami, R.; Bayer, R.; Galea, S. Precision medicine from a public health perspective. *Ann. Rev. Public Health* **2018**, *39*, 153–168. [CrossRef] [PubMed]

7. Biesecker, L.G.; Mullikin, J.C.; Facio, F.M.; Turner, C.; Cherukuri, P.F.; Blakesley, R.W.; Bouffard, G.G.; Chines, P.S.; Cruz, P.; Hansen, N.F.; et al. The Clinseq project: Piloting large-scale genome sequencing for research in genomic medicine. *Genet. Res.* **2009**, *19*, 1665–1674. [CrossRef] [PubMed]

8. Grant, M.J.; Booth, A. A typology of reviews: An analysis of 14 review types and associated methodologies. *Health Inf. Libr. J.* **2009**, *26*, 91–108. [CrossRef] [PubMed]

9. Facio, F.M.; Brooks, S.; Loewenstein, J.; Green, S.; Biesecker, L.G.; Biesecker, B.B. Motivators for participation in a whole-genome sequencing study: Implications for translational genomics research. *Eur. J. Hum. Genet.* **2011**, *19*, 1213–1217. [CrossRef] [PubMed]

10. Sanderson, S.C.; Linderman, M.D.; Suckiel, S.A.; Diaz, G.A.; Zinberg, R.E.; Ferryman, K.; Wasserstein, M.; Kasarskis, A.; Schadt, E.E. Motivations, concerns and preferences of personal genome sequencing research participants: Baseline findings from the Healthseq project. *Eur. J. Hum. Genet.* **2016**, *24*, 14–20. [CrossRef] [PubMed]

11. Gollust, S.E.; Gordon, E.S.; Zayac, C.; Griffin, G.; Christman, M.F.; Pyeritz, R.E.; Wawak, L.; Bernhardt, B.A. Motivations and perceptions of early adopters of personalized genomics: Perspectives from research participants. *Public Health Genet.* **2012**, *15*, 22–30. [CrossRef] [PubMed]

12. Kauffman, T.L.; Irving, S.A.; Leo, M.C.; Gilmore, M.J.; Himes, P.; McMullen, C.K.; Morris, E.; Schneider, J.; Wilfond, B.S.; Goddard, K.A.B. The Nextgen study: Patient motivation for participation in genome sequencing for carrier status. *Mol. Genet. Genom. Med.* **2017**, *5*, 508–515. [CrossRef] [PubMed]

13. Bollinger, J.M.; Joan, S.; Dvoskin, R.; Kaufman, D. Public preferences regarding the return of individual genetic research results: Findings from a qualitative focus group study. *Genet. Med.* **2012**, *14*, 451–457. [CrossRef] [PubMed]

14. Murphy, J.; Scott, J.; Kaufman, D.; Geller, G.; Leroy, L.; Hudson, K. Public expectations for return of results from large-cohort genetic research. *Am. J. Bioeth.* **2008**, *8*, 36–43. [CrossRef] [PubMed]

15. Allen, N.L.; Karlson, E.W.; Malspeis, S.; Lu, B.; Seidman, C.E.; Lehmann, L.S. Biobank participants' preferences for disclosure of genetic research results: Perspectives from the Ourgenes, Ourhealth, Ourcommunity project. *Mayo Clin. Proc.* **2014**, *89*, 738–746. [CrossRef] [PubMed]

16. Facio, F.M.; Eidem, H.; Fisher, T.; Brooks, S.; Linn, A.; Kaphingst, K.A.; Biesecker, L.G.; Biesecker, B.B. Intentions to receive individual results from whole-genome sequencing among participants in the Clinseq study. *Eur. J. Hum. Genet.* **2013**, *21*, 261–265. [CrossRef] [PubMed]

17. Wright, M.F.; Lewis, K.L.; Fisher, T.C.; Hooker, G.W.; Emanuel, T.E.; Biesecker, L.G.; Biesecker, B.B. Preferences for results delivery from exome sequencing/genome sequencing. *Genet. Med.* **2014**, *16*, 442–447. [CrossRef] [PubMed]

18. Hitch, K.; Joseph, G.; Guiltinan, J.; Kianmahd, J.; Youngblom, J.; Blanco, A. Lynch syndrome patients' views of and preferences for return of results following whole exome sequencing. *J. Genet. Couns.* **2014**, *23*, 539–551. [CrossRef] [PubMed]

19. Lupo, P.J.; Robinson, J.O.; Diamond, P.M.; Jamal, L.; Danysh, H.E.; Blumenthal-Barby, J.; Lehmann, L.S.; Vassy, J.L.; Christensen, K.D.; Green, R.C. Patients' perceived utility of whole-genome sequencing for their healthcare: Findings from the Medseq project. *Personal. Med.* **2016**, *13*, 13–20. [CrossRef] [PubMed]

20. Aronson, S.J.; Rehm, H.L. Building the foundation for genomics in precision medicine. *Nature* **2015**, *526*, 336–342. [CrossRef] [PubMed]

21. Collins, F.S.; Varmus, H. A new initiative on precision medicine. *N. Engl. J. Med.* **2015**, *372*, 793–795. [CrossRef] [PubMed]

22. Jarvik, G.P.; Amendola, L.M.; Berg, J.S.; Brothers, K.; Clayton, E.W.; Chung, W.; Evans, B.J.; Evans, J.P.; Fullerton, S.M.; Gallego, C.J. Return of genomic results to research participants: The floor, the ceiling, and the choices in between. *Am. J. Hum. Genet.* **2014**, *94*, 818–826. [CrossRef] [PubMed]

23. Piliavin, J.A.; Charng, H.-W. Altruism: A review of recent theory and research. *Ann. Rev. Sociol.* **1990**, *16*, 27–65. [CrossRef]

24. Batson, C.D. *The Altruism Question: Toward a Social-Psychological Answer*; Psychology Press: Hove, UK, 2014.

25. Feigin, S.; Owens, G.; Goodyear-Smith, F. Theories of human altruism: A systematic review. *Ann. Neurosci. Psychol.* **2014**, *1*, 1–9.

26. Presidential Commission for the Study of Bioethical Issues. *Anticipate and Communicate: Ethical Management of Incidental and Secondary Findings in the Clinical, Research, and Direct-to-Consumer Contexts*; Washington, DC, USA, 2013. Available online: https://bioethicsarchive.georgetown.edu/pcsbi/sites/default/files/FINALAnticipateCommunicate_PCSBI_0.pdf (accessed on 17 May 2018).

27. National Academies of Sciences, Engineering, and Medicine. *Returning Individual Research Results to Participants: Guidance for a New Research Paradigm*; The National Academies Press Health and Medicine Division: Washington, DC, USA, 2018.

28. Green, R.C.; Berg, J.S.; Grody, W.W.; Kalia, S.S.; Korf, B.R.; Martin, C.L.; McGuire, A.; Nussbaum, R.L.; O'Daniel, J.M.; Ormond, K.E.; et al. ACMG recommendations for reporting of incidental findings in clinical exome and genome sequencing. *Gen. Med.* **2013**, *15*, 565–574. [CrossRef] [PubMed]

29. Kalia, S.S.; Adelman, K.; Bale, S.J.; Chung, W.K.; Eng, C.; Evans, J.P.; Herman, G.E.; Hufnagel, S.B.; Klein, T.E.; Korf, B.R. Recommendations for reporting of secondary findings in clinical exome and genome sequencing, 2016 update (acmg sf v2. 0): A policy statement of the American college of medical genetics and genomics. *Genet. Med.* **2017**, *19*, 249–255. [CrossRef] [PubMed]

30. Ensenauer, R.E.; Michels, V.V.; Reinke, S.S. Genetic testing: Practical, ethical, and counseling considerations. *Mayo Clin. Proc.* **2005**, *80*, 63–73. [CrossRef]

31. Middleton, A.; Morley, K.I.; Bragin, E.; Firth, H.V.; Hurles, M.E.; Wright, C.F.; Parker, M. Attitudes of nearly 7000 health professionals, genomic researchers and publics toward the return of incidental results from sequencing research. *Eur. J. Hum. Genet.* **2016**, *24*, 21–29. [CrossRef] [PubMed]

32. Knoppers, B.M.; Ma'n, H.Z.; Sénécal, K. Return of genetic testing results in the era of whole-genome sequencing. *Nat. Rev. Genet.* **2015**, *16*, 553–559. [CrossRef] [PubMed]

33. Mackley, M.P.; Fletcher, B.; Parker, M.; Watkins, H.; Ormondroyd, E. Stakeholder views on secondary findings in whole-genome and whole-exome sequencing: A systematic review of quantitative and qualitative studies. *Genet. Med.* **2017**, *19*, 283–293. [CrossRef] [PubMed]

34. Amendola, L.M.; Lautenbach, D.; Scollon, S.; Bernhardt, B.; Biswas, S.; East, K.; Everett, J.; Gilmore, M.J.; Himes, P.; Raymond, V.M.; et al. Illustrative case studies in the return of exome and genome sequencing results. *Personal. Med.* **2015**, *12*, 283–295. [CrossRef] [PubMed]

35. Wolf, S.M. The past, present, and future of the debate over return of research results and incidental findings. *Genet. Med.* **2012**, *14*, 355–357. [CrossRef] [PubMed]

36. Gliwa, C.; Berkman, B.E. Do researchers have an obligation to actively look for genetic incidental findings? *Am. J. Bioeth.* **2013**, *13*, 32–42. [CrossRef] [PubMed]

37. Evans, J.P.; Rothschild, B.B. Return of results: Not that complicated? *Genet. Med.* **2012**, *14*, 358–360. [CrossRef] [PubMed]

38. Lewis, K.L.; Hooker, G.W.; Connors, P.D.; Hyams, T.C.; Wright, M.F.; Caldwell, S.; Biesecker, L.G.; Biesecker, B.B. Participant use and communication of findings from exome sequencing: A mixed-methods study. *Genet. Med.* **2015**, *18*, 577–583. [CrossRef] [PubMed]

39. Johnson, V.A.; Powell-Young, Y.M.; Torres, E.R.; Spruill, I.J. *A systematic Review of Strategies That Increase the Recruitment and Retention of African American Adults in Genetic and Genomic Studies*; The ABNF Journal: Official Journal of the Association of Black Nursing Faculty in Higher Education, Inc.: Lisle, IL, USA, 2011; Volume 22, p. 84.

40. Ramirez, A.G.; Thompson, I.M. How will the 'cancer moonshot' impact health disparities? *Cancer Causes Control* **2017**, *28*, 907–912. [CrossRef] [PubMed]

41. Landry, L.G.; Ali, N.; Williams, D.R.; Rehm, H.L.; Bonham, V.L. Lack of diversity in genomic databases is a barrier to translating precision medicine research into practice. *Health Aff.* **2018**, *37*, 780–785. [CrossRef] [PubMed]

42. Hollands, G.J.; French, D.P.; Griffin, S.J.; Prevost, A.T.; Sutton, S.; King, S.; Marteau, T.M. The impact of communicating genetic risks of disease on risk-reducing health behaviour: Systematic review with meta-analysis. *BMJ* **2016**, *352*, i1102. [CrossRef] [PubMed]

43. Janz, N.K.; Becker, M.H. The health belief model: A decade later. *Health Educ. Q.* **1984**, *11*, 1–47. [CrossRef] [PubMed]

44. Witte, K. Putting the fear back into fear appeals: The extended parallel process model. *Commun. Monogr.* **1992**, *59*, 329–349. [CrossRef]

45. Prochaska, J.O.; Velicer, W.F.; Rossi, J.S.; Goldstein, M.G.; Marcus, B.H.; Rakowski, W.; Fiore, C.; Harlow, L.L.; Redding, C.A.; Rosenbloom, D. Stages of change and decisional balance for 12 problem behaviors. *Health Psychol.* **1994**, *13*, 39–46. [CrossRef] [PubMed]

8

Precision Medicine for Alzheimer's Disease Prevention

Cara L. Berkowitz ⓘ, Lisa Mosconi, Olivia Scheyer, Aneela Rahman, Hollie Hristov and Richard S. Isaacson *

Department of Neurology, Weill Cornell Medicine, New York, NY 10021, USA; cab2040@med.cornell.edu (C.L.B.); lim2035@med.cornell.edu (L.M.); ols2011@med.cornell.edu (O.S.); anr2781@med.cornell.edu (A.R.); how2005@med.cornell.edu (H.H.)
* Correspondence: rii9004@med.cornell.edu

Abstract: Precision medicine is an approach to medical treatment and prevention that takes into account individual variability in genes, environment, and lifestyle and allows for personalization that is based on factors that may affect the response to treatment. Several genetic and epigenetic risk factors have been shown to increase susceptibility to late-onset Alzheimer's disease (AD). As such, it may be beneficial to integrate genetic risk factors into the AD prevention approach, which in the past has primarily been focused on universal risk-reduction strategies for the general population rather than individualized interventions in a targeted fashion. This review discusses examples of a "one-size-fits-all" versus clinical precision medicine AD prevention strategy, in which the precision medicine approach considers two genes that can be commercially sequenced for polymorphisms associated with AD, apolipoprotein E (APOE), and methylenetetrahydrofolate reductase (MTHFR). Comparing these two distinct approaches provides support for a clinical precision medicine prevention strategy, which may ultimately lead to more favorable patient outcomes as the interventions are targeted to address individualized risks.

Keywords: Alzheimer's disease prevention; precision medicine; clinical precision medicine; apolipoprotein ε4; APOE; methylenetetrahydrofolate reductase; MTHFR

---

1. Introduction to Precision Medicine

The National Institute of Health (NIH), along with several other research centers, has created the Precision Medicine Initiative as a new way of approaching medicine with a targeted and patient-centered focus [1]. Specifically, they have defined precision medicine as an "emerging approach for disease treatment and prevention that takes into account individual variability in genes, environment, and lifestyle for each person" [1]. This approach to the practice of medicine has a high potential for treating the nuances of individuals with different genetics, lifestyle factors, and medical comorbidities that may affect their response to treatment. Since its initiation, many fields, including oncology [2] and cardiology [3], have begun refocusing their efforts to more precision-based approaches to practicing medicine. The role that genetics plays in the development of late-onset Alzheimer's disease (AD) has been widely studied, with one study estimating genetics to account for more than 50% of the phenotypic variance [4]. However, the field of AD prevention has yet to fully advance intervention strategies from universal risk-reduction approaches to targeted interventions based on personalized risk factors, including genetics. In the following discussion, we review examples of a universal "one-size-fits-all" prevention strategy without any distinction that is based on genetics or other personalized risk factors versus a clinical precision medicine approach. From a practical clinical perspective, we have focused on two genes that can be commercially sequenced for polymorphisms that are associated with AD and that physicians may order to help better inform patient care. These include the most well-characterized genetic influencer on late-onset AD risk, apolipoprotein E (APOE), and another potential genetic influencer, methylenetetrahydrofolate reductase (MTHFR). With the increasing ease of both clinical lab-based, as well as direct-to-consumer genetic sequencing, a precision medicine approach that incorporates established genetic factors may be feasible and may also favorably affect patient outcomes by addressing individualized risks as well as pharmacogenomics and nutrigenomic considerations for AD.

2. "One-Size-Fits-All" Approach to AD Prevention

Randomized studies in AD prevention have traditionally used either single or multiple interventions to determine efficacy across a host of clinical outcome measures (e.g., cognitive function, serum biomarkers, brain imaging). The vast majority of these studies have used a "one-size-fits-all" approach to targeting diet, exercise, and other lifestyle factors without accounting for any individual genetic variables. Two large-scale randomized control trials (RCTs), the Multidomain Alzheimer Prevention Trial (MAPT) and Prevention of Dementia by Intensive Vascular Care (PreDIVA) trial did not show improvements in cognitive functioning with lifestyle interventions, including nutrition, physical activity, cognitive engagement, and management of comorbidities [5–7]. However, these studies used populations that were already experiencing some degree of cognitive decline or dementia. As AD starts developing in the brain decades before clinical symptoms become apparent [8], these study populations may not have been optimized to benefit from lifestyle modifications since individuals experiencing cognitive decline may already be beyond a critical window for AD prevention [9].

The Finnish Geriatric Intervention Study to Prevent Cognitive Impairment and Disability (FINGER) was the first multicenter RCT to investigate the effects of similar lifestyle interventions on cognitive functioning in non-impaired individuals at risk for cognitive decline [10]. The results of the FINGER trial demonstrated that all individuals, regardless of baseline cognition, cardiovascular risk, demographics, or socioeconomic status improved with lifestyle interventions [11,12]. While not included in the initial study, a sub-analysis of the FINGER trial further explored the impact of a particular genetic factor, APOE, on lifestyle interventions in this cohort. This sub-analysis is further discussed in the 'Precision Medicine Approach to AD Prevention' section.

Several other prevention studies have shown improvement in cognitive function by implementing universal lifestyle interventions in non-impaired individuals, but with highly variable results. The two categories of interventions with the most robust evidence thus far include nutrition (including dietary patterns and single or multi-nutrients) and physical exercise. The Mediterranean diet is one example of a dietary pattern that has been extensively studied for AD prevention. A recent meta-analysis investigating the impact of the Mediterranean diet on cognitive functioning showed that there was a lower risk of cognitive decline and conversion to mild cognitive impairment (MCI) or AD in subjects with higher adherence to the diet [13]. However, there are also studies that have failed to demonstrate benefits of diet-specific interventions for AD prevention as well as various studies with mixed findings about which particular dietary interventions are the most beneficial [14–16].

Another well-studied dietary intervention focusing on single or multi-nutrients in the area of AD prevention has aimed to optimize levels of omega-3 polyunsaturated fatty acids (n-3 PUFA), most specifically, docosahexaenoic acid (DHA) [17–23]. Epidemiological evidence indicates that regular fish consumption and higher n-3 PUFA levels may reduce the risk for age-associated cognitive decline and AD [24]. Also, higher blood n-3 PUFA levels are protective of cortical structures [25], and chronic fish oil supplementation is associated with increased posterior cingulate activation in non-demented older adults [26]. Additional studies have shown improvement in cognitive function or decreased risk of AD in healthy individuals with DHA supplementation [18–20] or with consumption of fish high in omega-3s once per week [20]. However, other studies have suggested that there is no benefit of omega-3 supplementation with regard to cognitive function and AD prevention [22,23].

Another lifestyle intervention that has been studied for AD prevention with variable results is physical activity. A meta-analysis on the role of physical activity in AD prevention concluded that physical activity significantly decreased the risk of developing AD [27]. In addition, an RCT that looked at the impact of physical activity on cognitive functioning demonstrated that individuals who participated in six months of physical activity showed improvement in cognitive functioning up to 18 months later [28]. Researchers have also investigated the timing and intensity of physical activity. One study found that light and vigorous activity in mid-life and light and moderate activity in late-life were associated with lower risks of developing MCI [29]. However, similar to the variations in the nutrition data, there have been varied findings and conclusions about the type and intensity of physical activity that are most effective at reducing the risk of AD, as well as studies demonstrating no risk reduction from physical activity [30–32].

The discrepancy in the data on nutritional interventions and physical activity may be related to a lack of a "one-size-fits-all" solution, and modifications in diet, exercise, and other lifestyle factors may need to be personalized to have maximum efficacy. Unlike universal risk reduction approaches, precision medicine strategies allow for incorporation of individual risk factors that may uniquely affect the response to interventions.

3. Precision Medicine Approach to AD Prevention

A precision medicine approach to AD prevention will need to fully utilize the genome in order to make personalized recommendations. In this section, we discuss some of the genetic influencers on late-onset AD that can currently be ordered by a practicing physician and provide examples of a targeted precision medicine approach based on these genetic factors.

4. APOE and AD Prevention

One of the most well-established genetic influencers on late-onset AD risk is APOE [33], which codes for the apolipoprotein E protein [34]. There are three major polymorphisms at the APOE loci: APOE ε2, ε3, and ε4. Studies have shown that APOE genotype significantly impacts the risk of AD. Specifically, the ε4 allele has been associated with an increased risk of AD [35], while the ε2 allele has been associated with a decreased risk [36]. In addition, the risk of developing AD is even greater in individuals with two copies of the ε4 allele when compared to those with only one copy [37].

Several pathophysiologic mechanisms may explain why APOE ε4 is associated with an increased risk of AD and APOE ε2 is associated with a decreased risk. First, the three major alleles code for proteins with different molecular properties that result in different binding properties of apolipoprotein E to β-amyloid. This difference in binding may contribute to the enhanced accumulation of β-amyloid plaques that was observed in ε4 individuals, which is one of the pathologic markers of AD [38]. Furthermore, their distinct molecular properties also result in differences in their ability to bind to and transport lipids. Studies have demonstrated that there are allele-specific interactions of APOE with both LDL and HDL receptors that play an important role in the development of atherosclerosis, which is one of the major risk factors for AD [34]. As the ε4 allele has been estimated to account for 27.3% of late-onset AD risk (with a heritability of 80%) and with emerging evidence that potential risk-reduction interventions may be preferentially effective (or less effective) depending on presence of the ε4 allele, it may be important to incorporate this genotype into the AD prevention approach [39].

There are several AD prevention interventions that can be personalized based on APOE genotype. Although the FINGER trial showed no significant differences in cognitive function between APOE genotypes with their multimodal lifestyle interventions, a within-group analysis of the APOE ε4 allele demonstrated that there was a significant difference in certain treatment versus control scores only for individuals with ε4 alleles [12]. This suggests that some inherent difference exists between individuals with and without APOE ε4 alleles that impacted the effectiveness of the interventions. Therefore, additional trials with larger sample sizes and more statistical power are important in order to discern the impact of APOE on these multimodal interventions.

Other single-factor studies have demonstrated that AD prevention interventions can be targeted based on APOE genotype. A systematic review of studies that altered dietary fat composition showed that changes in total cholesterol, LDL, and HDL were most significant in individuals with APOE ε4 alleles in 15 of the studies [40]. In another study, researchers found that, in response to a Mediterranean diet, both individuals with and without APOE ε4 alleles showed improvements in cognitive functioning, as measured by the Mini Mental State Exam (MMSE), but only individuals without ε4 alleles showed improvement in the clock drawing test, a measure of executive functioning and spatial reasoning [41]. Tailoring strategies to APOE genotype can also be effective for physical activity interventions. For example, one study demonstrated that sedentary individuals with ε4 alleles were at greater risk of developing MCI, whereas physically active individuals without ε4 alleles were at decreased risk [29]. Another study demonstrated that aerobic fitness was correlated with higher cognitive performance in ε4 homozygotes [42]. Similarly, with regard to omega-3 fatty acids, three recent RCTs showed an improvement in cognitive function with DHA supplementation in non-impaired individuals with ε4 alleles [43].

While a comprehensive review of the literature is beyond the scope of this manuscript, these studies demonstrate that, based on APOE genotype, individuals may exhibit more significant responses to different lifestyle interventions. For example, individuals with ε4 alleles may experience greater changes in total cholesterol, LDL, and HDL in response to reductions in dietary fat, whereas individuals without an ε4 allele might show greater improvement in certain cognitive functions from the Mediterranean diet. In addition, physical activity may benefit all individuals but may have increased efficacy for those with ε4 alleles. Similarly, DHA supplementation may also lead to greater improvement in cognitive function in those with at least one ε4 allele. Overall, genotype-specific strategies such as these may benefit patients by using an evidence-based approach and utilizing specific targeted interventions that were shown to be the most effective for individuals with their same genotype. Additional research to further elucidate the role of APOE genotype on different dietary, physical activity, and other lifestyle interventions will be important in the future as the precision medicine approach to AD prevention continues to develop.

5. MTHFR and AD Prevention

The MTHFR gene, which codes for the methylenetetrahydrofolate reductase protein, is another potential genetic contributor to AD and is also readily available for physicians to order in commercial labs. Several MTHFR polymorphisms have been described in the literature [44], but two polymorphisms, C677T and A1298C, have had the greatest investigation as to their association with AD [45]. These polymorphisms also appear to have a high prevalence in the general population [46], and one study reported that 92.5% of its AD subjects had at least one of these MTHFR polymorphisms [45].

The association between MTHFR polymorphisms and AD may relate to the catalytic role that the MTHFR protein plays as the rate-limiting step in the conversion of homocysteine into methionine, with the B-vitamins folate and cobalamin serving as cofactors [47]. Homocysteine is an amino acid that is involved in inflammation and has been associated with cognitive decline and an increased risk of AD [48,49]. One study in cognitively healthy individuals found that baseline homocysteine levels inversely correlated with cognitive testing scores and rates of cognitive decline over a five-year period [48]. Similarly, another study of 1000 individuals from the Framingham cohort looked at non-impaired individuals at baseline and showed a strong positive correlation between baseline homocysteine and the risk of dementia up to 11 years later [49]. Another longitudinal study showed there was an 88% increased rate of cognitive decline over ten years associated with doubling the homocysteine level from 10 mg/L to 20 mg/L [50].

Changes in the MTHFR protein that alter its catalytic function, such as seen in the C677T and A1298C polymorphisms, result in higher levels of serum homocysteine [51], and therefore, have the potential to increase the risk of AD. Several studies have shown an association between the A1298C polymorphism and an increased risk of AD [52], but not with the C677T polymorphism [52,53].

However, another study showed that the combination of these two polymorphisms with a third A1793G polymorphism, together known as Haplotype C, was associated with a decreased risk of AD [54]. Therefore, further research into the relationship between these polymorphisms and the risk of AD is warranted.

Similar to APOE, MTHFR genotype status may allow for targeted AD prevention interventions. B-vitamin supplementation (cyanocobalamin, folic acid, and B6) has been shown to slow cognitive decline in individuals with elevated homocysteine levels [55,56]. Several trials have studied a combination of B vitamins to determine whether lowering homocysteine can impact cognitive function and/or brain pathology [55]. While there is limited evidence thus far, individuals with one or more MTHFR polymorphisms may potentially benefit from genotype-specific recommendations. For example, as individuals with certain MTHFR polymorphisms have decreased catalytic ability of the MTHFR protein, replacing the traditional B-vitamins with their methylated counterparts (methylcobalamin for cyanocobalamin and methyltetrahydrofolate [5-MTH] for folic acid) that do not require hepatic conversion to active forms may increase the outcomes. One study demonstrated that 5-MTH supplementation in individuals with C677T and A1298C polymorphisms significantly increased the serum folate concentration when compared to folic acid, but it did not result in differences in the serum homocysteine concentration [57]. Additional studies evaluating the impact of methylated B-vitamins for specific MTHFR polymorphisms and AD risk may therefore help to advance the field of precision medicine for AD prevention.

6. Other Genetic Influencers on AD Prevention

In addition to the discussed polymorphisms in the APOE and MTHFR genes, recent genome-wide association studies (GWAS) have identified several other single nucleotide polymorphisms (SNPs) that are associated with an increased risk of AD: CLU, CR1, and PICALM. Although these genes are not yet routinely available for sequencing commercially, the impact of polymorphisms at these loci on dietary interventions for AD prevention has recently been investigated [58,59]. One study demonstrated that improvements in cognitive function in response to the Mediterranean diet differed depending on which polymorphisms an individual had [41]. These findings provide further evidence that genetics may modify the effectiveness of AD prevention interventions. As this trial only investigated the impact of the Mediterranean diet on polymorphisms at these loci, other dietary interventions as well as other lifestyle interventions should be explored in a similar manner. In addition, there are many other known genetic risk factors for AD, such as TOMM40, which have yet to be explored regarding their impact on lifestyle interventions for AD prevention [60]. However, these genes are also not yet routinely commercially available for sequencing. A discussion of all of the genes that are involved in AD risk is beyond the scope of this paper, but it is discussed further in an Alzgene meta-analysis [61].

7. Conclusions and Future Directions

This review considered examples of two approaches to AD prevention: a universal "one-size-fits-all" approach, which uses generalized prevention strategies for all individuals, and a clinical precision medicine approach, which factors in genotype-specific intervention strategies. While both approaches have merit, utilizing a precision medicine approach offers the opportunity to personalize interventions that are based on factors that may impact the efficacy of the interventions. Genotype-specific intervention strategies, in particular, hold a great deal of promise for advancing the field of AD prevention toward more personalized and effective intervention strategies.

Investigation into the impact of different genetic factors on AD prevention will continue to become more practicable through online genetic repositories that are available to the scientific community. For example, the Alzheimer's Disease Sequencing Project (ADSP) and Alzheimer's Disease Neuroimaging Initiative (ADNI) are ongoing large-scale whole-exome and whole-genome sequencing projects in individuals with AD available through the NIA Genetics of Alzheimer's Disease Data Storage Site (NIAGADS) and the database of Genotypes and Phenotypes (dbGaP) [62]. This increased availability of genetic data will provide additional resources to investigate the impact of various genetic factors on AD prevention interventions in the future.

In addition, there has been an exponential growth in the ability of consumers to order personal genomic testing on their own via a number of commercially available testing kits. In the United States, the Food and Drug Administration approved the first direct-to-consumer tests that provide genetic risk information for a subset of medical conditions, including APOE [63]. Further, despite these commercial tests not being meant for clinical purposes, it has also become more common for patients (and even some physicians) to use a number of online tools to further investigate the raw data provided by these tests. Websites such as Promethiase.com and Snpedia.com may be utilized, although there are currently no professional guidelines and/or standards on how to do this [64].

We should also be mindful of the ethical implications of integrating genetic risk factors into clinical practice. While the Risk Evaluation and Education for Alzheimer's Disease (REVEAL) study demonstrated that APOE ε4 disclosure to adult children of AD patients did not result in significant short-term psychological effects, the long-term effects have not been evaluated [65,66]. Clinicians should weigh the potential risks and benefits of disclosing genetic risk factors to their patients and should counsel patients accordingly prior to disclosing genotype status [67]. Referral to a certified genetic counselor should also be considered when clinically indicated. Over the last five years at the Alzheimer's Prevention Clinic (APC) at Weill Cornell Medicine and NewYork-Presbyterian, the majority of patients (over 95%) have consented to receive APOE and MTHFR testing [68]. Counseling is initially provided in person by either of the two treating clinicians (a board-certified Neurologist or Family Nurse Practitioner). Patients are also asked to complete an online course via AlzU.org that explains genetic risk for AD and limitations of these tests [69]. In select cases, when patients have additional questions or concerns about testing, patients may be referred to a genetic counselor. In all patients with a family history that is highly suggestive of early-onset (autosomal dominant) AD, patients are referred to a genetic counselor prior to any genetic testing. Studies are ongoing to determine whether APOE and MTHFR polymorphism disclosure to APC patients impacts outcomes (e.g., compliance with recommendations, psychological measures including anxiety and depression). Furthermore, additional analyses are planned to determine whether clinical outcomes (e.g., cognitive performance, blood biomarkers of AD risk) are differentially impacted by APOE and MTHFR genotype. Generally speaking, the use of genetic testing as a part of clinical evaluation and patient care has been a favorable addition in the opinion of the treating clinicians, although further study is warranted in a broader subset of clinicians and in diverse patient cohorts.

Finally, it is important to consider the limitations of a genetic-based precision medicine approach to AD prevention. The genomic-centered foundation that forms the core of precision medicine reduces diseases to their molecular and cellular processes. However, there are many risk factors for AD in which the exact pathogenesis is not fully understood. A precision medicine approach that relies solely on genetics may miss some of the underlying mechanisms that are important for AD prevention but as of yet are not fully established. In addition to genetics, there are many other important aspects of a precision medicine approach to AD prevention, including medical comorbidities such as hypertension [70,71], diabetes [72], and hyperlipidemia [73,74], which have been associated with an increased risk of developing AD. There are also other lifestyle factors in addition to diet, exercise, and omega-3 fatty acids, such as smoking status, alcohol consumption, and cognitive engagement, which may play a role in AD prevention. Therefore, a precision medicine approach should also encompass recommendations to target these lifestyle factors and medical comorbidities on an individual basis. All of these factors need to be considered together to maximize a precision medicine approach that targets AD prevention strategies to the individual. Ultimately, genetics should be incorporated as one part of an overarching precision medicine approach to individualize AD prevention strategies.

Author Contributions: Conceptualization, C.L.B. and R.S.I.; Writing-Original Draft Preparation, C.L.B.; Writing-Review & Editing, C.L.B., R.S.I., L.M., O.S., A.R., and H.W.; Visualization, C.L.B., R.S.I., and L.M.; Supervision, R.S.I.; Project Administration, O.S. and A.R.; Funding Acquisition, R.S.I. and L.M.

Funding: This research was funded by philanthropic support by the Zuckerman Family Foundation, Women's Alzheimer's Movement, David G. Kabiller Charitable Foundation (In Memory of Adele Rubin Tunick and In Memory of Kaisu Ilmanen), Rimora Foundation, the Washkowitz Family in Memory of Alan Washkowitz, proceeds from the Annual Memories for Mary fundraiser organized by David Twardock, and contributions from grateful patients of the Alzheimer's Prevention Clinic, Weill Cornell Memory Disorders Program; Grant funding by the Weill Cornell Medicine Clinical and Translational Science Center (NIH/NCATS #UL1TR002384), and NIH PO1AG026572. The funders had no role in the study design, data collection or analysis, decision to publish, or preparation of the manuscript.

References

1. U.S. National Library of Medicine. What is the Precision Medicine Initiative? 2018. Available online: https://ghr.nlm.nih.gov/primer/precisionmedicine/initiative (accessed on 10 April 2018).

2. Shin, S.H.; Bode, A.M.; Dong, Z. Precision medicine: The foundation of future cancer therapeutics. *npj Precis. Oncol.* **2017**, *1*, 12. [CrossRef] [PubMed]

3. Antman, E.M.; Loscalzo, J. Precision medicine in cardiology. *Nat. Rev. Cardiol.* **2016**, *13*, 591–602. [CrossRef] [PubMed]

4. Ridge, P.G.; Hoyt, K.B.; Boehme, K.; Mukherjee, S.; Crane, P.K.; Haines, J.L.; Mayeux, R.; Farrer, L.A.; Pericak-Vance, M.A.; Schellenberg, G.D.; et al. Assessment of the genetic variance of late-onset Alzheimer's disease. *Neurobiol. Aging* **2016**, *41*, 200.e13–200.e20. [CrossRef] [PubMed]

5. Carrié, I.; van Kan, G.A.; Gillette-Guyonnet, S.; Andrieu, S.; Dartigues, J.F.; Touchon, J.; Dantoine, T.; Rouaud, O.; Bonnefoy, M.; Robert, P.; et al. Recruitment strategies for preventive trials. The MAPT study (MultiDomain Alzheimer Preventive Trial). *J. Nutr. Health Aging* **2012**, *16*, 355–359. [CrossRef] [PubMed]

6. Gillette-Guyonnet, S.; Andrieu, S.; Dantoine, T.; Dartigues, J.F.; Touchon, J.; Vellas, B. Commentary on "A roadmap for the prevention of dementia II. Leon Thal Symposium 2008." The Multidomain Alzheimer Preventive Trial (MAPT): A new approach to the prevention of Alzheimer's disease. *Alzheimer's Dement.* **2009**, *5*, 114–121. [CrossRef] [PubMed]

7. Richard, E.; Van den Heuvel, E.; Moll van Charante, E.P.; Achthoven, L.; Vermeulen, M.; Bindels, P.J.; Van Gool, W.A. Prevention of dementia by intensive vascular care (PreDIVA): A cluster-randomized trial in progress. *Alzheimer Dis. Assoc. Disord.* **2009**, *23*, 198–204. [CrossRef] [PubMed]

8. Morris, J.C. Early-stage and preclinical Alzheimer disease. *Alzheimer Dis. Assoc. Disord.* **2005**, *19*, 163–165. [PubMed]

9. Schelke, M.W.; Hackett, K.; Chen, J.L.; Shih, C.; Shum, J.; Montgomery, M.E.; Chiang, G.C.; Berkowitz, C.; Seifan, A.; Krikorian, R.; et al. Nutritional interventions for Alzheimer's prevention: A clinical precision medicine approach. *Ann. N. Y. Acad. Sci.* **2016**, *1367*, 50–56. [CrossRef] [PubMed]

10. Kivipelto, M.; Solomon, A.; Ahtiluoto, S.; Ngandu, T.; Lehtisalo, J.; Antikainen, R.; Backman, L.; Hanninen, T.; Jula, A.; Laatikainen, T.; et al. The Finnish Geriatric Intervention Study to Prevent Cognitive Impairment and Disability (FINGER): Study design and progress. *Alzheimer's Dement.* **2013**, *9*, 657–665. [CrossRef] [PubMed]

11. Rosenberg, A.; Ngandu, T.; Rusanen, M.; Antikainen, R.; Backman, L.; Havulinna, S.; Hanninen, T.; Laatikainen, T.; Lehtisalo, J.; Levalahti, E.; et al. Multidomain lifestyle intervention benefits a large elderly population at risk for cognitive decline and dementia regardless of baseline characteristics: The FINGER trial. *Alzheimer's Dement.* **2018**, *14*, 263–270. [CrossRef] [PubMed]

12. Solomon, A.; Turunen, H.; Ngandu, T.; Peltonen, M.; Levalahti, E.; Helisalmi, S.; Antikainen, R.; Backman, L.; Hanninen, T.; Jula, A.; et al. Effect of the Apolipoprotein E Genotype on Cognitive Change During a Multidomain Lifestyle Intervention: A Subgroup Analysis of a Randomized Clinical Trial. *JAMA Neurol.* **2018**, *75*, 462–470. [CrossRef] [PubMed]

13. Singh, B.; Parsaik, A.K.; Mielke, M.M.; Erwin, P.J.; Knopman, D.S.; Petersen, R.C.; Roberts, R.O. Association of mediterranean diet with mild cognitive impairment and Alzheimer's disease: A systematic review and meta-analysis. *J. Alzheimer's Dis.* **2014**, *39*, 271–282. [CrossRef] [PubMed]

14. Kesse-Guyot, E.; Andreeva, V.A.; Lassale, C.; Ferry, M.; Jeandel, C.; Hercberg, S.; Galan, P. Mediterranean diet and cognitive function: A French study. *Am. J. Clin. Nutr.* **2018**, *97*, 369–376.

15. Wahl, D.; Cogger, V.C.; Solon-Biet, S.M.; Waern, R.V.; Gokarn, R.; Pulpitel, T.; Cabo, R.; Mattson, M.P.; Raubenheimer, D.; Simpson, S.J.; et al. Nutritional strategies to optimise cognitive function in the aging brain. *Ageing Res. Rev.* **2016**, *31*, 80–92. [CrossRef] [PubMed]

16. Mosconi, L.; McHugh, P.F. Let Food Be Thy Medicine: Diet, Nutrition, and Biomarkers' Risk of Alzheimer's Disease. *Curr. Nutr. Rep.* **2015**, *4*, 126–135. [CrossRef] [PubMed]

17. Kulzow, N.; Witte, A.V.; Kerti, L.; Grittner, U.; Schuchardt, J.P.; Hahn, A.; Floel, A. Impact of Omega-3 Fatty Acid Supplementation on Memory Functions in Healthy Older Adults. *J. Alzheimer's Dis.* **2016**, *51*, 713–725. [CrossRef] [PubMed]

18. Abubakari, A.R.; Naderali, M.M.; Naderali, E.K. Omega-3 fatty acid supplementation and cognitive function: Are smaller dosages more beneficial? *Int. J. Gen. Med.* **2014**, *7*, 463–473. [PubMed]

19. Yurko-Mauro, K.; Alexander, D.D.; van Elswyk, M.E. Docosahexaenoic acid and adult memory: A systematic review and meta-analysis. *PLoS ONE* **2015**, *10*, e0120391. [CrossRef] [PubMed]

20. Zhang, Y.; Chen, J.; Qiu, J.; Li, Y.; Wang, J.; Jiao, J. Intakes of fish and polyunsaturated fatty acids and mild-to-severe cognitive impairment risks: A dose-response meta-analysis of 21 cohort studies. *Am. J. Clin. Nutr.* **2016**, *103*, 330–340. [CrossRef] [PubMed]

21. Morris, M.C.; Brockman, J.; Schneider, J.A.; Wang, Y.; Bennett, D.A.; Tangney, C.C.; van de Rest, O. Association of Seafood Consumption, Brain Mercury Level, and APOE epsilon4 Status with Brain Neuropathology in Older Adults. *JAMA* **2016**, *315*, 489–497. [CrossRef] [PubMed]

22. Sydenham, E.; Dangour, A.D.; Lim, W.S. Omega 3 fatty acid for the prevention of cognitive decline and dementia. *Cochrane Database Syst. Rev.* **2012**, *13*, CD005379.

23. Jiao, J.; Li, Q.; Chu, J.; Zeng, W.; Yang, M.; Zhu, S. Effect of n-3 PUFA supplementation on cognitive function throughout the life span from infancy to old age: A systematic review and meta-analysis of randomized controlled trials. *Am. J. Clin. Nutr.* **2014**, *100*, 1422–1436. [CrossRef] [PubMed]

24. Cunnane, S.C.; Plourde, M.; Pifferi, F.; Begin, M.; Feart, C.; Barberger-Gateau, P. Fish, docosahexaenoic acid and Alzheimer's disease. *Prog. Lipid Res.* **2009**, *48*, 239–256. [CrossRef] [PubMed]

25. McNamara, R.K.; Asch, R.H.; Lindquist, D.M.; Krikorian, R. Role of polyunsaturated fatty acids in human brain structure and function across the lifespan: An update on neuroimaging findings. *Prostaglandins Leukot Essent. Fatty Acids* **2017**. [CrossRef] [PubMed]

26. Boespflug, E.L.; McNamara, R.K.; Eliassen, J.C.; Schidler, M.D.; Krikorian, R. Fish Oil Supplementation Increases Event-Related Posterior Cingulate Activation in Older Adults with Subjective Memory Impairment. *J. Nutr. Health Aging* **2016**, *20*, 161–169. [CrossRef] [PubMed]

27. Hamer, M.; Chida, Y. Physical activity and risk of neurodegenerative disease: A systematic review of prospective evidence. *Psychol. Med.* **2009**, *39*, 3–11. [CrossRef] [PubMed]

28. Lautenschlager, N.T.; Cox, K.L.; Flicker, L.; Foster, J.K.; van Bockxmeer, F.M.; Xiao, J.; Greenop, K.R.; Almeida, O.P. Effect of physical activity on cognitive function in older adults at risk for Alzheimer disease: A randomized trial. *JAMA* **2008**, *300*, 1027–1037. [CrossRef] [PubMed]

29. Krell-Roesch, J.; Pink, A.; Roberts, R.O.; Stokin, G.B.; Mielke, M.M.; Spangehl, K.A.; Bartley, M.M.; Knopman, D.S.; Christianson, T.J.; Petersen, R.C.; et al. Timing of Physical Activity, Apolipoprotein E epsilon4 Genotype, and Risk of Incident Mild Cognitive Impairment. *J. Am. Geriatr. Soc.* **2016**, *64*, 2479–2486. [CrossRef] [PubMed]

30. Sink, K.M.; Espeland, M.A.; Castro, C.M.; Church, T.; Cohen, R.; Dodson, J.A.; Guralnik, J.; Hendrie, H.C.; Jennings, J.; Katula, J.; et al. Effect of a 24-Month Physical Activity Intervention vs Health Education on Cognitive Outcomes in Sedentary Older Adults: The LIFE Randomized Trial. *JAMA* **2015**, *314*, 781–790. [CrossRef] [PubMed]

31. Sachs, B.C.; Skinner, J.S.; Sink, K.M.; Craft, S.; Baker, L.D. High intensity aerobic exercise improves performance on computer tests of executive function in adults with mild cognitive impairment: implications for cognitive assessment in clinical trials. *Alzheimer's Dement. J. Alzheimer's Assoc.* **2016**, *12*, 428. [CrossRef]

32. Chang, Y.K.; Pan, C.Y.; Chen, F.T.; Tsai, C.L.; Huang, C.C. Effect of resistance-exercise training on cognitive function in healthy older adults: A review. *J. Aging Phys. Act.* **2012**, *20*, 497–517. [CrossRef] [PubMed]

33. Ballard, C.; Gauthier, S.; Corbett, A.; Brayne, C.; Aarsland, D.; Jones, E. Alzheimer's disease. *Lancet* **2011**, *377*, 1019–1031. [CrossRef]

34. Mahley, R.W. Apolipoprotein E: Cholesterol transport protein with expanding role in cell biology. *Science* **1988**, *240*, 622–630. [CrossRef] [PubMed]

35. Corder, E.H.; Saunders, A.M.; Strittmatter, W.J.; Schmechel, D.E.; Gaskell, P.C.; Small, G.W.; Roses, A.D.; Haines, J.L.; Pericak-Vance, M.A. Gene dose of apolipoprotein E type 4 allele and the risk of Alzheimer's disease in late onset families. *Science* **1993**, *261*, 921–923. [CrossRef] [PubMed]

36. Talbot, C.; Lendon, C.; Craddock, N.; Shears, S.; Morris, J.C.; Goate, A. Protection against Alzheimer's disease with apoE epsilon 2. *Lancet* **1994**, *343*, 1432–1433. [CrossRef]

37. Farrer, L.A.; Cupples, L.A.; Haines, J.L.; Hyman, B.; Kukull, W.A.; Mayeux, R.; Myers, R.H.; Pericak-Vance, M.A.; Risch, N.; van Duijn, C.M. Effects of age, sex, and ethnicity on the association between apolipoprotein E genotype and Alzheimer disease. A meta-analysis. APOE and Alzheimer Disease Meta Analysis Consortium. *JAMA* **1997**, *278*, 1349–1356. [CrossRef] [PubMed]

38. Strittmatter, W.J.; Weisgraher, K.H.; Huang, D.Y.; Dong, L.M.; Salvesen, G.S.; Pericak-Vance, M.; Schmechel, D.; Saunders, A.M.; Goldgaber, D.; Roses, A.D. Binding of human apolipoprotein E to synthetic amyloid beta peptide: Isoform-specific effects and implications for late-onset Alzheimer disease. *Proc. Natl. Acad. Sci. USA* **1993**, *90*, 8098–8102. [CrossRef] [PubMed]

39. Van Cauwenberghe, C.; Vab Broeckhoven, C.; Sleegers, K. The genetic landscape of Alzheimer disease: clinical implications and perspectives. *Genet. Med.* **2016**, *18*, 421–430. [CrossRef] [PubMed]

40. Masson, L.F.; McNeill, G.; Avenell, A. Genetic variation and the lipid response to dietary intervention: A systematic review. *Am. J. Clin. Nutr.* **2003**, *77*, 1098–1111. [CrossRef] [PubMed]

41. Martinez-Lapiscina, E.H.; Galbete, C.; Corella, D.; Toledo, E.; Buil-Cosiales, P.; Salas-Salvado, J.; Ros, E.; Martinez-Gonzalez, M.A. Genotype patterns at CLU, CR1, PICALM and APOE, cognition and Mediterranean diet: The PREDIMED-NAVARRA trial. *Genes Nutr.* **2014**, *9*, 393. [CrossRef] [PubMed]

42. Etnier, J.L.; Caselli, R.J.; Reiman, E.M.; Alexander, G.E.; Sibley, B.A.; Tessier, D.; McLemore, E.C. Cognitive performance in older women relative to ApoE-epsilon4 genotype and aerobic fitness. *Med. Sci. Sports Exerc.* **2007**, *39*, 199–207. [CrossRef] [PubMed]

43. Yassine, H.N.; Braskie, M.N.; Mack, W.J.; Castor, K.J.; Fonteh, A.N.; Schneider, L.S.; Harrington, M.G.; Chui, H.C. Association of Docosahexaenoic Acid Supplementation with Alzheimer Disease Stage in Apolipoprotein E ε4 Carriers: A Review. *JAMA Neurol.* **2017**, *74*, 339–347. [CrossRef] [PubMed]

44. Sibani, S.; Christensen, B.; O'Ferrall, E.; Saadi, I.; Hiou-Tim, F.; Rosenblatt, D.S.; Rozen, R. Characterization of six novel mutations in the methylenetetrahydrofolate reductase (MTHFR) gene in patients with homocystinuria. *Hum. Mutat.* **2000**, *15*, 280–287. [CrossRef]

45. Roman, G.C. MTHFR Gene Mutations: A Potential Marker of Late-Onset Alzheimer's Disease? *J. Alzheimer's Dis.* **2015**, *47*, 323–327. [CrossRef] [PubMed]

46. Romero-Sánchez, C.; Gomez-Gutierrez, A.; Gomez, P.E.; Casas-Gomez, M.C.; Briceno, I. C677T (RS1801133) MTHFR gene polymorphism frequency in a colombian population. *Colomb. Med.* **2015**, *46*, 75–79. [PubMed]

47. Online Mendelian Inheritance in Man (OMIM). An Online Catalog of Human Genes and Genetic Disorders. 2018. Available online: https://www.omim.org/ (accessed on 5 May 2018).

48. McCaddon, A.; Hudson, P.; Davies, G.; Hughes, A.; Williams, J.H.; Wilkinson, C. Homocysteine and cognitive decline in healthy elderly. *Dement. Geriatr. Cogn. Disord.* **2001**, *12*, 309–313. [CrossRef] [PubMed]

49. Seshadri, S.; Beiser, A.; Selhub, J.; Jacques, P.F.; Rosenberg, I.H.; D'Agostino, R.B.; Wilson, P.W.; Wolf, P.A. Plasma homocysteine as a risk factor for dementia and Alzheimer's disease. *N. Engl. J. Med.* **2002**, *346*, 476–483. [CrossRef] [PubMed]

50. Clarke, R.; Birks, J.; Nexo, E.; Ueland, P.M.; Schneede, J.; Scott, J.; Molloy, A.; Evans, J.G. Low vitamin B-12 status and risk of cognitive decline in older adults. *Am. J. Clin. Nutr.* **2007**, *86*, 1384–1391. [CrossRef] [PubMed]

51. Weisberg, I.; Tran, P.; Christensen, B.; Sibani, S.; Rozen, R. A Second Genetic Polymorphism in Methylenetetrahydrofolate Reductase (MTHFR) Associated with Decreased Enzyme Activity. *Mol. Genet. Metab.* **1998**, *64*, 169–172. [CrossRef] [PubMed]

52. Mansouri, L.; Fekih-Mrissa, N.; Klai, S.; Mansour, M.; Gritli, N.; Mrissa, R. Association of methylenetetrahydrofolate reductase polymorphisms with susceptibility to Alzheimer's disease. *Clin. Neurol. Neurosurg.* **2013**, *115*, 1693–1696. [CrossRef] [PubMed]

53. Seripa, D.; Forno, G.D.; Matera, M.G.; Gravina, C.; Margaglione, M.; Palermo, M.T.; Wekstein, D.R.; Antuono, P.; Avis, D.G.; Daniele, A.; et al. Methylenetetrahydrofolate reductase and angiotensin converting enzyme gene polymorphisms in two genetically and diagnostically distinct cohort of Alzheimer patients. *Neurobiol. Aging* **2003**, *24*, 933–939. [CrossRef]

54. Wakutani, Y.; Kowa, H.; Kusumi, M.; Nakaso, K.; Yasui, K.; Isoe-Wada, K.; Yano, H.; Urakami, K.; Takeshima, T.; Nakashima, K. A haplotype of the methylenetetrahydrofolate reductase gene is protective against late-onset Alzheimer's disease. *Neurobiol. Aging* **2004**, *25*, 291–294. [CrossRef]

55. Smith, A.D.; Smith, S.M.; de Jager, C.A.; Whitbread, P.; Johnston, C.; Agacinski, G.; Oulhaj, A.; Bradley, K.M.; Jacoby, R.; Refsum, H. Homocysteine-lowering by B vitamins slows the rate of accelerated brain atrophy in mild cognitive impairment: A randomized controlled trial. *PLoS ONE* **2010**, *5*, e12244. [CrossRef] [PubMed]

56. Douaud, G.; Refsum, H.; de Jager, C.A.; Jacoby, R.; Nichols, T.E.; Smith, S.M.; Smith, A.D. Preventing Alzheimer's disease-related gray matter atrophy by B-vitamin treatment. *Proc. Natl. Acad. Sci. USA* **2013**, *110*, 9523–9528. [CrossRef] [PubMed]

57. Hekmatdoost, A.; Vahid, F.; Yari, Z.; Sadeghi, M.; Eini-Zinab, H.; Lakpour, N.; Arefi, S. Methyltetrahydrofolate vs Folic Acid Supplementation in Idiopathic Recurrent Miscarriage with Respect to Methylenetetrahydrofolate Reductase C677T and A1298C Polymorphisms: A Randomized Controlled Trial. *PLoS ONE* **2015**, *10*, e0143569. [CrossRef] [PubMed]

58. Harold, D.; Abraham, R.; Hollingworth, P.; Sims, R.; Gerrish, A.; Hamshere, M.L.; Pahwa, J.S.; Moskvina, V.; Dowzell, K.; Williams, A.; et al. Genome-wide association study identifies variants at CLU and PICALM associated with Alzheimer's disease. *Nat. Genet.* **2009**, *41*, 1088–1093. [CrossRef] [PubMed]

59. Lambert, J.C.; Heath, S.; Even, G.; Campion, D.; Sleegers, K.; Hiltunen, M.; Combarros, O.; Zelenika, D.; Bullido, M.J.; Tavernier, B.; et al. Genome-wide association study identifies variants at CLU and CR1 associated with Alzheimer's disease. *Nat. Genet.* **2009**, *41*, 1094–1099. [CrossRef] [PubMed]

60. Lutz, M.W.; Crenshaw, D.G.; Saunders, A.M.; Roses, A.D. Genetic variation at a single locus and age of onset for Alzheimer's disease. *Alzheimer's Dement.* **2010**, *6*, 125–131. [CrossRef] [PubMed]

61. Bertram, L.; McQueen, M.B.; Mullin, K.; Blacker, D.; Tanzi, R.E. Systematic meta-analyses of Alzheimer disease genetic association studies: The AlzGene database. *Nat. Genet.* **2007**, *39*, 17–23. [CrossRef] [PubMed]

62. Reitz, C. Genetic diagnosis and prognosis of Alzheimer's disease: Challenges and opportunities. *Expert Rev. Mol. Diagn.* **2015**, *15*, 339–348. [CrossRef] [PubMed]

63. U.S. Food Drug Administration. *Press Announcements—FDA Allows Marketing of First Direct-to-Consumer Tests that Provide Genetic Risk Information for Certain Conditions*; U.S. Food Drug Administration: Silver Spring, MD, USA, 2018.

64. Watershed DNA. Filtering a Promethease Report: One Genetic Counselor's Strategy. 2018. Available online: https://www.watersheddna.com/blog-and-news/filtering-a-promethease-report-one-genetic-counselors-strategy (accessed on 25 June 2018).

65. Cupples, L.A.; Farrer, L.A.; Sadovnick, A.D.; Relkin, N.; Whitehouse, P.; Green, R.C. Estimating risk curves for first-degree relatives of patients with Alzheimer's disease: The REVEAL study. *Genet. Med.* **2004**, *6*, 192–196. [CrossRef] [PubMed]

66. Green, R.C.; Roberts, J.S.; Cupples, L.A.; Relkin, N.R.; Whitehouse, P.J.; Brown, T.; Eckert, S.L.; Butson, M.; Sadovnick, A.D.; Quaid, K.A.; et al. Disclosure of APOE genotype for risk of Alzheimer's disease. *N. Engl. J. Med.* **2009**, *361*, 245–254. [CrossRef] [PubMed]

67. Stites, S. Cognitively Healthy Individuals Want to Know Their Risk for Alzheimer's Disease: What Should We Do? *J. Alzheimer's Dis.* **2018**, *62*, 499–502. [CrossRef] [PubMed]

68. Seifan, A.; Isaacson, R. The Alzheimer's Prevention Clinic at Weill Cornell Medical College/New York—Presbyterian Hospital: Risk Stratification and Personalized Early Intervention. *J. Prev. Alzheimer's Dis.* **2015**, *2*, 254–266.

69. Isaacson, R.S.; Haynes, N.; Seifan, A.; Larsen, D.; Christiansen, S.; Berger, J.C.; Safdieh, J.E.; Lunde, A.M.; Luo, A.; Kramps, M.; et al. Alzheimer's Prevention Education: If We Build It, Will They Come? www.AlzU.org. *J. Prev. Alzheimer's Dis.* **2014**, *1*, 91–98.

70. Gabin, J.M.; Tambs, K.; Saltvedt, I.; Sund, E.; Holmen, J. Association between blood pressure and Alzheimer disease measured up to 27 years prior to diagnosis: The HUNT Study. *Alzheimer's Res. Ther.* **2017**, *9*, 37. [CrossRef] [PubMed]

71. Morris, M.C.; Scherr, P.A.; Hebert, L.E.; Glynn, R.J.; Bennett, D.A.; Evans, D.A. Association of incident Alzheimer disease and blood pressure measured from 13 years before to 2 years after diagnosis in a large community study. *Arch. Neurol.* **2001**, *58*, 1640–1646. [CrossRef] [PubMed]

72. De Nazareth, A.M. Type 2 diabetes mellitus in the pathophysiology of Alzheimer's disease. *Dement. Neuropsychol.* **2017**, *11*, 105–113. [CrossRef] [PubMed]

73. Kivipelto, M.; Helkala, E.L.; Laakso, M.P.; Hanninen, T.; Hallikainen, M.; Alhainen, K.; Soininen, H.; Tuomilehto, J.; Nissinen, A. Midlife vascular risk factors and Alzheimer's disease in later life: Longitudinal, population based study. *BMJ* **2001**, *322*, 1447–1451. [CrossRef] [PubMed]

74. Solomon, A.; Kivipelto, M.; Wolozin, B.; Zhou, J.; Whitmer, R.A. Midlife serum cholesterol and increased risk of Alzheimer's and vascular dementia three decades later. *Dement. Geriatr. Cogn. Disord.* **2009**, *28*, 75–80. [CrossRef] [PubMed]

9

Does Medical Students' Personality Traits Influence Their Attitudes toward Medical Errors?

Chia-Lun Lo [1] 🆔, Hsiao-Ting Tseng [2,*] 🆔 and Chi-Hua Chen [3] 🆔

[1] Department of Health Business Administration, Fooyin University, Daliao District, Kaohsiung 831, Taiwan; allenlo.tw@gmail.com

[2] Department of Information Management, Tatung University, Zhongshan District, Taipei 104, Taiwan

[3] College of Mathematics and Computer Science, Fuzhou University, Minhou County, Fuzhou 350100, China; chihua0826@gmail.com

* Correspondence: appleapple928@gmail.com

Abstract: This study examined medical students' perceptions towards medical errors and the policy of the hospital within the internship curriculum, and explored how aspects of personality traits of medical students relate to their attitude toward medical errors. Based on the theory of the Five-Factor-Model (FFM) and related literature review, this study adopted a self-devised structured questionnaire to distribute to 493 medical students in years five to seven in the top three medical schools, representing a 56.7% valid questionnaire response rate. Results showed that agreeableness is more important than other personality traits, and medical students with high agreeableness are good communicators and have a more positive attitude to avoid errors in the future. On the contrary, students with low neuroticism tended to be more relaxed and gentle. If medical educators can recruit new students with high agreeableness, these students will be more likely to effectively improve the quality of medical care and enhance patient safety. This study anticipates that this method could be easily translated to nearly every medical department entry examination, particularly with regards to a consciousness-based education of future physicians.

Keywords: medical errors; personality; attitude; medical students

1. Background

Patients receive health care to improve their health. However, since the increase of medical error events, medical errors have caused media coverage and public concern about patient safety. Medical errors will greatly affect the safety of patients. Hence, how to reduce the severity and frequency of medical errors has become an important issue in fields related to medical care. The teaching material known as Tomorrow's Doctors [1] emphasizes that improving communication between physicians and patients may reduce medical errors. Usherwood [2] empirically showed that communication skills can have positive effects on students' learning of listening skills and compassion; such skills can also improve physician-patient relationships and patient satisfaction [3]. Therefore, worldwide healthcare institutions emphasize that clinicians can reduce the probability of medical errors by improving their communication with patients. Meanwhile, more and more studies [4–16] highlight the importance of attitude toward medical errors in medical students' education.

Physician training takes a considerable amount of time. Medical students, especially those in the later years of medical school, should be taught good communication skills to reduce the obstacles in physician-patient relationships during their education. Internship systems were expected to increase physicians' efficiency and value attached to patient safety [17]. To reach these goals, Taiwan launched a comprehensive medical education reform in 2002. Educators in Taiwan adopted multiple approaches—interviews, personality tests, entrance examinations, etc.—to identify new medical students with both high academic ability and suitable personalities for clinical work, and help them become qualified physicians in the future, so as to further reduce medical errors.

The National Patient Safety Foundation (NPSF) proposed that helping medical school students understand medical errors can help them avoid similar mistakes [18]. Lester and Tritter [19] also mentioned that training medical students in communication skills could improve their future behavior as physicians. Seiden [20] suggested that medical students play important roles in the prevention of medical errors, and that teaching them to understand possible medical errors can effectively enhance patient safety. However, although suitable personality traits and good communication skills in medical students have been valued by healthcare institutions in various countries, medical students are often neglected in studies on the improvement of patient safety education [20]. Studies pointed out that most physicians agree that the reduction of medical errors is an important issue, but the number of medical errors actually reported is much lower than expected [10]. This is because most medical education programs attach importance to practical, professional techniques, and do not focus on educating students about medical errors. Flin et al. [21] investigated medical students' attitude towards medical errors and found that most students had insufficient knowledge about how to report errors. Muller [16] proposed that irreversible medical errors might make interns experience a loss of self-confidence or self-esteem, and feel guilt or other negative emotions. Fischer et al. [22], using resident doctors as subjects, found that subjects' personality traits affected how they reported errors and learned. Lievens [23] found that in past studies, when people have more positive and cheerful personality traits, their attitudes towards learning outcomes, self-efficacy, behaviors, performance, etc., are more positive. Other research has also pointed out that when medical staff members have higher self-efficiency for avoiding medical errors, they are less likely to make such errors [24]. Self-efficiency is defined as staff members' belief in reducing errors and enhancing patient safety [25]. In other words, when medical staff have positive, strong feelings of confidence about their own roles and possess attitudes towards avoiding errors and being competent, they will avoid making errors.

In the past, relevant research pointed out that the younger the doctor, the more likely they are to make medical errors [26]. However, this does not mean that the occurrence of medical errors is a necessary route in the process of medical service development. The National Patient Safety Foundation (NPSF) has said that educating medical students about medical errors can help future physicians avoid similar mistakes [18]. Seiden [20] also believes that medical students play an important role in the prevention of medical errors; educating them to understand medical errors can effectively improve patient safety. In the face of medical errors, it is very important to have a positive attitude of learning from mistakes. For example, in the aviation industry and the energy industry, for example, employees are encouraged to report on possible errors and adverse events, and learn from mistakes to avoid making similar mistakes in the future [27,28]. There is a lack of research on medical errors in medical students in Taiwan, and we have no way of knowing what attitudes and ideas they have. However, attitudes will affect behavior. After a period of time, this group of medical students will be put into the workplace and become important members of the medical industry. Therefore, it is necessary to understand their attitudes toward medical errors.

As seen in the above research, physicians' personality traits may affect their attitude towards facing medical errors, and it is very important that they have appropriate concepts of and attitudes towards patient safety. For medical educators, the purpose of medical education is to cultivate future medical personnels' ability to grasp the overall picture of their patient's health. The Harvard College of Medicine considers the cultivation of an appropriate personality and the ability to make effective value judgments to be the most important educational outcomes (or aims of education). If this study is able to teach medical students how to view and understand medical errors, this study would likely be able to correct their misconceptions, which is especially important for medical students about to become interns in hospitals. Therefore, identifying the appropriate personality traits for being an efficient medical student is one of the important factors of the reform and improvement of current medical education. However, this study does not know how various personality traits influence medical students' responses to medical errors. Therefore, this study examined the relationship between personality traits and attitudes toward medical errors in a sample of students with internship experience from their final years of medical school. The results could inform the recruitment of future medical students.

2. Methods

2.1. Participants

A questionnaire survey was sent to 866 medical students (in their 5th, 6th and 7th years), from three medical schools in Taiwan. This study chose this group for the survey because in Taiwan, medical students in their final three years must attend practical training in hospitals. In the end, there were total of 493 (56.9%) valid questionnaires. Demographic data was also collected to obtain accurate backgrounds for all of the participating students. Among them, there were 343 males (71.0%) and 140 females (29.0%); most of the respondents were 21 to 25 years old, with 272 (56.8%); followed by 198 (41.3%) from 26 to 30 years old, and seven (1.5%) from 31 to 35 years old. There were two (1.7%) over 36 years old and four respondents who did not fill in this field. The average age of respondents was 24.66 years old, with a standard deviation of 1.67. The youngest respondents were 22 years old, and the oldest were 38 years old. There were 224 (46.7%) in fifth year, 207 (43.1%) in sixth year, and 49 (10.2%) in seventh year. There were three respondents who did not fill out this field.

The research was approved by the dean of each department at each medical school, and after compiling a list of all students, this study sent the questionnaire via email. Students were asked to complete the questionnaire and send it back to us if they were interested in taking part in the study.

2.2. Instruments

The study used a cross-sectional design, and the questionnaire had three sections. The first and second sections were based on a review of the medical error literature, and questions employed a six-point Likert-like scale, ranging from not at all agree (1) to agree completely (6). Except for the personality section, the main sections included the following items:

2.2.1. First Section: Attitudes Towards Medical Errors

- Disclosing and reporting medical errors covered respondents' attitudes towards disclosing and reporting medical errors after they have occurred (five items).
- Reacting to and learning about medical errors measured respondents' attitudes towards how they react to and learn about medical errors (four items).
- Emotional reaction covers respondents' emotional reactions to errors after they have occurred (four items).
- Self-efficacy measured respondents' level of self-awareness and perceived competence in avoiding medical errors (four items).
- Safety promotion covered respondents' attitudes towards promoting safety (three items).
- Self-ability asked respondents to rate how well they believe they can do their job (three items).

2.2.2. Second Section: Factors Affect the Occurrence of Medical Errors

- Training and communication asked respondents to indicate their level of agreement with employee training and the effectiveness of communication for avoiding medical errors (six items).
- Management system also measured respondents' degree of recognition for avoiding medical errors (six items).

A factor analysis was conducted to determine whether student responses were in line with the themes outlined above. In addition, this study measured respondents' personality traits according to the Five-Factor-Model (FFM). The FFM is a model for describing human personality, which proposes that various personality characteristics can be grouped under five higher-order personality domains: Extraversion, Agreeableness, Conscientiousness, Emotional Stability, and Openness [29]. The research tool contains 43 items employing a six-point Likert scale ranging from 1 (strongly disagree) to 6 (strongly agree). Focus groups and a pilot study was carried out using 15 interns. Demographic data was also covered in the questionnaire. The internal consistency in the pilot study was acceptable (Cronbach's $\alpha > 0.7$).

2.3. Data Analysis

This study first excluded invalid questionnaires, and used descriptive statistics, including mean, to represent a central location where the results were relatively concentrated. Standard deviation (SD) was used to represent the degree of discreteness of the results. This study then examined how differences in the personality traits of medical students related to differences in their attitudes towards medical errors. In addition to the Pearson correlation coefficient, this study used multiple regression analyses to test the relationship between personality traits and attitudes towards medical errors.

3. Results

3.1. Experimental Environments

The questionnaires were distributed to 866 medical students with internship experience, and 493 valid questionnaires were received across the three years (valid response rate = 56.9%). The goodness of fit test of the questionnaires showed significant differences. The final sample contained 213 respondents in medical school A, 113 in medical school B, and 167 in medical school C, as shown in Table 1.

Table 1. Survey response rate.

School	Total	Surveys Completed	Response Rate
"A" medical school	447	213	47.7%
"B" medical school	128	113	88.3%
"C" medical school	291	163	57.4%
Grand total	866	493	56.9%

Seventy-one percent of respondents were male, and the mean (SD) age was 24.66 (1.67) years old. Four hundred and sixty-one (96%) respondents had interned in medical centers, and among them, 126 (26.7%) had been in the surgical department, 11 (23.5%) in internal medicine, 77 (16.3%) in the gynecological department, 70 (14.8%) in pediatrics, and 88 (18.6%) respondents in the remaining departments including X-rays, family medicine, otolaryngology (ENT), neurology, psychiatry, etc.

The personality traits investigated in this study were Extraversion, Openness, Conscientiousness, Agreeableness, and Neuroticism. The relationships between these dimensions and students' attitudes towards medical errors are summarized in Table 2.

Medical students tended to have high Conscientiousness (4.18, SD = 0.75) and Agreeableness (4.16, SD = 0.59), but low Neuroticism (3.58, SD = 0.64). Regarding attitudes towards medical errors, most showed high scores on reacting to and learning about medical errors (6.64, SD = 1.01), while they tended to have lower scores on disclosing and reporting medical errors (5.23, SD = 1.20) and self-ability (4.93, SD = 1.22). For the factors that might affect the occurrence of medical errors, students agreed significantly more with training and communication (7.02, SD = 0.89) compared with management systems (6.39, SD = 1.00).

Regarding to the relationships between personality traits and attitudes toward medical errors, the results show that disclosing and reporting medical errors showed significant positive correlations with the personality traits of Extraversion, Openness, and Conscientiousness; reacting to and learning about medical errors showed significant positive correlations with Extraversion, Openness, Conscientiousness, and Agreeableness; emotional reaction showed a significant positive correlation with only Agreeableness; self-efficiency showed a significant positive correlation with Agreeableness, and a significant negative correlation with Neuroticism; and finally, self-ability showed a significant positive correlation with Extraversion, Openness, Conscientiousness, and Agreeableness. Regarding the factors that might affect the occurrence of medical errors, both training and communication and management systems had significant positive correlations with Extraversion, Openness, Conscientiousness, and Agreeableness, while training and communication also showed a significant negative correlation with Neuroticism.

3.2. Comparison of Personality Traits with High Identification and Attitudes Towards Medical Errors

This study determined the standard deviations of the average values of students' personality traits to denote which traits students showed high or low identification with, and analyzed how the personality traits that students highly identified with influenced their attitudes towards medical errors, as shown in Table 3.

For disclosing and reporting medical errors, the gender of medical students could have explained the statistically significant differences in variance between personality traits and attitudes towards medical errors ($F = 4.454$, $p < 0.001$). The coefficient of determination was $R^2 = 0.074$, adjusted $R^2 = 0.073$. After controlling for gender using the regression coefficient test, this study found a significant relationship between Conscientiousness and disclosing and reporting medical errors ($\beta = 0.178$, $p < 0.05$), indicating that respondents with higher Conscientiousness may also have more positive attitudes towards disclosing and reporting medical errors.

For reacting to and learning about medical errors, gender could again account for statistically significant differences ($F = 5.991$, $p < 0.001$). The coefficient of determination was $R^2 = 0.096$, adjusted $R^2 = 0.093$. After controlling for gender, this study found a statistically significant relationship between Agreeableness ($\beta = 0.197$, $p < 0.01$) and reacting to and learning about medical errors.

For emotional reaction, gender could explain statistically significant differences ($F = 2.560$, $p < 0.05$). The coefficient of determination was $R^2 = 0.043$, adjusted $R^2 = 0.032$. After controlling for gender, this study found no statistically significant relationship between personality traits and emotional reaction.

For self-efficiency, gender could explain statistically significant differences ($F = 12.114$, $p < 0.001$). The coefficient of determination was $R^2 = 0.177$, adjusted $R^2 = 0.160$. After controlling for gender, this study found a statistically significant relationship between Conscientiousness ($\beta = 0.267$, $p < 0.001$) and self-efficiency.

For safety promotion, gender could explain the statistically significant difference. After controlling for gender, this study found a statistically significant relationship between Agreeableness ($\beta = -0.145$, $p < 0.05$) and safety promotion.

For self-ability, gender could explain statistically significant differences ($F = 7.839$, $p < 0.001$). The coefficient of determination was $R^2 = 0.121$, adjusted $R^2 = 0.118$. After controlling for gender, this study found that Extraversion ($\beta = 0.138$, $p < 0.05$) and Agreeableness ($\beta = 0.216$, $p < 0.001$) had statistically significant relationships with self-ability.

For training and communication, gender could explain the statistically significant difference ($F = 10.960$, $p < 0.001$). The coefficient of determination was $R^2 = 0.163$, adjusted $R^2 = 0.154$. After controlling for gender, this study found that Extraversion ($\beta = 0.233$, $p < 0.01$) and Agreeableness ($\beta = 0.234$, $p < 0.001$) had statistically significant relationships with training and communication.

Finally, for management systems, genders could again explain statistically significant differences ($F = 8.282$, $p < 0.001$). The coefficient of determination was $R^2 = 0.163$, adjusted $R^2 = 0.123$. After controlling for gender, this study found a statistically significant relationship between Agreeableness ($\beta = 0.136$, $p < 0.001$) and management systems.

Table 2. Means, standard deviations and correlation matrices for combined data with $n = 493$.

Dimensions		Scale (Number of Items)	Mean	SD	a1	a2	a3	a4	a5	b1	b2	b3	b4	b5	b6	b7	b8
Personality traits	a1	Extraversion	3.94	0.67	—												
	a2	Openness	4.17	0.74	0.75***	—											
	a3	Conscientiousness	4.18	0.75	0.70***	0.72***	—										
	a4	Agreeableness	4.61	0.59	0.55***	0.59***	0.58***	—									
	a5	Neuroticism	3.58	0.64	-0.16***	-0.26***	-0.27***	-0.23***	—								
Medical students' attitude towards medical errors	b1	Disclosing and reporting medical errors (5)	5.23	1.20	0.19***	0.20***	0.26***	0.22***	-0.06	—							
	b2	Reacting to and learning about medical errors (4)	6.64	1.01	0.25***	0.17***	0.24***	0.41***	-0.09	0.34***	—						
	b3	Emotional reaction (4)	5.96	1.10	0.06	0.01	0.02	0.11*	0.07	-0.02	0.18***	—					
	b4	Self-efficiency (4)	4.81	1.24	0.39***	0.41***	0.40***	0.29***	-0.15**	0.33***	0.03	-0.08	—				
	b5	Safety promotion (3)	6.24	1.22	-0.09*	-0.07	-0.07	-0.17***	-0.04	-0.12*	-0.30***	-0.25***	0	—			
	b6	Self-ability (3)	4.93	1.22	0.26***	0.27***	0.26***	0.29***	-0.06	0.25***	0.10*	-0.01	0.36***	-0.09	—		
	b7	Training and communication (6)	7.02	0.89	0.30***	0.19***	0.19***	0.41***	-0.12**	0.12**	0.55***	0.30***	0.06	-0.29***	0.09*	—	
	b8	Management systems (6)	6.39	1.00	0.35***	0.31***	0.26***	0.33***	-0.08	0.18***	0.35***	0.17***	0.17***	-0.19***	0.14**	0.69***	—

*: $p < 0.05$; **: $p < 0.01$; ***: $p < 0.001$; SD = Standard Deviation

Table 3. Regression between the attitude of medical error and medical students' personality traits for combined data with $n = 493$.

Variables	Disclosing and Reporting Medical Errors β	t-Value	Reacting to and Learning about Medical Errors β	t-Value	Emotional Reaction β	t-Value	Self-Efficiency β	t-Value	Safety Promotion β	t-Value	Self-Ability β	t-Value	Training and Communication β	t-Value	Management Systems β	t-Value
Gender	0.032	0.59	-0.041	0-.775	0.120	2.224*	0.135	2.680**	-0.032	-0.584	-0.065	-1.246	-0.075	-1.474	-0.076	-1.471
Openness	-0.031	-0.424	0.127	1.764	-0.056	-0.763	0.169	2.495*	0.019	0.257	0.138	1.973*	2.330	3.313**	0.128	1.831
Extraversion	0.067	0.908	-0.015	0-.202	-0.076	-1.016	-0.045	-0.648	-0.058	-0.761	0.023	0.322	-0.070	-0.990	0.140	1.942
Conscientiousness	0.178	2.496*	0.045	0.642	0.026	0.360	0.267	3.995***	-0.021	-0.297	0.057	0.828	0.013	0.196	0.024	0.340
Agreeableness	0.072	1.145	0.197	3.216**	-0.104	-1.662	0.068	1.155	-0.145	-2.296*	0.216	3.550***	0.234	3.972***	0.136	2.268***
Neuroticism	-0.060	-1.103	-0.033	0-0.602	-0.092	-1.677	-0.007	-0.14	-0.083	-1.499	0.080	1.500	-0.080	-1.53	-0.012	-0.226
F-value	4.454***		5.991***		2.560*		12.114***		1.957		7.839***		10.960***		8.282***	
R^2	0.074		0.096		0.043		0.177		0.033		0.121		0.163		0.127	
∆F	5.270***		6.974***		2.280*		13.136***		2.238		9.124***		12.376***		9.631***	
∆R^2	0.073		0.093		0.032		0.16		0.031		0.118		0.154		0.123	

*: $p < 0.05$; **: $p < 0.01$; ***: $p < 0.001$

4. Discussions

4.1. Experiment Result Discussions

The training process that medical students undergo is very strict, and after they graduate, they must obtain a medical license in order to become fully-fledged medical practitioners. Despite this, physicians seem unable to cope with or resolve medical errors even when they often encounter them. Mizahi [30] found that when hospital staff members made a medical error, they typically adopted three coping strategies: denial, discounting, and distancing. Medical students' learning attitudes typically develop during their internship, passed down by supervising physicians. If medical school students are given an inaccurate understanding of the disclosure of medical errors and have unsuitable personality traits, they are more likely to conceal medical errors. Previous studies on this issue have discussed its fundamental causes, including notification platforms [31,32], disclosure [33,34], personality traits or gender [16], and emotions [33]. This study discussed the basic personality dimensions, attempted to identify the attitudes of interning medical students toward medical errors, and examined the influences of personality traits on these attitudes.

The results of this study showed that medical students scored highest on Agreeableness, followed by Conscientiousness, Openness, and Extraversion; they scored the lowest on Neuroticism. These differed from the results of Lievens et al.'s [23] study on medical students, which also used the FFM; Vohra et al. [25] pointed out that effective medical students often have personality traits of Agreeableness or Extraversion according to the well-known "Big Five" Inventory (Five Factor Model (FFM)). Moreover, these researchers found that students scored highest on Extraversion, followed by Agreeableness. These differences related to the educational system in Taiwan. Lievens et al. [23] found that Conscientiousness might affect medical students' grades on their written examinations before graduation; however, medical students in Taiwan enrolled in universities according to their grades on written examinations, and thus most of them are relatively diligent and hardworking. This study can see from the various characteristics of these personality traits [35] that high Agreeableness should be helpful for medical students in communicating with patients and cooperating with other hospital staff; in addition, the cautiousness, sense of responsibility, and drive that accompanies individuals with high Conscientiousness would be helpful for avoiding medical errors.

The majority of interns believe that medical errors are avoidable, and that training can effectively reduce the occurrence of these errors [36]. This study arrived at a similar conclusion: nearly 70% of respondents believed errors to be avoidable, and more than half regarded training and education to be the most important factors that affect medical errors. Furthermore, more than 90% of respondents attached importance to training and communication. According to Singh et al. [37], among the common medical errors made by interns, 70% are caused by miscommunication with team members and 58% are due to a lack of technical expertise and knowledge. Thus, the likelihood that interns would make a medical error due to a lack of education or miscommunication with team members is very high.

Active disclosure of possible errors might help patients and their family members understand an error situation and reduce the occurrence of litigations [38]. Gallagher [39] divided medical errors into three categories: near-miss, relatively not serious, and relatively serious. When medical errors are relatively serious, physicians tend to support error disclosure. While the present study was only concerned with categorizing errors according to whether they caused injury, the results were similar to those of Gallagher and colleagues in that when errors caused injury, students tended to view disclosure more positively than when errors did not cause injury. In this study, the emotional reaction attitude dimension was found to be the most negatively viewed, with around 90% of respondents having worry that being accused might affect their future employment; this is similar to the findings of Muller and Ornstein's [16] study, wherein they discussed the issues that resident physicians and interns tend to worry about after errors occur.

This study found that Agreeableness and Conscientiousness have the greatest influence on medical students' attitude towards medical errors. Students with high Agreeableness tend to pay more attention to organization management and systems for avoiding errors, and have more positive attitudes toward personnel communication and coping with medical errors; these features may be determined by their high empathy. Medical students with high Conscientiousness are more likely to be confident in avoiding errors and have a greater sense of justice, often wanting to disclose the error after they have made it. Compared with other personality traits, Agreeableness is more likely to have a significant influence on feelings of responsibility towards and learning of errors, promotion of safety, self-ability, training and communication, and the health care management system.

Previous studies investigated the attitudes of medical students towards medical errors and patient safety, but only those of first-year medical students. Thus, the samples provided less knowledge about medical errors and how physicians report them [21]. The subjects of this study were medical students in their final three years, who had already entered hospitals for internships, and the results were generally positive, as in Flin's [21] study. However, this study provides more comprehensive evidence showing that medical students who have high Agreeableness tend to have more positive attitudes toward medical errors in general.

4.2. Study Limitations

This study faces the following research limitations. Firstly, this study chose medical students who were in their 5th, 6th, or 7th year as subjects, and while the overall response rate was acceptable, there were fewer students in their 7th year. This may be because 7th year students are too busy with their internships, and spend less time in school, which would lead to a lower response rate. In addition, because samples were taken from only three hospitals, it is not clear whether these results can be extrapolated to the entire medical student population.

Secondly, the main problem with this research is to understand the personality traits of medical students and their attitudes towards medical errors. Hopefully, effective interventions can be put in place in the medical education process to reduce the incidence of medical errors. However, medical errors are sometimes caused by poor medical communication, but this study has not discussed medical communication. In addition, there may be individual biases in the personality traits of medical students. In other words, there may be systematic errors in communication between physicians, medical students, and support teams, mainly because of the lack of openness.

5. Conclusions and Future Work

From the results of the present study and those of previous studies, it is clear that medical students with high Agreeableness have more positive attitudes towards medical errors, and are more likely to avoid errors in the future; in addition, in encountering such errors, they will be well equipped to face and solve them. Finally, if medical educators can recruit new students with high Agreeableness, these students will be more likely to effectively improve the quality of medical care and enhance patient safety. Therefore, the results of this study can inform the future recruitment of medical school students. Further research is required with larger sample sizes, including other medical personnel or subjects from other academic backgrounds. By comparing these other groups, this study will be able to further generalize the results.

Author Contributions: C.-L.L. and H.-T.T. proposed and evaluated the methods. The experiments results were performed and discussed by C.-L.L. and H.-T.T. C.-L.L., H.-T.T. and C.-H.C. wrote the manuscript.

Funding: This research was funded by the Ministry of Science and Technology of Taiwan grant number MOST 106-2410-H-242-001.

References

1.   General Medical Council, Education Committee. *Tomorrow's Doctor: Recommendations on Undergraduate Medical Education*; General Medical Council: London, UK, 1993.

2. Usherwood, T. Subjective and behavioural evaluation of the teaching of patient interview skills. *Méd. Educ.* **1993**, *27*, 41–47. [CrossRef] [PubMed]

3. Coulter, A. Partnerships with patients: The pros and cons of shared clinical decision-making. *J. Health Serv. Res. Policy* **1997**, *2*, 112–121. [CrossRef] [PubMed]

4. Dudas, R.A.; Bundy, D.G.; Miller, M.R.; Barone, M. Can teaching medical students to investigate medication errors change their attitudes towards patient safety? *BMJ Qual. Saf.* **2011**, *20*, 319–325. [CrossRef] [PubMed]

5. Varjavand, N.; Bachegowda, L.S.; Gracely, E.; Novack, D.H. Changes in intern attitudes toward medical error and disclosure. *Méd. Educ.* **2012**, *46*, 668–677. [CrossRef] [PubMed]

6. Paxton, J.H.; Rubinfeld, I.S. Medical errors education for students of surgery: A pilot study revealing the need for action. *J. Surg. Educ.* **2009**, *66*, 20–24. [CrossRef] [PubMed]

7. Paxton, J.H.; Rubinfeld, I.S. Medical errors education: A prospective study of a new educational tool. *Am. J. Méd. Qual.* **2010**, *25*, 135–142. [CrossRef] [PubMed]

8. Gunderson, A.; Tekian, A.; Mayer, D. Teaching interprofessional health science students medical error disclosure. *Méd. Educ.* **2008**, *42*, 531. [CrossRef] [PubMed]

9. Gunderson, A.J.; Smith, K.M.; Mayer, D.B.; McDonald, T.; Centomani, N. Teaching medical students the art of medical error full disclosure: Evaluation of a new curriculum. *Teach. Learn. Med.* **2009**, *21*, 229–232. [CrossRef] [PubMed]

10. Kaldjian, L.C.; Jones, E.W.; Wu, B.J.; Forman-Hoffman, V.L.; Levi, B.H.; Rosenthal, G.E. Disclosing medical errors to patients: Attitudes and practices of physicians and trainees. *J. Gen. Intern. Med.* **2007**, *22*, 988–996. [CrossRef] [PubMed]

11. Martinez, W.; Lo, B. Medical students' experiences with medical errors: An analysis of medical student essays. *Méd. Educ.* **2008**, *42*, 733–741. [CrossRef] [PubMed]

12. Newell, P.; Harris, S.; Aufses, A., Jr.; Ellozy, S. Student perceptions of medical errors: Incorporating an explicit professionalism curriculum in the third-year surgery clerkship. *J. Surg. Educ.* **2008**, *65*, 117–119. [CrossRef] [PubMed]

13. White, A.A.; Gallagher, T.H.; Krauss, M.J.; Garbutt, J.; Waterman, A.D.; Dunagan, W.C.; Fraser, V.J.; Levinson, W.; Larson, E.B. The attitudes and experiences of trainees regarding disclosing medical errors to patients. *Acad. Med.* **2008**, *83*, 250–256. [CrossRef] [PubMed]

14. Halbach, J.L.; Sullivan, L.L. Teaching medical students about medical errors and patient safety: Evaluation of a required curriculum. *Acad. Med.* **2005**, *80*, 600–606. [CrossRef] [PubMed]

15. Kaldjian, L.C.; Jones, E.W.; Wu, B.J.; Forman-Hoffman, V.; Levi, B.H.; Rosenthal, G.E. Disclosing medical errors to patients: A survey of faculty, residents, and students. *J. Gen. Intern. Med.* **2006**, *21*, 36.

16. Muller, D.; Ornstein, K. Perceptions of and attitudes towards medical errors among medical trainees. *Méd. Educ.* **2007**, *41*, 645–652. [CrossRef] [PubMed]

17. Coombes, I.D.; Mitchell, C.A.; Stowasser, D.A. Safe medication practice: Attitudes of medical students about to begin their intern year. *Méd. Educ.* **2008**, *42*, 427–431. [CrossRef] [PubMed]

18. *Annual Report 1999*; National Patient Safety Foundation: Washington, DC, USA, 2000.

19. Lester, H.; Tritter, J.Q. Medical error: A discussion of the medical construction of error and suggestions for reforms of medical education to decrease error. *Méd. Educ.* **2001**, *35*, 855–861. [CrossRef] [PubMed]

20. Seiden, S.; Galvan, C.; Lamm, R. Role of medical students in preventing patient harm and enhancing patient safety. *Qual. Saf. Health Care* **2006**, *15*, 272–276. [CrossRef] [PubMed]

21. Flin, R.; Yule, S.; McKenzie, L.; Paterson-Brown, S.; Maran, N. Attitudes to teamwork and safety in the operating theatre. *Surgeon* **2006**, *4*, 145–151. [CrossRef]

22. Fischer, M.A.; Mazor, K.M.; Baril, J.; Alper, E.; DeMarco, D.; Pugnaire, M. Learning from mistakes: Factors that influence how students and residents learn from medical errors. *J. Gen. Intern. Med.* **2006**, *21*, 419–423. [CrossRef] [PubMed]

23. Lievens, F.; Coetsier, P.; De Fruyt, F.; De Maeseneer, J. Medical students' personality characteristics and academic performance: A five-factor model perspective. *Méd. Educ.* **2002**, *36*, 1050–1056. [CrossRef] [PubMed]

24. Katz-Navon, T.; Naveh, E.; Stern, Z. Safety self-efficacy and safety performance: Potential antecedents and the moderation effect of standardization. *Int. J. Health Care Qual. Assur.* **2007**, *20*, 572–584. [CrossRef] [PubMed]

25. Vohra, P.D.; Johnson, J.K.; Daugherty, C.K.; Wen, M.; Barach, P. Housestaff and medical student attitudes toward medical errors and adverse events. *Jt. Comm. J. Qual. Patient Saf.* **2007**, *33*, 493–501. [CrossRef]

26. Chang, B.J. The Physician's Knowledge, Attitude and Responses toward Patient Safety Issues—Case Studies from Hospitals in Northern Taiwan. Master's Thesis, National Taiwan University, Taipei, Taiwan, 2003.

27. Robert, L.H.; Merritt, A.C. *Culture at Work in Aviation and Medicine: National, Organizational and Professional Influences*; Routledge: London, UK, 2017.

28. Roberts, K.H.; Rousseau, D.M. Research in nearly failure-free, high-reliability organizations: Having the bubble. *IEEE Trans. Eng. Manag.* **1989**, *36*, 132–139. [CrossRef]

29. Goldberg, L.R. The development of markers for the Big-Five factor structure. *Psychol. Assess.* **1992**, *4*, 26. [CrossRef]

30. Mizrahi, T. Managing medical mistakes: Ideology, insularity and accountability among internists-in-training. *Soc. Sci. Med.* **1984**, *19*, 135–146. [CrossRef]

31. Wu, A.W.; Folkman, S.; McPhee, S.J.; Lo, B. Do house officers learn from their mistakes? *JAMA* **1991**, *265*, 2089–2094. [CrossRef] [PubMed]

32. Schenkel, S.M.; Khare, R.K.; Rosenthal, M.M.; Sutcliffe, K.M.; Lewton, E.L. Resident perceptions of medical errors in the emergency department. *Acad. Emerg. Med.* **2003**, *10*, 1318–1324. [CrossRef]

33. Hevia, A.; Hobgood, C. Medical error during residency: To tell or not to tell. *Ann. Emerg. Med.* **2003**, *42*, 565–570. [CrossRef]

34. Crook, E.D.; Stellini, M.; Levine, D.; Wiese, W.; Douglas, S. Medical errors and the trainee: Ethical concerns. *Am. J. Med. Sci.* **2004**, *327*, 33–37. [PubMed]

35. Pilpel, D.; Schor, R.; Benbassat, J. Barriers to acceptance of medical error: The case for a teaching program (695). *Méd. Educ.* **1998**, *32*, 3–7. [CrossRef] [PubMed]

36. McCrae, R.R.; Costa, P.T., Jr. Validation of the five-factor model of personality across instruments and observers. *J. Pers. Soc. Psychol.* **1987**, *52*, 81–90. [CrossRef] [PubMed]

37. Sorokin, R.; Riggio, J.M.; Hwang, C. Attitudes about patient safety: A survey of physicians-in-training. *Am. J. Méd. Qual.* **2005**, *20*, 70–77. [CrossRef] [PubMed]

38. Singh, H.; Thomas, E.J.; Petersen, L.A.; Studdert, D.M. Medical errors involving trainees: A study of closed malpractice claims from 5 insurers. *Arch. Intern. Méd.* **2007**, *167*, 2030. [CrossRef] [PubMed]

39. Gallagher, T.H.; Waterman, A.D.; Garbutt, J.M.; Kapp, J.M.; Chan, D.K.; Dunagan, W.C.; Fraser, V.J.; Levinson, W. US and Canadian physicians' attitudes and experiences regarding disclosing errors to patients. *Arch. Intern. Méd.* **2006**, *166*, 1605. [CrossRef] [PubMed]

10

Use of Real Patients and Patient-Simulation-Based Methodologies for Teaching Gastroenterology to Pre-Clinical Medical Students

Joshua DeSipio [1], John Gaughan [2], Susan Perlis [3] and Sangita Phadtare [4],* [iD]

[1] Department of Medicine, Gastroenterology/Liver Diseases Division, Cooper University Health, Camden, NJ 08103, USA; DeSipio-Joshua@CooperHealth.edu
[2] Cooper Research Institute, Cooper University Health, Camden, NJ 08103, USA; gaughan-john@CooperHealth.edu
[3] Office of Medical Education, Cooper Medical School of Rowan University, Camden, NJ 08103, USA; perliss@rowan.edu
[4] Department of Biomedical Sciences, Cooper Medical School of Rowan University, Camden, NJ 08103, USA
*   Correspondence: phadtare@rowan.edu

Abstract: In recent years, there has been an increasing focus on the need to integrate formal knowledge with clinical experience in the pre-clinical years since the initial years of medical education play an important role in shaping the attitudes of medical students towards medicine and support the development of clinical reasoning. In this study, we describe approaches that involve real patients and patient-simulation-based methodologies to teach gastroenterology to second year medical students. Our goals were to (i) demonstrate bio-psychosocial aspects of clinical practice, (ii) demonstrate commonality of gastrointestinal ailments, and (iii) help understand complex gastroenterology concepts. We used two main approaches including brief, pre-prepared questions and answers discussing with the patients in various sessions throughout the course and a two-hour session that included patient participation, patient simulation modalities with high fidelity mannequins, a lightening round of interactive cases, and a Patient Oriented Problem Solving (POPS) session. The approaches improved the effectiveness of the delivery of the content-heavy, fast-paced GI course and provided opportunities for the students to think about gastroenterology from both basic and clinical points of view. The approaches involved peer teaching, which supports knowledge acquisition and comprehension. Very positive feedback and overall engagement of students suggested that these approaches were well-received.

Keywords: gastroenterology; patient participation; patient simulation; active learning; peer teaching

1. Introduction

The initial years of medical education play an important role in shaping the attitudes of medical students towards medicine and training them for their future role as a physician [1,2]. The Carnegie Foundation for the Advancement of Teaching report [3,4] emphasized the need to integrate formal knowledge with clinical experience in the learning environment. Numerous studies have shown the benefits of exposing students to patients prior to traditional clerkship rotations [5,6]. Benefits of early exposure to patient care include developing comfort with patients, developing efficient clinical skills, encouraging active learning, making learning more relevant, and reducing difficulty with the transition to clinical practice [7–11]. Therefore, for the past three decades, there has been a push to integrate clinical experiences into pre-clinical education. The growing consideration to provide some opportunities for integrating pre-clinical and clinical phases have resulted in implementing various types of vertically and horizontally integrated practical experiences into the early years of curricula in medical schools [12–14].

The Cooper School of Rowan University (CMSRU) received full LCME (Liaison Committee on Medical Education) accreditation in 2016 and graduated its third cohort of students in 2018. The pre-clinical curriculum integrates basic and clinical sciences and includes a mix of lectures, laboratories, and active learning activities. Our pre-clinical courses are comprised of approximately six hours with each Active Learning Group sessions (ALG), lectures, and afternoon lab sessions. Some courses also include team-based learning (TBL), jigsaws, or other interactive sessions. Attendance for the ALGs and some afternoon sessions is mandatory. Each ALG group consists of eight students and two faculty facilitators (one basic science and one clinician) and meets for two hours, three times per week. Students are given opportunities involving patient interaction such as the courses, Week on Wards (WOW), and an Ambulatory Clerkship at the Cooper Rowan Clinic. The Gastroenterology (GI) course is taught in the fall semester of the second year of medical school. It is a four-week course that integrates the biochemistry, pathophysiology, anatomy, histology, and embryology along with the signs and symptoms, diagnostic methods, and treatment modalities of GI, hepatic, and biliopancreatic diseases and nutrition.

The sheer volume of information that had to be presented to the students during the GI course made it a very fast-paced and somewhat daunting course. In response, we incorporated several methodologies in the course, which allow the students the opportunity to pause and reflect on the content being taught within the context of the big picture. Previously, we described the reception and efficacy of an interactive activity on nutritional pathology that was introduced in this course. The activity included discussion about various nutrition pathologies based on real-life cases, which made the exercise very clinically relevant to the students. The activity was very well received and helped enhance competency in nutrition for the students [15]. In this study, we described another activity that we used in this course, which involved real patients and patient-simulation-based methodologies. Our goals were to demonstrate bio-psychosocial aspects of clinical practice, demonstrate commonality of gastrointestinal aliments, and help students understand complex gastroenterology concepts.

2. Experimental Section

We used two main approaches: inclusion of (i) brief, pre-prepared question-and-answer sessions with patients in various sessions throughout the course and a two-hour session that included various elements such as patient participation, patient simulation modalities with high fidelity mannequins for demonstration of upper endoscopy and colonoscopy, a lightening round of interactive cases with questions and answers, and a new activity that is reminiscent of the Patient Oriented Problem Solving (POPS) methodology [15–19]. However, only half of this session was based on the POPS structure. It was collectively referred to as POPS (or POPS 2) for course scheduling and evaluation purposes and is described below as such.

2.1. Selection and Participation of Patients Throughout the GI Course

We selected six patients with each suffering from a different gastrointestinal disorder to participate in the course activities. The disorders were infection with *Helicobacter pylori*, gallstones, celiac disease, liver cirrhosis, ulcerative colitis, and irritable bowel syndrome. Most of the patients who participated were people who the students saw every day such as faculty and staff. The course directors met with the patients to learn about their disease, the symptoms they experienced, the treatments they were undergoing, the biopsychosocial aspects including the challenges they faced, and how these diseases influenced them and their families. We then prepared the key features from each of these discussions in the form of questions and answers and shared these with the respective participating patients for accuracy. We also included a note for the GI concept that we wanted to emphasize for each disease. This pre-preparation allowed the patient participants to be brief yet effective with respect to time and delivery in the specific class sessions. The patients participated in various sessions throughout the course. Two patients participated as content experts in ALGs with one of the course directors. Two patients participated during lectures and in the interactive session on diarrhea described below. The entire class met the patients who participated in the ALGs or in the diarrhea interactive session since attendance for these sessions is mandatory. Attendance at lectures is not mandatory. Since the lectures are recorded and the recordings are accessible to the entire class, those students who did not attend the lecture in person were able to watch the questions and answers sessions with the patients. Table 1 describes the patients who participated along with the sessions in which they participated and the main aspects of the respective GI diseases discussed.

Table 1. Highlights of the patient participation.

GI Disease	Session	Highlighted Points of Discussion
Helicobacter pylori infection	ALG * about *H. pylori*, acid-peptic disease	Recurrent infection due to antibiotic resistance of *H. pylori*, importance of confirmation of eradication, symptoms, diagnostic methods, treatment received, understanding the challenges patients face with the side effects of the treatment for this disease, life style changes.
Gallstone	Lecture on biliary diseases	Symptoms, demographic attributes of vulnerable population, treatment (type of surgery), pathophysiology of changing from chronic to acute to chronic disease states, life style changes, emphasis on talking to gallstone patients about seeking help in a timely manner.
Liver cirrhosis	Lecture on non-viral hepatitis	Underlying cause-alcoholism-pathophysiology, symptoms, treatment received, effect on overall quality of life, challenges faced due to dietary restrictions, importance of family support.
Celiac disease	Interactive session on diarrhea	Symptoms, how disease was diagnosed, treatment, dietary changes, overall effect on quality of life, family history of the disease-role of genetics, relationship to other autoimmune diseases (e.g., Graves Disease), inadequacy of screening methods.
Irritable bowel syndrome	Interactive session on diarrhea	Symptoms, demographic attributes of vulnerable population, triggers, challenges involved in diagnosis particularly colonoscopy, treatment options, dietary modifications, life style changes.
Ulcerative colitis	ALG * about inflammatory bowel syndrome	Symptoms, diagnosis, pathophysiology, challenges and life style changes after surgeries (colectomy and ileostomy), advice to the students as future physicians about how talking to these patients will be beneficial.

* ALG: Active Learning Group.

2.2. Interactive Session on Diarrhea Cases

Diarrhea is caused by a variety of gastroenterology disorders including both with infectious and non-infectious etiology. Our main goals were clinical aspects and physiological manifestations of different GI diseases that cause diarrhea and to demonstrate to the students how endoscopy and colonoscopy can be used for the diagnosis of some of these diseases.

2.2.1. Structure of the Diarrhea Session

The session was carried out in a large lecture hall with two faculty facilitators who are the course directors of the GI course. It was two-hours in duration and was divided in two major parts. The first part focused on non-infectious diarrhea and included a virtual upper endoscopy and colonoscopy demonstration, question-and-answer time with real patients, and a lightening round of upper endoscopy/colonoscopy-based interactive diarrhea cases. The gastroenterologist, serving as the GI co-course director, used simulation modalities such as standardized patients and high fidelity mannequins that realistically replicate the clinical environment to demonstrate how upper endoscopy and colonoscopy is carried out. The demonstration was also shown on the computer screens using screen-in screen projection. Students were able to see the gastroenterologist carrying out these procedures and, at the same time, were able to see what he observed in the simulated patient on the computer screen. The lecture hall in which this activity was carried out has computer screens on all the walls, which allows the students optimal viewing regardless of their location in the classroom. The gastroenterologist provided live commentary as the scope was travelling down the simulated patient's GI tract. He also asked the students questions about different regions of the GI tract when the procedure progressed. This was followed by a question-and-answer session with real patient who suffered from irritable bowel syndrome (IBS). The last component of the demonstration was a lightening round in which four case stems were displayed individually with their endoscopy/colonoscopy presentations and discussions followed about what the underlying diseases were. The diseases represented non-infectious GI diseases with diarrhea as one of the main symptoms including IBS, Crohns, Celiac disease, and VIPoma. The second part of the session included a group activity and a post-quiz. The students learned about four infectious diseases causing diarrhea (Enterotoxigenic *Escherichia coli, Giardia lamblia, Vibrio cholerae, Clostridium difficile*) during the group activity, which was based on the Patient Oriented Problem Solving (POPS) methodology [15–17,20]. Details of the POPS session are described below. Except for Celiac disease, the diarrhea session introduced the students to all of these diseases for the first time in the GI course. Discussions of other aspects of these diseases occurred in later lectures. The timeline of this entire session is below.

- Demonstration of endoscopy and colonoscopy using simulation modalities (25 min)
- Questions and answers session with real patient suffering from IBS (20 min)
- Lightening round of four, non-infectious GI diseases with diarrhea (15 min)
- POPS session with four infectious diarrhea cases and post-quiz (60 min)

2.2.2. Preparation Required before the Diarrhea Session

The students were given a brief description of the main goals and format of the two-hour session in the course introduction lecture. Detailed instructions for the session were posted in advance on the course website. The only preparation required was for the second part of the session, which entails the POPS activity. The students were asked to read one page containing four stems that described clinical presentation of the four GI POPS cases, but were not required to study these cases or carry out research about these. Additionally, 80 students were randomly assigned to 20 groups of four students each. Each student was given a group number and a color (blue/green/purple/yellow) that corresponded to one of the four infectious diarrhea cases. They were asked to sit in their group when they arrived for the session.

2.2.3. POPS Cases and Quiz

Each student within the group was assigned to learn about one of the four infectious diarrhea cases. Each case was assigned a color such as green (Enterotoxigenic *Escherichia coli*), purple (*Giardia lamblia*), yellow (*Vibrio cholerae*), or purple (*Clostridium difficile*). Having colored sheets was very useful for fast distribution during the session. During this part of the session, the students were given one colored page containing the information about their stem with the clinical presentation and patient history as well as laboratory data for one of the four diseases. The underlying cause, physiology and treatment options for each disease was presented in question-and-answer form to facilitate thought-provoking discussions among students. Important concepts were underlined or bolded. Highlights of each case are given in Table 2. All of these were actual cases modified to suit the purpose of the activity. The students were given approximately 10 min for reading their respective case materials. Each student then presented highlights of his/her material to the other three students in the group. They were allowed to carry out additional research on any aspects they wished to know more about and also allowed to ask the faculty facilitators for help if needed. After each of the four students at each table finished discussing their cases, the students took a post-quiz as a group, which contributed towards 3% of the final course grade.

Since the materials covered in the diarrhea session was not taught before this session, we felt that it was not appropriate to have the students take a pre-quiz. They were only asked to take a post-quiz. The quiz consisted of eight, USMLE Step 1-style questions. An example of one question is shown in Table 3.

Table 2. Highlights of the infectious diarrhea cases used in the session.

Deficiency	Case	Major Points Discussed
Clostridium difficile	Patient acquired *C. difficile* infection after treatment with clindamycin at the hospital for a different issue.	Diagnosis, risk factors for *C. difficile infection*, microbiology, and pathophysiology of *C. difficile-mechanism of action of exotoxins*.
Enterotoxigenic *Escherichia coli* (ETEC)	Large scale outbreak of diarrhea in an office picnic.	Differentiating the different types of *E. coli* that cause diarrhea, symptoms, pathophysiology-mechanism of heat-labile and heat-stable *E. coli* toxins, treatments.
Giardia lamblia	*Giardia lamblia* infection after pancreas-kidney transplantation.	Epidemiology of *Giardia* infections including the unusual mode of acquiring infection, diagnosis-biopsy presentation, symptoms and treatment, life cycle of *Giardia*.
Vibrio cholerae	A patient with watery diarrhea.	Symptoms, diagnosis, pathophysiology-mechanism of action of enterotoxin, reasoning behind treatment options.

Table 3. Example of a quiz question.

Question. A 50-year-old man has to undergo a dental procedure. He has an artificial heart valve. Therefore, he was given clindamycin to prevent bacterial endocarditis. A week later, he has discomfort in the lower abdomen and develops watery diarrhea. Which one of the following explains the mechanism of action of toxin that is responsible for his condition?
A.   Activation of enterocyte cyclic GMP (guanosine monophosphate)
B.   Stimulation of the vagus nerve in the abdominal viscera
C.   Inactivation of regulatory pathways mediated by Rho family proteins
D.   Activation of Gsα through an ADP (adenosine diphosphate)—ribosylation reaction

2.3. Outcome Measures of the Approaches Used

2.3.1. Evaluation of Reception of the Approaches

We assessed the efficacy of the approaches described here using three modes of evaluation by the students. The CMSRU Office of Medical Education (OME) collects students' overall evaluation of the course as well as the evaluation of each of the course sessions (lectures, ALGs, TBLS, POPS, jigsaws, and labs) as a standard practice. These evaluations are collected anonymously following the school policies and are distributed to the course directors and participating respective faculty in an aggregate manner. We also carried out an additional evaluation of the approaches described here via a paper survey. The standard, electronic evaluation of the diarrhea session carried out by the CMSRU OME is designated here as Evaluation A. The additional paper survey collected after the completion of the diarrhea session is designated as Evaluation B. The comments pulled from the two questions asked in the standard, electronic overall course evaluation as described below are designated as Evaluation C.

Evaluation A

The students are asked to evaluate each session in a course. Since the students have to complete a large number of surveys, the school has adapted a policy that reduces the number of surveys each student has to complete in a course. According to this policy, about half of the class is asked to evaluate each interactive session. Therefore, 37 students completed the survey for the diarrhea POPS session. We have observed that the outcomes of these surveys are representative of the perception of the entire class. The standard evaluation form that is used for any interactive session (e.g., TBLs, jigsaws, POPS) includes eleven Likert scale questions: (i) the objectives of the session were clear, (ii) the session was well organized, (iii) the session was relevant to my education, (iv) the content helped me meet session objectives, (v) the session content was related to course objectives, (vi) the session stimulated me to want to learn more about the subject, (vii) the faculty maintained my interest, (viii) the faculty demonstrated appropriate knowledge, (ix) the faculty explained the material clearly, (x) the faculty used questions and student participation effectively, and (xi) the faculty demonstrated professionalism. Students are also asked to provide qualitative comments on the session.

Evaluation B

As mentioned above, the evaluation form A is a common form used for any interactive session in any given course by the CMSRU OME. To maintain consistency for evaluation across various courses in the curriculum, the evaluation forms are not modified for individual courses/sessions. We, therefore, decided to include an additional evaluation in the form of a paper survey to assess the reception of the inclusion of patients throughout the GI course along with the inclusion of the patient simulation in the diarrhea session. The authors have used additional paper surveys to assess efficacy of individual interactive sessions before [15,16]. The paper survey was distributed to the students at the end of the diarrhea session. Since this session is scheduled towards the end of the GI course, it provided the last opportunity to have the entire class in one place. The paper survey contained three Likert style questions and one open-ended question. The Likert scale questions were: (i) Was the inclusion of GI patient(s) during this exercise and throughout the GI course informative with respect to the biopsychosocial aspects of the GI disorders? (ii) Did the inclusion of GI patient(s) during this exercise and throughout the GI course enhance your empathy towards them? and (iii) Did you find working with your peers and the interactive nature of this activity conducive to learning about the GI system? The fourth question asked for any comment on the activity with respect to its structure and usefulness and inclusion of patient simulation elements. We received prior approval from the Rowan Institutional Review Board (IRB) (project ID: Pro2016001014) to conduct the paper surveys and also to use the data from the surveys and quizzes for publication. The anonymous paper surveys were administered as per the guidelines set by Rowan Institutional Review Board and did not contain personal identification markers. The students were informed that the evaluation of this activity was voluntary and anonymous and did not influence their grades.

Evaluation C

As mentioned above, in addition to the evaluation of each of the course sessions, the CMSRU OME collects students' overall evaluation of the course as a routine practice. The entire class is asked to complete the overall evaluation for the course. Two of the several questions included in this form are: (i) Were there any sessions that were particularly outstanding? and (ii) What was the most vivid/thought-provoking, useful, or otherwise memorable information they learned in the course? We used comments received for these two questions as evaluation C for this study.

2.3.2. Evaluation of Efficacy of the POPS Activity via Student Performance in Post-Quiz

In order to do well in the post-quiz, each student in a group needed to be a responsible member of his/her group and effectively present the respective material to his/her teammates. The students also needed to carefully read and synthesize the information and understand the underlying concepts. This was especially imperative since this was the first time the diarrhea cases were presented to them. The efficacy of the session as evidenced by post-quiz scores demonstrated that the session was highly effective as only one group got one question wrong. The concepts were further reviewed and consolidated in a one-hour lecture the following week.

3. Results

3.1. Evaluation of Reception of the Approaches

The students' reception of these approaches was very positive. All the comments received for the open-ended questions in evaluations A, B, and C are given collectively in Table 4. The origin of each comment is given as a superscript at the end as [A], [B], or [C]. The thematic analysis of the comments suggests that the main aspects liked by the students were team work, peer learning, helpful for understanding, and enjoyable, engaging involvement of patients including humanizing medicine, retention of concepts, and patient simulation. There were several additional positive comments on the inclusion of the patients, patient simulation, and also about this POPS in the various other evaluations collected for the GI course. It is also interesting to note that there were no negative comments about these approaches in any of the evaluations collected, which suggests their very positive reception in general.

Table 4. Students comments received.

Team Work

1. I think these sessions are really helpful in learning the material. By reading the article and teaching it to our fellow team members, I feel we are learning the information even better than if we read it alone on our own. You need to really know something before you can teach it to someone else. Additionally, the cases that present the different material help me to remember the information even more. During the exam, I found myself thinking back and saying "Oh that was the blue case in the pops session." It really helped with recall of the information. [A]

2. I think the POPS really helps the students more than a normal TBL session. Learning from peers helps to make the material easier to understand and remember. [B]

3. The POP sessions because of the method of learning it involved and required. [C]

4. The POPS sessions were very helpful to discuss topics with other students. I was able to remember the material better through these discussions. [C]

Helpful for Understanding

5. These are always excellent! I learn so much! [A]

6. SO HELPFUL. [A]

7. Helpful to have this before the diarrhea lecture. [A]

8. Interactive sessions were helpful. However, visual simulation was not the greatest quality in MRP small screens. Perhaps (Faculty name) can show real pictures/videos from actual cases. [A]

9. Great and helpful session. [A]

10. POPS are very helpful! [B]

11. POPS are great for learning. [B]

12. I thought that the lightening round questions were super helpful!! [B]

13. All aspects of the activity are very effective and a great aspect to the course that I enjoy. [B]

14. Well-orchestrated and effective learning environment. [B]

Table 4. *Cont.*

Enjoyable, Engaging

15.	Perfect! [A]
16.	Very helpful and enjoyable! [A]
17.	Thank you Dr. (Faculty name) for consistently engaging us in the learning process! We appreciate the work you put into pulling this together! [A]
18.	Keep doing a great job. [A]
19.	Great course. [B]
20.	I love Pop! [B]
21.	Well done course. [B]
22.	These are awesome. Pop never looked or sounded so good. [B]
23.	This is the best Pop I've ever had!! I hope every pop is like this pop! [B]
24.	Love these sessions. [B]
25.	Very helpful. [B]
26.	Replaces TBLs with this. [B]
27.	I liked. [B]
28.	It is great!! [B]
29.	I love (faculty name)'s POPS. [B]
30.	It was great. [B]
31.	Love it!!! [B]
32.	Great! [B]
33.	Please expand this to all blocks! [B]
34.	Good activity. [B]
35.	I love this format!!! [B]
36.	POPs are much better than TBLs. [B]
37.	I really enjoyed the POPS sessions. [C]
38.	POPs session number 2. [C]
39.	Really enjoyed the POPS 2 session! [C]
40.	I loved the pop sessions. [C]
41.	The POPS were great. [C]
42.	Pops. [C]

Involvement of Patients: Humanizing Medicine, Retention of Concepts

43.	It brings perspective to the concepts we learn and puts a face to a story. [B]
44.	Really helped being able to walk through different clinical scenarios and having the patients helps humanize it. [B]
45.	Nice to get the patient perspectives. [B]

Table 4. *Cont.*

46.	I LOVE it—I strongly believe this should happen in <u>all</u> courses in order to increase our understanding of the patients. We are treating <u>people</u>, not disease! I think it would also go a long way toward promoting empathy. [B]
47.	I really appreciated the real patient experiences. [B]
48.	I think every course should bring in patients. Not only does it enhance our clinical understanding, but it also helps us. [B]
49.	POPs are awesome! Great experience. Patient experiences are vital! Include them in (another course name)! [B]
50.	Loved the Alcoholic liver patient's story, the clinical correlation, and the human aspect of the session. It is so important that med students learn <u>NOT</u> to blame patients even if they are somewhat responsible for their disease course. [B]
51.	The addition of patients is a good idea. [B]
52.	It would be helpful to have good/bad interactions the patients experienced with their doctors plus the frustrations of suffering from symptoms while waiting to determine diagnosis. [B]
53.	I loved hearing from the patients. I wish every course did this. [B]
54.	Helps to understand how patients react to illness. Gives me a 10000 feet view of the disease process. [B]
55.	I LOVED having the patients come in and share their experiences. I thought that was a really powerful part of the course and I hope they continue to do this. [C]
56.	Enjoy the patient stories and POP sessions. [C]
57.	I thought the real life cases were a great way to integrate the course with the clinic. [C]
58.	I loved the POPs sessions and the personal stories from patients. They both helped solidify a lot of information.
59.	Hearing patient stories. [C]
60.	I enjoyed having the real patients coming in and telling their stories. [C]
61.	I also enjoyed hearing from the patients. [C]
62.	I loved the session with the patient who had liver cirrhosis due to chronic alcohol consumption. It was a very "human" perspective and story. It really touched me and helped me apply the information I was learning in the lecture environment to the real life experience of patients. [C]
63.	The guests that were brought in throughout the block were really thoughtful and well related to the topics of the day. [C]
64.	I loved when (Faculty name) brought in patients to talk to us about their experiences. Very thoughtful! [C]
65.	I really liked the personal patient stories. Additionally, it was easier to remember the material from the POPs session.
66.	Physical exam and patient experiences. [C]
67.	Personally enjoyed the patient profiles the most. I think that adds a much needed piece to the puzzle that is often lost during the first and second year. Reading an ALG case about a fictional person is one thing but being presented with actual people reminds you that these diseases affect actual people. [C]
68.	Patient stories. [C]
69.	Hearing stories from the real-life patients was very, very helpful and insightful. [C]

Table 4. *Cont.*

70.	All of the stories told to help give context to the information were very useful. [C]
71.	I really enjoyed having the volunteer patients come and talk with us. It gave a different perspective on "cases" that we were learning about and helped us to have a better appreciation for the topics we were discussing. [C]
72.	Meeting patients and having them share the way these illnesses affect their everyday life. Sometimes it's easy to skip over that or not even think about it during lectures. [C]
73.	Honestly, the most thought-provoking information came from the visiting patients. [C]
74.	It was very interesting to learn how GI issues are so common in society and how greatly they can affect a patient's quality of life. [C]
75.	I LOVED THE USE OF PATIENT STORY-TELLING. It was incredibly meaningful and enriching to hear the patient experiences and it incorporated psychosocial elements into our curriculum. This was an excellent idea. Please continue. [C]
76.	Including the patient sessions. [C]
77.	Please have more POPS sessions. I learn so much more from this active learning session than from TBL quizzes. This is a great component of the curriculum. It really helps us retain information. [A]
78.	The patients added a face to the diseases and disorders. This also makes it easier to remember because it is a story as opposed to a lecture. [B]
79.	Hearing patient stories helps solidify the information we are learning. [B]

Patient Simulation

80.	The demo was informative and I enjoyed the patient story. [A]
81.	One of my favorites of the block! Seeing the colonoscopy was awesome. [A]
82.	This was a great session! The endoscopy/colonoscopy demonstration with cases was interesting. I really enjoyed learning about IBS from (patient name) as well. [B]
83.	I really enjoyed seeing how a colonoscopy is done. [B]
84.	Really liked the endoscopy/colonoscopy. [B]
85.	All the times we had patients come to class/pops—I'll never forget! Additionally, the virtual colonoscopy was so cool. [C]
86.	Learning about the different causes of diarrhea and the poop visual has really stood out. [C]

[A] Comments about diarrhea session (Patient-Oriented-Problem-Solving; POPS 2) (question in the standard electronic survey). [B] Any comment on the activity with respect to POPS 2 structure and usefulness and inclusion of patient simulation elements (question in the paper survey). [C] Were there any sessions that were particularly outstanding? What's the most vivid/ thought-provoking, useful, or otherwise memorable information you've learned so far in this class? (questions in the electronic overall course evaluation survey).

Results of the eleven Likert scale questions in the Evaluation A are presented in Figure 1.

The results of the responses received for the three Likert scale questions in evaluation B are presented in Table 5. Out of the 80 students who participated in the interactive session, 77 chose to complete the paper surveys. The electronic data in Evaluation form A was provided to us in an aggregate form. However, the paper surveys allowed tabulation of the data for each response. Therefore, we were able to calculate Cronbach's Alpha for evaluating the involvement of patients in the course. The Cronbach's Alpha was 0.7, which suggests that there is a strong internal consistency and reliability of the items in the survey measurement [21].

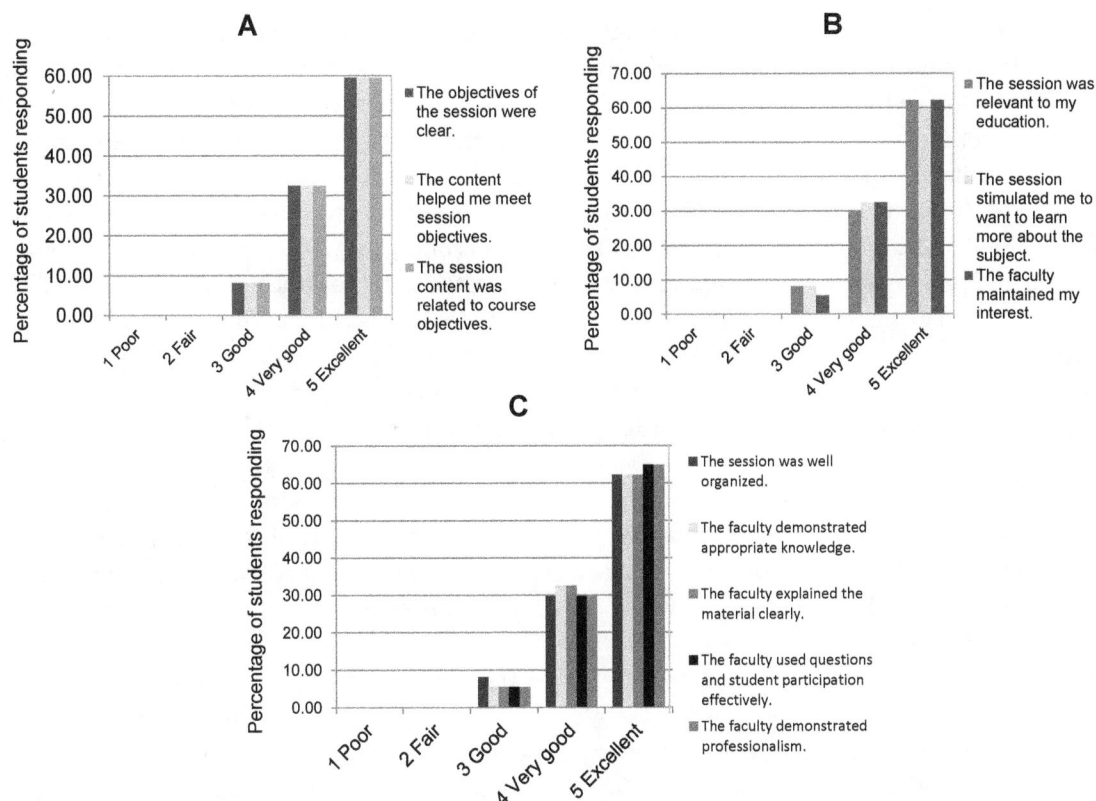

Figure 1. Quantitative representation of the student evaluation data of the interactive session with respect to (**A**) usefulness of the learning objectives, (**B**) relevancy and interest, and (**C**) structure and execution. The students evaluated the activity, which contained eleven Likert scale questions (five choices are shown) regarding these aspects.

Table 5. Quantitative presentation of students' responses to the involvement of patients in the gastroenterology course.

Item	Percent Responding					
	Strongly Disagree	**Disagree**	**Neutral**	**Agree**	**Stronly Agree**	**Mean Score**
Likert Scale	1	2	3	4	5	
Informative	0.00	1.30	5.19	10.39	83.12	4.8
Enhance empathy	1.30	0.00	2.60	15.58	80.52	4.7
Conducive to learning	0.00	0.00	1.30	28.57	70.13	4.7

3.2. Student Performance in the Post-POPS Session Quiz

There were a total of 20 groups with 80 students in groups of four who took the post-quiz. 19 groups answered all of the eight questions in the post-quiz correctly while one group got one question wrong. This was remarkable since the students were exposed to new material for the first time during this session. The concepts discussed in the POPS session were briefly reviewed and consolidated in lectures following the session. The students did very well on the questions based on these topics in the final course exam.

4. Discussion

Early clinical exposure (ECE) integrates the knowledge of basic and clinical sciences and the psychosocial aspects of the medical practice [22]. This approach helps to facilitate the transition from pre-clinical years to clinical years. It also enhances students' motivation and supports their appreciation of the relevance of basic sciences in clinical practice [2,8,11,23]. A study based on reflective essays written by fourth-year medical students [24] showed the influence of two pre-clinical education aspects that students noted on their conceptions of altruism, compassion, and respect. They perceived that the classes that allowed them to consider biopsychosocial aspects of patients' lives before implementing a course of action in their medical care had a positive influence while the academic environment or culture itself that emphasizes their performance on exams to be anti-altruistic. Different types of early patient experiences may provide unique learning outcomes and acculturation for preclinical medical students [8]. An education model proposed by Dornan and colleagues [25] emphasized the importance of supported participation in clinical learning and suggested that the educational environment that supports and challenges learners can increase their participation within it. This, in turn, helps them develop additional competencies such as study strategies and clinical skills, which motivates them and may also help students to develop confidence and professional identity. This model emphasized that participation is central to student learning and that learning is shaped by human interactions.

High-fidelity patient simulation has been increasingly used as a teaching modality for health professional students. Life-size manikins that mimic real patients are used to simulate normal and disease conditions. These have been mainly used for residents or medical students in their clinical years. However, some studies indicate that patient simulators have been successfully used for first-year medical students coupled with problem-based learning to reinforce curricular concepts while bringing the cases to life [26–31].

We had given careful consideration in selecting patients for participation in the GI course and the aspects we wanted to emphasize for each disease. Important points include prior preparation of question-and-answer-based, patient-doctor scripts allowing the information to be delivered in a very succinct and time-efficient manner. Most of these patients in our learning activity were people the students encountered at the school every day. This emphasized the point about how common gastroenterology diseases are. Additionally, since the students knew these 'patients,' they were very comfortable asking them questions. The patients were chosen to emphasize specific aspects of GI disease. For example, we were able to discuss the genetics of and cross-relationship between different autoimmune disorders using the celiac disease patient while the gallstone patient was able to demonstrate how the gallstone disease can switch between acute and chronic phases, which is an aspect that the students usually find difficult to grasp. Patient participation encounters were brief given the time-constraints of the course, which were dispersed in different sessions throughout the course and aligned with the materials taught during respective weeks and ensured that all the students were exposed to the patient interviews. Each patient interview included the challenges they face living with a GI disease, which humanized the experience for the students.

Important considerations for the two-hour diarrhea session include the patient simulation that was designed to demonstrate the healthy state versus the disease state of the GI system using scoping methodologies. Students were asked questions during this demonstration about which area of the GI tract they were observing along with comments on what they expect to see in that organ for a particular disease. This created further engagement in the demonstration and encouraged them to think about and build on the GI concepts they had learned in the course. The interactive lightening round cases and questions further consolidated the diagnostic role of endoscopy and colonoscopy in various GI disorders. The POPS cases were designed to promote team work and peer teaching to learn new materials in a time-efficient manner, which is consistent with the notion that peer teaching enhances comprehension since it depends on sharing both cognitive and social congruence [32–34]. The complexity and length of all the case materials were comparable and appropriate for the duration of the session along with the highlighting of important points to reduce the need for additional guidance during the session and to ensure consistency for all groups. The session was facilitated in a single large room with two faculty members, which eliminated the need for additional faculty time or multiple rooms. The session did not require much prior preparation from the students, which suited the fast pace and time constraints of this very content-heavy course. Being able to take the post-quiz in a group further enforced reliance on peers and reduced the stress of test-taking, which allowed the students to focus on thinking critically about the concepts rather than worrying about performance on the quizzes. This, in turn, allowed them to enjoy the activity as an education experience. The quiz questions required the students to know the underlying mechanisms and employ higher-level thinking to apply that knowledge to clinical scenarios.

As evidenced by the very positive student reception of these approaches and their detailed comments, our goals for these approaches were achieved. Students stated that inclusion of patients in the course allowed them to put a 'face' on the disease and gave a practical connection that helped them to visualize it. They experienced patients in real time with respect to their needs and challenges, which provided them with better insight into the pathophysiology of the case at hand. These approaches gave them an opportunity to ask questions, which consolidated their learning and enhanced their connection to the patients. Since the interactions were designed in the form of questions and answers with the gastroenterologist course director of the GI course, the students had the experience of how a physician might interact with a patient and create a doctor-patient bond rather than solely looking at the patient as a case to treat. This may contribute to them becoming more invested in their future patients' welfare. They also stated that the interactive approaches helped make the concepts more memorable and easier to understand.

One limitation of this study is that we examined a cohort of medical students in one medical school. However, benefits of early patient exposure have been reported in various healthcare disciplines such as nurse anesthesia students, dental students, and optometry students [7,35,36]. Although our evaluation strategies primarily focus on student satisfaction with the learning experience and post-quiz, these prior studies suggest that early experiences help students understand and align with patient and community perspectives and generate evidence for perceived and actual benefits of preclinical experience in front-loaded clinical programs. Another limitation of this study is that, while the POPS part of the activity works well with small groups (4–5 students), it limits how many diseases can be taught in a specific learning session. Assigning more than one case per student may not work well since it will require the students learn a large volume of material and teach it to their peers in a short amount of time.

5. Conclusions

We designed and implemented several approaches that involved real patients and patient simulation in the M2 GI course to stimulate student interest in gastroenterology, help them understand complex GI concepts, and demonstrate the bio-psychosocial aspects of the clinical practice. The approaches improved the effectiveness of the delivery of the GI course in that these learning activities provided opportunities for the students to think about gastroenterology from both basic and clinical perspectives. The POPS activity was based on peer teaching that involves cognitive development as well as social collegiality and, therefore, plays an important role in enhancing knowledge acquisition and comprehension. The excellent overall class performance in the post-quiz demonstrated that the students were able to learn and effectively apply new concepts in a short amount of time. Extremely positive feedback about the experience and the overall engagement of students suggested that these approaches were well received, which encourages us to implement them in other courses in our curriculum.

Author Contributions: S.P. (Sangita Phadtare) conceived and designed the study. J.D. provided further expertise. S.P. (Sangita Phadtare) and J.D. carried out the study. J.G. carried out the statistical analysis. S.P. (Sangita Phadtare) wrote the manuscript and J.D. and S.P. (Susan Perlis) provided editorial suggestions on the manuscript.

Funding: This research received no external funding.

Acknowledgments: The authors thank Gregory Staman, Lisa Fecteau and John Dill for their help in using the simulation modalities.

References

1. Mafinejad, M.K.; Mirzazadeh, A.; Peiman, S.; Hazaveh, M.M.; Khajavirad, N.; Allamed, S.-F.; Naderi, N.; Foroumando, M.; Afsahari, A.; Asghari, F. Medical students' attitudes towards early clinical exposure in Iran. *Int. J. Med. Educ.* **2016**, *7*, 195–199. [CrossRef] [PubMed]

2. Littlewood, S.; Ypinazar, V.; Margolis, S.A.; Scherpbier, A.; Spencer, J.; Dornan, T. Early practical experience and the social responsiveness of clinical education: Systematic review. *BMJ* **2005**, *331*, 387–391. [CrossRef] [PubMed]

3. Saba, T.G.; Hershenson, M B.; Arteta, M.; Ramirez, I.A.; Mullan, P.B.; Owens, S.T. Pre-clinical medical student experience in a pediatric pulmonary clinic. *Med. Educ. Online* **2015**, *20*, 28654. [CrossRef] [PubMed]

4. Irby, D. Educating physicians for the future: Carnegie's calls for reform. *Med. Teach.* **2011**, *33*, 547–550. [CrossRef] [PubMed]

5. Dornan, T.; Littlewood, S.; Margolis, S.A.; Scherpbier, A.; Spencer, J.; Ypinazar, V. How can experience in clinical and community settings contribute to early medical education? A BEME systematic review. *Med. Teach.* **2006**, *28*, 3–18. [CrossRef] [PubMed]

6. Yardley, S.; Littlewood, S.; Margolis, S.A.; Scherpbier, A.; Spencer, J.; Ypinazar, V.; Dornan, T. What has changed in the evidence for early experience? Update of a BEME systematic review. *Med. Teach.* **2010**, *32*, 740–746. [CrossRef] [PubMed]

7. Fuensanta, A.; Vera-Diaz; Johnson, C. Perceived Enhanced Clinical Readiness for Second-Year Optometry Interns. *Optom. Educ.* **2017**, *43*, 1–13.

8. Wenrich, M.D.; Jackson, M.B.; Wolfhagen, I.; Ramsey, P.G.; Scherpbier, A.J. What are the benefits of early patient contact? A comparison of three preclinical patient contact settings. *BMC Med. Educ.* **2013**, *13*, 80. [CrossRef] [PubMed]

9. Dornan, T.; Tan, N.; Boshuizen, H.; Gick, R.; Isba, R.; Mann, K.; Scherpbier, A.; Spencer, J.; Timmins, E. How and what do medical students learn in clerkships? Experience based learning (ExBL). *Adv. Health Sci. Educ.* **2014**, *19*, 721–749. [CrossRef] [PubMed]

10. Godfrooji, M.B.; Diemers, A.D.; Scherpbier, A. Students' perceptions about the transition to the clinical phase of a medical curriculum with preclinical patient contacts; a focus group study. *BMC Med. Educ.* **2010**, *10*, 28. [CrossRef] [PubMed]

11. Diemers, A.D.; Dolmans, D.H.; Verwijnen, M.G.; Heineman, E.; Scherpbier, A.J. Students' opinions about the effects of preclinical patient contacts on their learning. *Adv. Health Sci. Educ.* **2008**, *13*, 633–647. [CrossRef] [PubMed]

12. Dahle, L.O.; Brynhildsen, J.; Behrbohm, F.M.; Rundquist, I.; Hammar, M. PROS and CONS of vertical integration between clinical medicine and basic science within a problem-based undergraduate medical curriculum: Examples and experiences from Linkoping, Sweden. *Med. Teach.* **2002**, *2*, 280–285. [CrossRef] [PubMed]

13. Dornan, T.; Bundy, C. What can experience add to early medical education? Consensus survey. *BMJ* **2004**, *329*, 834. [CrossRef] [PubMed]

14. Başak, O.; Yaphe, J.; Spiegel, W.; Wilm, S.; Carelli, F.; Metsemakers, J.F. Early clinical exposure in medical curricula across Europe: An overview. *Eur. J. Gen. Pract.* **2009**, *15*, 4–10. [CrossRef] [PubMed]

15. DeSipio, J.; Phadtare, S. An Interactive Session on Nutritional Pathologies for Health Professional Students. *Healthcare* **2015**, *3*, 519–528. [CrossRef] [PubMed]

16. Lopez, H.; Goldman, E.; Gaughan, J.; Phadtare, S. From Anatomical Knowledge to Clinical Comprehension: A Peer-Oriented Learning Session to Help Medical Students Make the Leap. *Med. Sci. Educ.* **2017**, *27*, 177–181. [CrossRef]

17. Ingenito, A.J.; Wooles, W.R. Survey results of POPS use in United States and Canadian schools of medicine and pharmacy. *J. Clin. Pharmacol.* **1995**, *35*, 117–127. [CrossRef] [PubMed]

18. Zhang, Z.; Liu, W.; Han, J.; Guo, S.; Wu, Y. A trial of patient-oriented problem-solving system for immunology teaching in China: A comparison with dialectic lectures. *BMC Med. Educ.* **2013**, *13*, 11. [CrossRef] [PubMed]

19. Lathers, C.M.; Smith, C.M. Development of innovative teaching materials: Clinical pharmacology problem-solving (CPPS) units: Comparison with patient-oriented problem-solving units and problem-based learning—A 10-year review. *J. Clin. Pharmacol.* **2002**, *42*, 477–491. [CrossRef] [PubMed]

20. Wolff, M.; Wagner, M.J.; Poznanski, S.; Schiller, J.; Santen, S. Not another boring lecture: Engaging learners with active learning techniques. *J. Emerg. Med.* **2015**, *48*, 85–93. [CrossRef] [PubMed]

21. Inuwa, I.M. Perceptions and Attitudes of First-Year Medical Students on a Modified Team-Based Learning (TBL) Strategy in Anatomy. *Sultan Qaboos Univ. Med. J.* **2012**, *12*, 336–343. [CrossRef]

22. Tayade, M.C.; Bhimani, N.; Kulkarni, N.B.; Dandekar, K.N. The impact of early clinical exposure on first MBBS students. *Int. J. Health Biomed. Res.* **2014**, *2*, 176–181.

23. Kachur, E.K. Observation during early clinical exposure—An effective instructional tool or a bore? *Med. Educ.* **2003**, *37*, 88–89. [CrossRef]

24. Wear, D.; Zarconi, J. Can compassion be taught? *Let's ask our students. J. Gen. Intern. Med.* **2008**, *23*, 948–953. [PubMed]

25. Dornan, T.; Boshuizen, H.; King, N.; Scherpbier, A. Experience-based learning: A model linking the processes and outcomes of medical students' workplace learning. *Med. Educ.* **2007**, *41*, 84–91. [CrossRef] [PubMed]

26. Wimmer, M.J.; Wilks, D.H.; Grammer, R.W.; Doerr, R.G.; Summers, D.E.; Ressetar, H.G. Use of Patient Simulation in Problem-Based Learning for First-Year Medical Students. *Med. Sci. Educ.* **2014**, *24*, 253–261. [CrossRef]

27. Gordon, J.A.; Oriol, N.E.; Cooper, J.B. Bringing good teaching cases "to life": A simulator-based medical education service. *Acad. Med.* **2004**, *79*, 23–27. [CrossRef] [PubMed]

28. Gordon, J.A.; Brown, D.F.; Armstrong, E.G. Can a simulated critical care encounter accelerate basic science learning among preclinical medical students? A pilot study. *Simul. Healthc.* **2006**, *1*, 13–17. [CrossRef] [PubMed]

29. Larson-Williams, L.M.; Youngblood, A.Q.; Peterson, D.T.; Zinkan, J.L.; White, M.L.; Abdul-Latif, H.; Matalka, L.; Epps, S.N.; Tofil, N.M. Simulation of diabetic ketoacidosis for cellular and molecular basics of medical practice. *Simul. Healthc.* **2009**, *4*, 232–236.

30. Winston, I.; Szarek, J.L. Problem-based learning using a human patient simulator. *Med. Educ.* **2005**, *39*, 526–527. [CrossRef] [PubMed]

31. Liaw, S.Y.; Chen, F.G.; Klainin, P.; Brammer, J.; O'Brien, A.; Samarasekera, D. D. Developing clinical competency in crisis event management: An integrated simulation problem-based learning activity. *Adv. Health Sci. Educ. Theory Pract.* **2010**, *15*, 403–413. [CrossRef] [PubMed]

32. Yu, T.C.; Wilson, N.C.; Singh, P.P.; Lemanu, D.P.; Hawken, S.J.; Hill, A.G. Medical students-as-teachers: A systematic review of peer-assisted teaching during medical school. *Adv. Med. Educ. Pract.* **2011**, *2*, 157–172. [PubMed]

33. Schmidt, H.G.; Moust, J.H. What makes a tutor effective? A structural-equations modeling approach to learning in problem-based curricula. *Acad. Med.* **1995**, *70*, 708–714. [CrossRef] [PubMed]

34. Ten Cate, O.; Durning, S. Dimensions and psychology of peer teaching in medical education. *Med. Teach.* **2007**, *29*, 546–552. [CrossRef] [PubMed]

35. Imus, F.S.; Burns, S.M.; Fisher, R.; Ranalli, L. Students perceptions on pre-clinical experience in a front-loaded nurse anesthesia program. *J. Nurs. Educ. Pract.* **2015**, *5*, 22–27.

36. Orsinia, C.; Binnieb, V.I.; Fuentesc, F.; Ledezmac, P.; Jerez, O. Implications of motivation differences inpreclinical-clinical transition of dental students: A one-year follow-up study. *Educ. Méd.* **2016**, *17*, 193–196. [CrossRef]

11

Importance of Patient–Provider Communication to Adherence in Adolescents with Type 1 Diabetes

Niral J. Patel, Karishma A. Datye and Sarah S. Jaser *

Department of Pediatrics, Vanderbilt University Medical Center, Nashville, TN 37232, USA;
niral.patel@vumc.org (N.J.P.); karishma.a.datye@vanderbilt.edu (K.A.D.)
* Correspondence: sarah.jaser@vanderbilt.edu

Abstract: Effective communication between pediatric diabetes patients and their providers has the potential to enhance patient satisfaction and health outcomes, as well as improve diabetes-related self-management. In this review, we highlight the importance of communication between patients and providers, focusing on the effect of communication on adherence in the high-risk population of adolescents with type 1 diabetes. We synthesize the literature describing patient–provider communication in pediatric populations and provide implications for practice that focus on the most relevant, modifiable factors for improving self-management in adolescents with type 1 diabetes.

Keywords: type 1 diabetes; adolescents; providers; self-management; patient-HCP communication; patient satisfaction

1. Introduction

Most adolescent patients with type 1 diabetes (T1D) do not meet treatment goals, which increases their risk for diabetes related complications [1]; therefore, finding ways to improve adherence to therapy is crucial. T1D affects more than 1 in 400 youth in the United States [2], making it one of the most common chronic childhood health conditions. The intensive treatment plan recommended for T1D requires a daily regimen of blood glucose checks, insulin administration, carbohydrate counting, and many other tasks (see Figure 1) that can become burdensome and challenging over time [3,4]. While the management of T1D is difficult at all ages, it can be particularly challenging during adolescence, when the interplay of physiologic and psychosocial changes can negatively affect glycemic control [5]. Maintaining good glycemic control can decrease the risk of complications such as retinopathy and nephropathy, but only 17% percent of adolescents with T1D meet American Diabetes Association targets for hemoglobin A1C [6], a surrogate for disease control. Additionally, while glycemic control is poorest during adolescence, it is better both before and after adolescence [7,8]. Adolescents with T1D are clearly a high-risk population; therefore, minimizing the challenges of diabetes management in this population is important. Recent reviews have examined various facilitators and barriers of adolescents' adherence to treatment, such as parental involvement [9], peer influence [10], psychological adjustment [11], and access to care [12]. A potentially important and modifiable factor that has received less attention in the pediatric diabetes arena is patient-provider communication, and how this communication is linked to adherence to therapy.

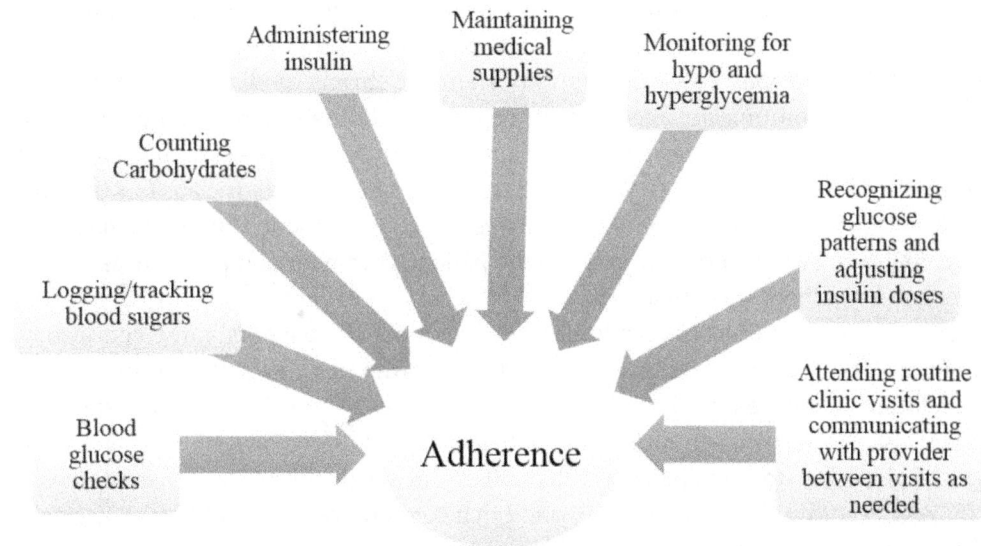

Figure 1. Type 1 Diabetes Treatment Regimen Tasks Associated with Adherence. Adapted from: Jaser et al. 2016 [4].

Adolescents experience significant physiological and psychosocial changes during this developmental stage, including increased insulin resistance related to pubertal hormones, significant weight gain, higher insulin needs [13], and increasing independence from parents. Unfortunately, this newfound autonomy often results in problems with adherence and may further exacerbate poor glycemic control [14]. In addition, adolescents with chronic conditions may be more likely to engage in high-risk behaviors, such as drug and alcohol use, cigarette smoking, and unprotected sexual activity, than their peers [15], and these risky behaviors have the potential for greater adverse health outcomes in youth with chronic health conditions [16]. In their most recent practice guidelines, the American Diabetes Association (ADA) noted the difficulties in managing diabetes during this period and recommended that providers discuss potential stressors during visits [3]. Thus, understanding the important role of communication between patients, their caregivers, and providers, and addressing challenges between these groups may help adolescents improve adherence and achieve optimal glycemic control. We use the term "adherence" as it acknowledges the active role of patients in developing and following a treatment plan [17,18]. In this review, we synthesize the recent literature on patient-provider communication in pediatric populations, with a focus on the factors that are developmentally relevant, modifiable, and may be addressed by providers, including time management, technology, health numeracy, and provider burnout. We also note implications for practice, by offering recommendations to improve communication between patients, caregivers, and providers.

2. Importance and Function of Communication

Communication can be an effective tool to create a connection and share information between healthcare providers, patients, and family members. Verbal communication in the healthcare arena is defined as the act of exchanging information in order to identify the medical issue [19]. Non-verbal communication is the emotional tone of an interaction between people and includes the signals given off by how a person speaks, stands, looks, and acts when speaking with another person. The functions of communication affect health outcomes either directly or indirectly [20]. For example, when a provider verbally discusses key concerns and sympathizes with patients about their specific symptoms, there is a positive influence on health outcomes and emotional well-being (i.e., direct pathway), as well as increased trust and understanding between the patient and provider (i.e., indirect pathway) [20].

The patient-provider relationship is strongly related to adherence to treatment (i.e., following the recommended regimen), health outcomes, and patient and provider satisfaction in all medical conditions [18,19], but it may be especially important for chronic pediatric conditions. Pediatric providers need to communicate effectively, not only with their patients, but also with their patients' caregivers, which may explain why, in a meta-analysis, the association between physician communication and patient adherence was found to be stronger for pediatricians ($r = 0.25$) than adult physicians ($r = 0.18$) [18]. By communicating effectively with the patient's family members, providers can obtain caregivers' insight and knowledge of the patient's behavior and preferences, which has the potential to increase adherence to treatment.

Successful communication between healthcare providers and patients' caregivers also improves satisfaction with care [21]. For example, in a study of youth with chronic conditions (e.g., asthma, diabetes mellitus, or sickle-cell disease) using videotapes of clinic visits, investigators found a significant association between clinic visit satisfaction (based on parent report) and observed friendliness of physicians towards parents [22]. Similarly, in a national survey of parents of youth with diabetes (SEARCH study), 43% of parents reported that communication was a barrier to care, and 48% of parents reported that getting information (defined by having questions discussed/answered) was a barrier to care [23]. These findings are concerning in that patients' caregivers report feeling unable to communicate with providers to allow their questions and concerns to be addressed and answered. But when providers communicate effectively, the result is enhanced transmission and retrieval of important clinical information (e.g., better description of symptoms) and improved understanding of the treatment plan [18], all of which have the potential to increase adherence and improve health outcomes.

Communication with patients is particularly important in pediatric diabetes, given the complexity of the recommended treatment plan and frequency of clinic visits [3]. However, many adolescents with diabetes perceive clinic visits as stressful and negative, describing concerns about confrontation regarding poor glycemic control [24]. Given this negative connotation around provider visits, adolescents are not always willing to exchange important information with providers. A qualitative study of adolescents' experiences of communicating with health professionals highlighted several barriers to good communication between patients and providers [25]. Specifically, adolescents with chronic illness described a reluctance to discuss personal or sensitive issues (especially when parents or other health professionals were in the room) and to ask questions that revealed problems with adherence. Further, adolescents reported feeling as though they were unable to exchange information when the provider had poor communication skills or when the provider focused on the adolescent's health condition without asking about other aspects of the adolescent's life. Similarly, adolescents say that they value health care professionals who take time to offer emotional support [24]. For example, deWit and colleagues demonstrated that asking adolescents about quality of life during clinic visits improved psychosocial well-being and diabetes-related family conflict, and adolescents reported greater satisfaction with care [26]. Providers can also improve outcomes by supporting patient autonomy in developing a treatment plan [20]. Thus, it is important for providers to acknowledge the needs of adolescents and treat them as a critical member of the decision-making process to achieve optimal adherence to the complex treatment regimen.

3. Essential Factors to Improve Communication

Adolescence is a high-risk time for patients with type 1 diabetes, as it is associated with poor glycemic control [6] and problems with adherence [5] as youth take over more responsibility for management. In the following sections, we identify potential factors to improve communication and note implications for practice, by offering recommendations to help providers communicate effectively with adolescents and their caregivers (see Table 1). Since a discussion of all of the factors that may influence communication is beyond the scope of this paper, we focused on time management, technology, health numeracy, and provider burnout as potentially modifiable, provider-led factors that may improve adherence in pediatric diabetes.

Table 1. Essential Factors for Improving Communication.

Factor	Recommendations
Time	■ Pre-visit computerized assessments ■ Use EMR Effectively ■ Group visits
Technology	■ Text messaging as communication tool ■ Integrate technology with interpersonal communication skills
Health Numeracy	■ Practice hypothetical situations during clinic visits ■ Simplify treatment recommendations based on patients' numeracy level
Provider Burnout	■ Practice stress reduction strategies (e.g., mindfulness training) ■ Seek out workplace resources

4. Time Management in the Era of the Electronic Medical Record

Successful communication requires time for providers to communicate with patients and their caregivers; however, with increased use of technology, providers are spending less time in direct patient care, and more time entering data into an electronic system of care [27,28]. This is especially concerning in the context of adolescent visits due to the amount of information providers need to discuss during visits, and the inherent differences in treating adolescents (compared to other developmental stages). The ADA identifies several issues specific to adolescence that need to be addressed by providers, including changes in insulin requirements due to puberty, concerns about self-image, risk of behavioral problems such as depression, transition to self-management, and transition to an adult diabetes provider [29]. In addition, the ADA recommends that providers spend part of each clinic visit alone with adolescents to address these issues [3]. Recent data from the preventive medicine field suggests that in visits that were "partially confidential," in which the adolescent was allowed private discussion time with the provider, there was a statistically significant increase in the number of issues discussed during the visit [30]. The authors of this study suggest that a "split-visit model," in which caregivers participate for a portion of the visit and allow adolescents time alone with their providers, is the most fruitful and allows the most discussion [30], particularly around risk behaviors such as drug and alcohol use, cigarette smoking, and unprotected sexual activity [15]. The unique challenges in caring for adolescents with T1D make time management even more critical to maximize time with patients and their caregivers.

With the mandate to use electronic medical records (EMR), it is especially important for providers to manage their time and maintain good communication throughout the clinic visit with each patient. In a review by Shachak and Reis [31], both positive and negative effects of the EMR on patient-provider communication emerged. Specifically, the authors noted a positive effect on information exchange, but a negative effect on "patient centeredness". The ways in which physicians used the computer during visits influenced their ability to communicate with their patients; while some (the "informational-ignoring physicians") lost rapport with patients because they relied too heavily on the computer at the expense of facing the patient and making regular eye contact, others (the "interpersonal style" physicians) focused more on the patient, spoke to patients without typing, and did not use the computer at the beginning of the encounter. Although this study was not specific to pediatric patients, the findings are relevant to pediatric providers who are communicating with patients and their adult caregivers.

Exploring the specifics of the patient encounter enriches our understanding of how to keep office visits patient centered. A recent study of adult patients examined videotaped patient-provider visits, in which providers used a computer and the electronic health record during the visit. In this sample, patient-centered communication decreased when providers spent more time looking at their computers and when there was increased conversational dead space (defined as time when neither the patient nor the provider was talking) [32]. These findings suggest that providers should learn strategies to maximize patient centeredness and avoid spending the entire patient encounter entering information into the medical record [31,32]. For example, researchers recommend that providers learn "blind typing" (i.e., typing while looking at the patient), start with patient concerns, learn to find patient resources rapidly online, separate data entry from the encounter, point to the screen and highlight data to show the patient, and look at patients during the clinic appointment (e.g., push the monitor away when listening).

Given the time constraints on pediatric providers during routine clinic visits, new time-saving strategies are being developed and tested. For example, conducting screenings prior to the actual patient-physician encounter may streamline patient visits. One study demonstrated that a computerized assessment of health behaviors completed by adolescents in the waiting room (before the visit) allowed physicians to focus on areas of concern with their patients, resulting in positive effects on adherence to recommendations for nutrition and physical activity level [33]. Pediatric diabetes providers could broaden the scope of such a tool to include other relevant information that could then facilitate a discussion during the patient-physician encounter, such as asking about quality of life [26]. For youth who are uncomfortable speaking with providers, creating a list of questions or topics to discuss prior to the visit may also be helpful [24]. Scheduling time for patients and caregivers to meet with a certified diabetes educator may also allow for greater discussion of barriers to adherence than can be addressed during a visit with the physician or nurse practitioner.

Providers have recently explored the use of group visits or shared medical appointments (appointments with multiple patients seen together) as a way to avoid repeating the same information to individual patients and increase direct point of care between the provider and patient [34]. With conditions such as T1D, many families are experiencing similar challenges, and a group setting may allow adolescents and caregivers to share strategies to overcome those challenges [35]. Thus, group appointments may have the indirect benefit of forming a support system for families of youth with T1D. Shared appointments may also present an opportunity for providers to model effective communication around diabetes management. For example, providers can teach and encourage caregivers to review logbooks with their adolescent and talk about "high" and "low" numbers calmly. Given the multiple demands on their time, providers should work to balance their time between direct and indirect patient care (e.g., note entry) and use available resources when possible to maximize time with adolescent patients for discussion of barriers and facilitators to self-management.

5. Technology as a Communication Tool

Providers are increasingly using technology as a tool to increase communication and help adolescents manage their diabetes. Health information technologies, such as automated messages and patient portals, have the potential to facilitate patient-provider communication, and may even improve delivery of care [36]. Adolescents are more likely than adults to use internet-based technologies, due to the flexibility, easy accessibility, and innovative strategies technology allows [37]; therefore, interventions that employ technology may serve as an excellent portal for patient-provider communication. Mobile phone-based options may be especially appealing to adolescents, since 88% of adolescents 13–17 have access to a mobile phone [38]. The use of technology is also an emerging option for patients that live far from medical centers or may not be able to come into diabetes clinic with concerns. For example, Carroll and colleagues [39] tested an intervention that used a cell phone device (Glucophone^{TM}) to automatically deliver adolescent patients' blood glucose values to providers' computers. This data allowed providers to evaluate and offer therapeutic consultations in real time and reduced the worry and concerns of parents. More recently, researchers tested the effects of a mobile app to improve self-management in adolescents with T1D. In a randomized clinical trial comparing adolescents who received the app to usual care, no differences were found in any of the outcomes, including frequency of blood glucose monitoring, glycemic control, or quality of life, and the study authors hypothesized that sharing blood glucose data with providers may have increased the effect of the intervention [40]. Similarly, the feasibility and acceptability of text messaging interventions for youth with T1D has been demonstrated, but the effects on diabetes-related outcomes have been inconsistent [41]. In short, it may be useful for providers of adolescent patients to include an online or technology-based option in their diabetes treatment plans. However, in order to maintain gains in adherence, technology must be integrated with other components of interpersonal communication [42].

6. Health Numeracy

Health numeracy is another important component of health communication in pediatric diabetes, where frequent interpretation of numbers is necessary. There are many skills involved in health numeracy, including the ability to compute basic and multistep math functions and interpret measurements, graphs, and time [43]. In pediatric diabetes, patients (and their caregivers) must be able to identify abnormal blood sugars, calculate correction doses of insulin based on blood sugars that are out of the target range, count carbohydrates and match their meal intake with insulin, and understand general trends of their blood sugars to adjust insulin doses as necessary. Assessing the health numeracy of adolescent patients and their caregivers has potential to improve adherence, given the complexity of the diabetes regimen in the setting of puberty (and changing insulin requirements), school, work, and social changes, and the increased independence of diabetes management.

In a recent study, lower health numeracy among adolescents with diabetes was related to caregivers taking greater responsibility for diabetes care and lower diabetes problem-solving skills in adolescents [44]. These findings support the need for providers to gauge patients' and caregivers' numeracy levels in order to provide appropriate information regarding nutrition, insulin adjustments, and glucose monitoring [45]. For example, if a patient or his/her caregivers cannot read food labels or interpret serving sizes (and therefore are unsure of how many carbohydrates they are eating), the treatment plan is doomed to fail [46]. Providers may find it valuable to provide a hypothetical situation (e.g., asking patients to calculate a mealtime insulin dose using a hypothetical blood sugar and number of carbohydrates eaten) to determine the health numeracy of the patient and/or caregiver, ensure that patients are able to calculate insulin doses correctly, and determine readiness for advanced technologies such as insulin pumps and continuous glucose monitoring systems. In addition, providers may consider using simpler ratios (10 g of carbohydrates: 1 unit of insulin vs. 7:1) when making treatment recommendations to help patients that are experiencing numeracy problems. Pediatric providers are crucial stakeholders in the health of adolescents with diabetes [47]; therefore, it is essential that they are able to successfully communicate the specific components of the treatment plan by taking into account patients' health numeracy.

7. Provider Burnout

Provider burnout may also contribute to poor communication among patients and providers. In recent years, the requirements and obligations of providers have increased; many providers are expected to see patients while meeting external obligations, such as conducting scientific research, mentoring medical students, and engaging in continuing education or career development programs [48]. Providers report stress related to increased workload, reduced control over work environment, and frustration with patients' poor adherence to treatment recommendations [49]. Studies show that 28% of health care providers show clinically significant distress levels [50], and these rates may be increasing. For example, Shenafelt et al. found that physicians' reports of burnout/satisfaction with work-life balance has increased from 45.5% in 2011 to 54.4% in 2014 ($p < 0.001$) [51]. Provider burnout is associated with impairment in patient interaction and communication, deteriorating productivity, and decreased empathy [49,52].

Taking care of adolescent patients with diabetes may be particularly stressful, given the frequency of problems with adherence and challenges meeting treatment goals in this age group. Therefore, stress-reduction programs are needed to alleviate provider burnout that may have a negative impact on communication. For example, mindfulness programs, which focus on "the ability to pay attention in a particular way; on purpose, in the present moment, and nonjudgmentally" [53] have proven effective for decreasing physician burnout and increasing personal accomplishment and empathy [54]. Further, medical centers have made efforts to address burnout by providing resources for providers. For example, a pilot program at Stanford University allowed faculty to trade time spent on committees and other administrative duties for in-home support, such as meal delivery and cleaning services, or work-related support, such as grant writing assistance. This program increased the feeling of being supported, especially among female faculty [55]. In order to increase positive health outcomes among both themselves and their patients, providers should monitor stress levels and seek out resources within the workplace or community for reducing and managing stress. By preventing and addressing burnout, providers may be more effective in their interactions with patients [52].

8. Implications for Practice

Communication between the patient, caregiver, and provider is an essential component of promoting adherence in pediatric diabetes. Fortunately, research supports the notion that communication skills are a modifiable factor [56]; a meta-analysis of communication training programs for physicians' demonstrated increases in collaborative communication, empathy, and improved attitudes toward psychosocial issues [56]. For example, a recent study used standardized patients to enact phone call counseling scenarios to improve physician (pediatrician or family physician) communication. Physicians were asked to call the "mother" (standardized patient) of a newborn who had specific newborn screening results that needed to be reviewed. After the baseline counseling phone call, the intervention group received a report card providing feedback and outlining various aspects of their communication. Both the intervention and control groups then performed another phone counseling session with a standardized patient. The authors found that the intervention group improved in certain areas of all four of the quality indicators studied ("assessment of understanding," "organizing behaviors," "precautionary empathy," and "jargon" use) [57]. These findings highlight specific ways that training could improve providers' communication in pediatric diabetes by providing autonomy support to patients and taking a more collaborative approach [58].

In addition, training in cultural competency has the potential to improve providers' communication skills. It is well established that a better understanding of patients' cultural beliefs, values, and traditions also improves communication and may increase disclosure of personal health information [59]. However, a recent review by Twomey [60] highlighted the lack of culturally competent communication among pediatric healthcare providers and their patients, concluding that many providers lack the training required to provide optimal care among culturally diverse populations. To address these deficits, many healthcare systems are gradually integrating training programs related to cultural sensitivity that helps providers to be more effective in communicating with ethnic minorities. In a systematic review of 34 studies on this topic, the authors determined that there is no one specific way to train providers about culture; however, there is substantial evidence that cultural competency training improves clinicians' knowledge and impacts the attitude and skills of healthcare providers [61].

Finally, the recent changes to the Medical College Admission Test (which is required for admission to medical school) to include a section on social and behavioral sciences is noteworthy in regards to provider communication [62]. The Association of American Medical Colleges hopes that the increased focus on social and health care issues will result in more well-rounded physicians. Changing the way providers are trained and requiring that providers understand the behavioral and socio-cultural issues of their patients, signals an important shift toward acknowledging the importance of provider communication. Similarly, the inclusion of patient-centered communication in the ADA's 2015 recommendation for care reflects this shift [63].

Effective communication between providers, patients, and caregivers is essential to mitigate the many challenges facing pediatric patients with T1D and has the potential to improve adherence in patients with T1D. In this review, we identified several potentially modifiable factors that can impede successful communication and offered recommendations for providers to address these barriers (see Table 1). More research is needed to determine the most effective, specific communication strategies for providers who care for adolescents with T1D. Given that adolescents with T1D are a high-risk sample, even small improvements in patient-provider communication have the potential to improve adherence and other outcomes.

Acknowledgments: Karishma A. Datye is supported by a generous gift from the Odom Family.

Author Contributions: N.J.P. researched the topic, wrote the paper, and created the table. K.A.D. wrote the discussion section, edited the paper and created the figure. S.S.J. wrote the introduction and edited the paper.

References

1. Diabetes Control and Complications Trial Research Group. The effect of intensive treatment of diabetes on the development and progression of long-term complications in insulin-dependent diabetes mellitus. *N. Engl. J. Med.* **1993**, *329*, 977–986.

2. Hamman, R.F.; Bell, R.A.; Dabelea, D.; D'Agostino, R.B.; Dolan, L.; Imperatore, G.; Lawrence, J.M.; Linder, B.; Marcovina, S.M.; Mayer-Davis, E.J.; et al. The SEARCH for Diabetes in Youth study: Rationale, findings, and future directions. *Diabetes Care* **2014**, *37*, 3336–3344. [CrossRef] [PubMed]

3. American Diabetes Association. Standards of Medical Care in Diabetes—2018. *Diabetes Care* **2018**, *41*, S1–S2.

4. Jaser, S.S.; Datye, K.A. Frequency of missed insulin boluses in type 1 diabetes and its impact on diabetes control. *Diabetes Technol. Ther.* **2016**, *18*, 341–342. [CrossRef] [PubMed]

5. Borus, J.S.; Laffel, L. Adherence challenges in the management of type 1 diabetes in adolescents: Prevention and intervention. *Curr. Opin. Pediatr.* **2010**, *22*, 405–411. [CrossRef] [PubMed]

6. Miller, K.M.; Foster, N.C.; Beck, R.W.; Bergenstal, R.M.; DuBose, S.N.; DiMeglio, L.A.; Maahs, D.M.; Tamborlane, W.V.; T1D Exchange Clinic Network. Current state of type 1 diabetes treatment in the U.S.: Updated data from the T1D Exchange clinic registry. *Diabetes Care* **2015**, *38*, 971–978. [CrossRef] [PubMed]

7. Pinhas-Hamiel, O.; Hamiel, U.; Boyko, V.; Graph-Barel, C.; Reichman, B.; Lerner-Geva, L. Trajectories of HbA1c Levels in Children and Youth with Type 1 Diabetes. *PLoS ONE* **2014**, *9*, e109109. [CrossRef] [PubMed]

8. Clements, M.A.; Foster, N.C.; Maahs, D.M.; Schatz, D.A.; Olson, B.A.; Tsalikian, E.; Lee, J.M.; Burt-Solorzano, C.M.; Tamborlane, W.V.; Chen, V.; et al. Hemoglobin A1c (HbA1c) changes over time among adolescent and young adult participants in the T1D exchange clinic registry. *Pediatr. Diabetes* **2016**, *17*, 327–336. [CrossRef] [PubMed]

9. Young, M.T.; Lord, J.H.; Patel, N.J.; Gruhn, M.A.; Jaser, S.S. Good cop, bad cop: Quality of parental involvement in type 1 diabetes management in youth. *Curr. Diabetes Rep.* **2014**, *14*, 546. [CrossRef] [PubMed]

10. Palladino, D.K.; Helgeson, V.S. Friends or foes? A review of peer influence on self-care and glycemic control in adolescents with type 1 diabetes. *J. Pediatr. Psychol.* **2012**, *37*, 591–603. [CrossRef] [PubMed]

11. Delamater, A.M.; de Wit, M.; McDarby, V.; Malik, J.; Acerini, C.L. Psychological care of children and adolescents with type 1 diabetes. *Pediatr. Diabetes* **2014**, *15*, 232–244. [CrossRef] [PubMed]

12. Naranjo, D.; Mulvaney, S.; McGrath, M.; Garnero, T.; Hood, K. Predictors of self-management in pediatric type 1 diabetes: Individual, family, systemic, and technologic influences. *Curr. Diabetes Rep.* **2014**, *14*, 544. [CrossRef] [PubMed]

13. Amiel, S.A.; Sherwin, R.S.; Simonson, D.C.; Lauritano, A.A.; Tamborlane, W.V. Impaired insulin action in puberty. *N. Engl. J. Med.* **1986**, *315*, 215–219. [CrossRef] [PubMed]

14. Comeaux, S.J.; Jaser, S.S. Autonomy and insulin in adolescents with type 1 diabetes. *Pediatr. Diabetes* **2010**, *11*, 498–504. [CrossRef] [PubMed]

15. Suris, J.C.; Michaud, P.A.; Akre, C.; Sawyer, S.M. Health risk behaviors in adolescents with chronic conditions. *Pediatrics* **2008**, *122*, e1113–e1118. [CrossRef] [PubMed]

16. Weitzman, E.R.; Ziemnik, R.E.; Huang, Q.; Levy, S. Alcohol and marijuana use and treatment nonadherence among medically vulnerable youth. *Pediatrics* **2015**, *136*, 450–457. [CrossRef] [PubMed]

17. Sarbacker, G.B.; Urteaga, E.M. Adherence to insulin therapy. *Diabetes Spectrum* **2016**, *29*, 166–170. [CrossRef] [PubMed]

18. Zolnierek, K.B.H.; DiMatteo, M.R. Physician communication and patient adherence to treatment: A meta-analysis. *Med. Care* **2009**, *47*, 826–834. [CrossRef] [PubMed]

19. Ong, L.M.; De Haes, J.C.; Hoos, A.M.; Lammes, F.B. Doctor-patient communication: A review of the literature. *Soc. Sci. Med.* **1995**, *40*, 903–918. [CrossRef]

20. Street, R.L.; Makoul, G.; Arora, N.K.; Epstein, R.M. How does communication heal? Pathways linking clinician–patient communication to health outcomes. *Patient Educ. Couns.* **2009**, *74*, 295–301. [CrossRef] [PubMed]

21. Nobile, C.; Drotar, D. Research on the quality of parent-provider communication in pediatric care: Implications and recommendations. *J. Dev. Behav. Pediatr.* **2003**, *24*, 279–290. [CrossRef] [PubMed]

22. Swedlund, M.P.; Schumacher, J.B.; Young, H.N.; Cox, E.D. Effect of communication style and physician–family relationships on satisfaction with pediatric chronic disease care. *Health Commun.* **2012**, *27*, 498–505. [CrossRef] [PubMed]

23. Valenzuela, J.M.; Seid, M.; Waitzfelder, B.; Anderson, A.M.; Beavers, D.P.; Dabelea, D.M.; Dolan, L.M.; Impatore, G.; Marcovina, S.; Reynolds, K.; et al. Prevalence of and disparities in barriers to care experienced by youth with type 1 diabetes. *J. Pediatr.* **2014**, *164*, 1369–1375. [CrossRef] [PubMed]

24. Lowes, L.; Eddy, D.; Channon, S.; McNamara, R.; Robling, M.; Gregory, J.W.; DEPICTED Study Team. The experience of living with type 1 diabetes and attending clinic from the perception of children, adolescents and carers: Analysis of qualitative data from the DEPICTED study. *J. Pediatr. Nurs.* **2015**, *30*, 54–62. [CrossRef] [PubMed]

25. Beresford, B.A.; Sloper, P. Chronically ill adolescents' experiences of communicating with doctors: A qualitative study. *J. Adolesc. Health* **2003**, *33*, 172–179. [CrossRef]

26. De Wit, M.; Delemarre-van de Waal, H.A.; Bokma, J.A.; Haasnoot, K.; Houdijk, M.C.; Gemke, R.J.; Snoek, F.J. Monitoring and Discussing Health-Related Quality of Life in Adolescents with Type 1 Diabetes Improve Psychosocial Well-Being: A randomized controlled trial. *Diabetes Care* **2008**, *31*, 1521–1526. [CrossRef] [PubMed]

27. Block, L.; Habicht, R.; Wu, A.W.; Desai, S.V.; Wang, K.; Silva, K.N.; Niessen, T.; Oliver, N.; Feldman, L. In the wake of the 2003 and 2011 duty hours regulations, how do internal medicine interns spend their time? *J. Gen. Intern. Med.* **2013**, *28*, 1042–1047. [CrossRef] [PubMed]

28. Friedberg, M.W.; Chen, P.G.; Aunon, F.M.; Van Busum, K.R.; Pham, C.; Caloyeras, J.P.; Mattke, S.; Pitchforth, E.; Quigley, D.D.; Brook, R.H.; et al. *Factors Affecting Physician Professional Satisfaction and Their Implications for Patient Care, Health Systems, and Health Policy*; RAND Corporation: Monica, CA, USA, 2014.

29. Chiang, J.L.; Kirkman, M.S.; Laffel, L.M.; Peters, A.L. Type 1 diabetes through the life span: A position statement of the American Diabetes Association. *Diabetes Care* **2014**, *37*, 2034–2054. [CrossRef] [PubMed]

30. Gilbert, A.L.; Rickert, V.I.; Aalsma, M.C. Clinical conversations about health: The impact of confidentiality in preventive adolescent care. *J. Adolesc. Health* **2014**, *55*, 672–677. [CrossRef] [PubMed]

31. Shachak, A.; Reis, S. The impact of electronic medical records on patient–doctor communication during consultation: A narrative literature review. *J. Eval. Clin. Pract.* **2009**, *15*, 641–649. [CrossRef] [PubMed]

32. Street, R.L.; Liu, L.; Farber, N.J.; Chen, Y.; Calvitti, A.; Zuest, D.; Gabuzda, M.T.; Bell, K.; Gray, B.; Rick, S.; et al. Provider interaction with the electronic health record: The effects on patient-centered communication in medical encounters. *Patient Educ. Couns.* **2014**, *96*, 315–319. [CrossRef] [PubMed]

33. Patrick, K.; Sallis, J.F.; Prochaska, J.J.; Lydston, D.D.; Calfas, K.J.; Zabinski, M.F.; Wilfley, D.E.; Saelens, B.E.; Brown, D.R. A multicomponent program for nutrition and physical activity change in primary care: PACE+ for adolescents. *Arch. Pediatr. Adolesc. Med.* **2001**, *155*, 940–946. [CrossRef] [PubMed]

34. Quiñones, A.R.; Richardson, J.; Freeman, M.; Fu, R.; O'Neil, M.E.; Motu'apuaka, M.; Kansagara, D. Educational group visits for the management of chronic health conditions: A systematic review. *Patient Educ. Couns.* **2014**, *95*, 3–29. [CrossRef] [PubMed]

35. Berget, C.; Lindwall, J.; Shea, J.J.; Klingensmith, G.J.; Anderson, B.J.; Cain, C.; Raymond, J.K. Team Clinic: An Innovative Group Care Model for Youth With Type 1 Diabetes—Engaging Patients and Meeting Educational Needs. *J. Nurse Pract.* **2017**, *3*, e269–e272. [CrossRef] [PubMed]

36. Wade-Vuturo, A.E.; Mayberry, L.S.; Osborn, C.Y. Secure messaging and diabetes management: Experiences and perspectives of patient portal users. *J. Am. Med. Inform. Assoc.* **2013**, *20*, 519–525. [CrossRef] [PubMed]

37. Harris, M.A.; Hood, K.K.; Mulvaney, S.A. Pumpers, skypers, surfers and texters: Technology to improve the management of diabetes in teenagers. *Diabetes Obes. Metab.* **2012**, *14*, 967–972. [CrossRef] [PubMed]

38. Lenhart, A. Teens, Social Media & Technology Overview. 2015. Available online: http://www.pewinternet. org/2015/04/09/teens-social-media-technology-2015 (accessed on 1 February 2018).

39. Carroll, A.E.; DiMeglio, L.A.; Stein, S.; Marrero, D.G. Using a cell phone–based glucose monitoring system for adolescent diabetes management. *Diabetes Educ.* **2011**, *37*, 59–66. [CrossRef] [PubMed]

40. Goyal, S.; Nunn, C.A.; Rotondi, M.; Couperthwaite, A.B.; Reiser, S.; Simone, A.; Katzman, D.K.; Cafazzo, J.A.; Palmert, M.R. A mobile app for the self-management of type 1 diabetes among adolescents: A randomized controlled trial. *JMIR mHealth uHealth* **2017**, *5*, e82. [CrossRef] [PubMed]

41. Herbert, L.; Owen, V.; Pascarella, L.; Streisand, R. Text message interventions for children and adolescents with type 1 diabetes: A systematic review. *Diabetes Technol. Ther.* **2013**, *15*, 362–370. [CrossRef] [PubMed]

42. Mulvaney, S.A.; Ritterband, L.M.; Bosslet, L. Mobile intervention design in diabetes: Review and recommendations. *Curr. Diabetes Rep.* **2011**, *11*, 486–493. [CrossRef] [PubMed]

43. Montori, V.M.; Rothman, R.L. Weakness in numbers. The Challenge of numeracy in health care. *J. Gen. Intern. Med.* **2005**, *20*, 1071–1072. [CrossRef] [PubMed]

44. Mulvaney, S.A.; Lilley, J.S.; Cavanaugh, K.L.; Pittel, E.J.; Rothman, R.L. Validation of the diabetes numeracy test with adolescents with type 1 diabetes. *J. Health Commun.* **2013**, *18*, 795–804. [CrossRef] [PubMed]

45. Rothman, R.L.; Montori, V.M.; Cherrington, A.; Pignone, M.P. Perspective: The role of numeracy in health care. *J. Health Commun.* **2008**, *13*, 583–595. [CrossRef] [PubMed]

46. Rothman, R.L.; Housam, R.; Weiss, H.; Davis, D.; Gregory, R.; Gebretsadik, T.; Shintani, A.; Elasy, T.A. Patient understanding of food labels: The role of literacy and numeracy. *Am. J. Prev. Med.* **2006**, *31*, 391–398. [CrossRef] [PubMed]

47. Drotar, D. Physician behavior in the care of pediatric chronic illness: Association with health outcomes and treatment adherence. *J. Dev. Behav. Pediatr.* **2009**, *30*, 246–254. [CrossRef] [PubMed]

48. Gabel, S. Demoralization in health professional practice: Development, amelioration, and implications for continuing education. *J. Contin. Educ. Health Prof.* **2013**, *33*, 118–126. [CrossRef] [PubMed]

49. Linzer, M.; Gerrity, M.; Douglas, J.A.; McMurray, J.E.; Williams, E.S.; Konrad, T.R. Physician stress: Results from the physician worklife study. *Stress Health* **2002**, *18*, 37–42. [CrossRef]

50. Firth-Cozens, J. Doctors, their wellbeing, and their stress. *BMJ* **2003**, *326*, 670–671. [CrossRef] [PubMed]

51. Shanafelt, T.D.; Hasan, O.; Dyrbye, L.N.; Sinsky, C.; Satele, D.; Sloan, J.; West, C.P. Changes in burnout and satisfaction with work-life balance in physicians and the general US working population between 2011 and 2014. *Mayo Clin. Proc.* **2015**, *90*, 1600–1613. [CrossRef] [PubMed]

52. Shanafelt, T.D.; West, C.; Zhao, X.; Novotny, P.; Kolars, J.; Habermann, T.; Sloan, J. Relationship between increased personal well-being and enhanced empathy among internal medicine residents. *J. Gen. Intern. Med.* **2005**, *20*, 559–564. [CrossRef] [PubMed]

53. Kabat-Zinn, J. *Wherever You Go, There You Are: Mindfulness Meditation in Everyday Life*; Hachette Books: New York, NY, USA, 2009.

54. Krasner, M.S.; Epstein, R.M.; Beckman, H.; Suchman, A.L.; Chapman, B.; Mooney, C.J.; Quill, T.E. Association of an educational program in mindful communication with burnout, empathy, and attitudes among primary care physicians. *JAMA* **2009**, *302*, 1284–1293. [CrossRef] [PubMed]

55. Wright, A.A.; Katz, I.T. Beyond burnout—Redesigning care to restore meaning and sanity for physicians. *N. Engl. J. Med.* **2018**, *378*, 309–311. [CrossRef] [PubMed]

56. Jenkins, V.; Fallowfield, L. Can communication skills training alter physicians' beliefs and behavior in clinics? *J. Clin. Oncol.* **2002**, *20*, 765–769. [PubMed]

57. Farrell, M.H.; Christopher, S.A.; Kirschner, A.L.P.; Roedl, S.J.; Faith, O.O.; Ahmad, N.Y.; Farrell, P.M. Improving the quality of physician communication with rapid-throughput analysis and report cards. *Patient Educ. Couns.* **2014**, *97*, 248–255. [CrossRef] [PubMed]

58. Delamater, A.M. Improving patient adherence. *Clin. Diabetes* **2006**, *24*, 71–77. [CrossRef]

59. Havranek, E.P.; Hanratty, R.; Tate, C.; Dickinson, L.M.; Steiner, J.F.; Cohen, G.; Blair, I.A. The effect of values affirmation on race-discordant patient-provider communication. *Arch. Intern. Med.* **2012**, *172*, 1662–1667. [CrossRef] [PubMed]

60. Twomey, T.C. Pediatricians and pediatric nurses in the delivery of culturally competent care: A scoping literature review to investigate progress and issues around culturally diverse care in pediatrics. *Pediatr. Neonatal Nurs. Open J.* **2014**, *1*, 19–25. [CrossRef]

61. Lie, D.A.; Lee-Rey, E.; Gomez, A.; Bereknyei, S.; Braddock, C.H., III. Does cultural competency training of health professionals improve patient outcomes? A systematic review and proposed algorithm for future research. *J. Gen. Intern. Med.* **2011**, *26*, 317–325. [CrossRef] [PubMed]

62. Mann, S. AAMC Approves New MCAT Exam with Increased Focus on Social, Behavioral Sciences. Available online: https://www.aamc.org/newsroom/reporter/march2012/276588/mcat2015.html (accessed on 1 February 2018).

63. American Diabetes Association. Strategies for Improving Care. *Diabetes Care* **2015**, *38*, S5–S7.

12

A Population-Based Conceptual Framework for Evaluating the Role of Healthcare Services in Place of Death

Wei Gao [1],* ⓘ, Sumaya Huque [1], Myfanwy Morgan [2] and Irene J. Higginson [1]

[1] Cicely Saunders Institute of Palliative Care, Policy and Rehabilitation, King's College London, Bessemer Road, Denmark Hill, London SE5 9PJ, UK; Sumaya.huque@gmail.com (S.H.); Irene.higginson@kcl.ac.uk (I.J.H.)

[2] Institute of Pharmaceutical Science, King's College London, London SE1 9NH, UK; Myfanwy.morgan@kcl.ac.uk

* Correspondence: wei.gao@kcl.ac.uk

Abstract: Background: There is a significant geographical disparity in place of death. Socio-demographic and disease-related variables only explain less than a quarter of the variation. Healthcare service factors may account for some (or much) of the remaining variation but their effects have never been systematically evaluated, partly due to the lack of a conceptual framework. This study aims to propose a population-based framework to guide the evaluation of the role of the healthcare service factors in place of death. Methods: Review and synthesis of health service models that include the impact of a service component on either place of death/end of life care outcomes or service access/utilization. Results: The framework conceptualizes the impact of healthcare services on the place of death as starting from the end of life care policies that in turn influence service commissioning and shape healthcare service characteristics, including service type, service capacity—facilities, service location, and workforce, through which service utilization and ultimately place of death are affected. Patient socio-demographics, disease-related variables, family and community support and social care also influence place of death, but they are not the focus of this framework and therefore are grouped as needs and other environmental factors. Information on service utilization, together with the place of death, creates loop feedback to inform policy and service commission. Conclusions: The framework provides guidance for analysis aiming to understand the role of healthcare services in place of death. It aids the interpretation of results in the light of existing knowledge and potentially identifies service factors that can be addressed to improve end of life care.

Keywords: place of death; healthcare services; conceptual framework; end of life care outcome; end of life care policies and commissioning; determinants

1. Background

Place of death has evolved over the past two decades from a quality indicator to an outcome measure in end of life care (EoLC) [1,2]. Although the majority of terminally ill patients prefer to die at home or in a home-like environment such as hospices, hospitals remain the most common place of death. In 2001–2010, of all deaths from non-accidental causes (N = 4.6 million) in England, 57% occurred in a hospital, 19% at home, 17% in a care home, and only 5% in hospice [3]. It is a national commitment of the United Kingdom (UK) policy to offer people who are approaching the end of life to die in a place of their choice [4,5] with national and local efforts directed to facilitating such a choice. However, without high-quality EoLC provision, the choice of place of death can never be a real one. A survey of 245 family physicians found that 94% of patients admitted to hospital with limited life expectancy was due to an inadequate care provision (i.e., an acute situation for which the care setting was not prepared) in their usual care setting [6]. Characterizing where people die and the factors that influence their site of death is important to inform the development and implementation of policy and EoLC services.

A systematic review [7] involving 58 studies, with over 1.5 million patients from 13 countries, concluded that place of death results from interactions between three main groups of factors: those related to the illness, the individual, and the environment. The GUIDE_Care project which investigated variations in place of death using routine death registry data found that individual patient level characteristics, such as age, marital status and diagnosis, were able to explain only a quarter of the variation in place of death [3]. These findings suggest that variables related to healthcare services may have a role in determining the place of death. However, there is a scarcity of empirical studies that have systematically assessed the influence of healthcare service provision on place of death. Two major reviews [7,8] on the determinants of place of death identified a total of 87 studies, few of which evaluated the role of healthcare services in place of death. A key barrier, as identified by Phillips et al., is the lack of a conceptual model [9].

The aim of this paper is to propose a conceptual framework to guide the planning, analysis, and interpretation of factors related to healthcare services that may influence place of death.

2. Methods

The development of this framework was built on a conceptual model of factors influencing death at home by Gomes & Higginson [7], identified through the search of published and peer-reviewed literatures (up to August 2018) in Ovid MEDLINE, EMBASE and PsycInfo. The details of the search are enclosed in Appendix A. It was also the only theoretical model on the determinants of place of death resulting from our literature search. However, this model was developed from empirical studies and contains limited information on healthcare variables. Hence, we identified six further health service models, which include the impact of a service component on either end of life care outcomes or service access/utilization [9–14]. Other than Laguna's model, which was selected on the basis of its close relevance to end of life care, the other models were generic but widely cited in health service research. The service components that may potentially influence place of death (Table 1) and their sequential organization were identified from and guided by these models.

Table 1. The components of the referenced models contributed.

Models	Contributed Components
Gomes & Higginson, 2006	Patient factors, other environmental factors
Phillips, et al., 1998	Policies, commissioning
Andersen & Newman, 2005	Service type, service capacity—facilities
Levesque et al., 2013	Service location, commissioning
Donabedian, 1988	Workforce
Kindig et al., 2008	Commissioning, service location
Laguna et al., 2012	Service type, workforce, commissioning

3. Results

3.1. The Conceptual Framework

Healthcare services in this framework refer to all health and care services related to end of life care; these include generic (e.g., hospital, general practice) and specialized (e.g., hospice) care services (Figure 1). The characteristics of such provision initially depend on the EoLC policies and their implementation through healthcare service commissioning, which, in turn, influences service utilization and ultimately where people die. Individual socio-demographic and disease-related characteristics (patient factors), together with social care, and family and community support (environmental factors), are not the focus of this framework; they are included as the variables to be controlled for when evaluating the service impact on the place of death. Information on service utilization and place of death create loop feedback to inform end of life care policies and service commissioning. The arrows indicate the direction of the impact. The solid and dotted lines represent direct and indirect effects (or feedback loop), respectively.

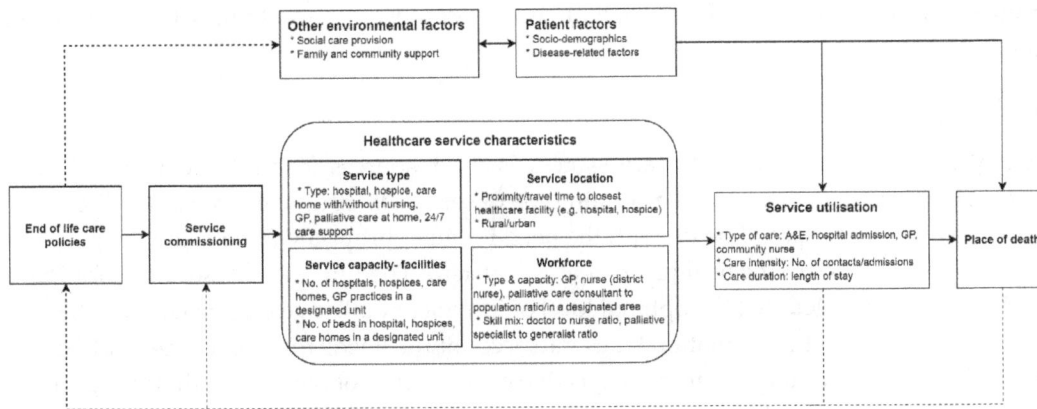

Figure 1. A conceptual framework for the role of healthcare service factors in place of death.

3.2. End of Life Care Policies

Variations in health care utilization and outcomes between geographic areas have been linked to broad health system policies and provision [15], although no formal research has evaluated the policy impact on the population-based end of life care outcomes. However, a series of large-scale natural experimental studies using the English death registry database provided some evidence for a causal link between national EoLC improvement efforts, which promote community based care and increased home deaths [2,16–18]. The addition of EoLC policies in our framework prompts the identification of concrete actions and policy levers that have been taken to improve EoLC quality [4].

3.3. Service Commissioning

Healthcare service planning and commissioning is the process of deciding what kinds of services should be provided to local populations, who should provide them, and how they should be paid for. The UK's End of Life Care Strategy (2008) focused on raising the profile of EoLC with strategic commissioning, delivery of high-quality services, and enhanced education, training and research in the field [4]. The strategy also emphasizes the importance of coordinated care and support for caregivers. This is supported by evidence from a study in the United States that spending on home and community-based services increases the chance of home death, through reducing the risk of the end of life relocation to a nursing home [19].

3.4. Healthcare Service Characteristics

Healthcare services are characterized by type, capacity (facilities and workforces) and location. These characteristics can be perceived as resulting from EoLC policies requiring service commissioning and service providers to take actions to improve EoLC and its outcomes. We put these characteristics in separate boxes, signifying that they are relatively independent of each other and cite some indicators that may be used to represent the corresponding service characteristics.

3.5. Service Type

The service options available to patients is a key determinant of where they die [7,8]. When hospital-based care dominated the healthcare system, most people died in hospitals [20].

However place of death has been slowly but steadily shifting to home or usual residence over the past two decades in countries with efforts to promote community-based palliative and end of life care [3,18,20–24]. Studies have shown that home-based care delivered at a patient's home is effective in enabling home deaths [25,26]. General practitioners' home visits during the last three months was positively associated with death at home [27]. Enrolment in palliative care programs was associated with lower odds of dying in hospitals [28]. For analysis purposes, type of care can be categorized into primary (General Practice—GP, care home), secondary (hospital) and tertiary (specialist palliative services) care.

3.6. Service Capacity—Facilities

A key component of the healthcare system is the resources (capital and labor) devoted to healthcare [10]. The mere presence of a certain type of service is insufficient to lead to the use of the service and a change in place of death with the need for an appropriate fit between the population's demand and the supplies of the healthcare delivery system. The European Association for Palliative Care (EAPC) recommended that the optimal level of in-patient palliative care provision is 80–100 bed per million population. This estimation takes into account the needs for both cancer and non-cancer conditions [29]. A 10-year large-scale retrospective cohort study of patients with lung cancer found that hospice death was more likely in areas with more hospice beds [30]. Similar supply-side (service provision and availability) effects were also seen in the pattern of hospice deaths in children and young people with cancer—overall, hospice death was low but more than doubled in the proportion from 6% to 13% during the study period, where hospice service provision was also improved [18]. Rates (number of facilities, beds in a defined unit, e.g., per 100,000 inhabitants) and densities (number of facilities, beds or staffing in a defined size of the area, e.g., per square kilometers) can be used to measure and compare service capacity of different regions.

3.7. Service Location

A growing body of research suggests that the geographical accessibility of healthcare facilities, and not merely the general level of provision of services in a geographic area, has a definitive role in service utilization and health outcomes [11,31,32]. Proximity to a specific healthcare facility, (e.g., hospital, hospice or nursing home) has been shown to increase the probability of cancer patients dying in that particular facility [33]. The geographical location of services has implication for resource allocation and optimization. We, therefore, included the location of healthcare services as a determinant of the place of death in our conceptual model. Geographical accessibility to services can be measured at the individual or area level. A commonly used measure is the distance from a patient's residential address to their closest hospital, hospice, and care home [34], or the average of the individually measured distances of a group of patients in an area of interests for an area level measure. With technology advancement, more sophisticated measures (e.g., travel time incorporating road attributes) have been proposed and developed [35]. Rural/urban settlement, which is often identified as an attributable factor for disparities in service usage and place of death [36,37], can also be used as a proxy measure for service availability and accessibility.

3.8. Workforce

Healthcare services can be viewed as complex and interdependent interventions that lead to changes in health and care outcomes. Delivering high-quality EoLC requires a well-developed and highly competent workforce [38,39]. The involvement of general practitioners in facilitating patients to achieve their preferred place of death is consistent across studies [27,40,41]. The mechanism through which the workforce exerts an impact on the place of death is yet unknown but may be related to the following aspects: the category of the workforce (e.g., general practitioner, nurse, palliative care consultant), staffing level, and skill mix. The staffing level can be measured by the number of full-time equivalent employees, such as the nurse-to-patient ratio [42].

Skill mix refers to the mix and breadth of staff, professions, and experience and/or qualifications [43]. The right skill mix is needed for both effective and efficient patient care, including the end of life care [44]; it is a quality statement (QS16) in the National Institute for Health and Care Excellence (NICE) guidance for End of Life Care for adults [45]. The EAPC recommended that the core team for palliative care should consist of doctors and nurses as a minimum [46], though no study has investigated whether and how skill mix is related to place of death. This needs to be addressed in future studies. A common measure for the skill mix is the ratio of the number of staff in selected (usually two) workforce categories. For example, palliative care consultant to nurse ratio.

As palliative and end of life care is a multidisciplinary approach encompassing not only physical but also psychological, social and spiritual components, future workforce evaluation studies should also consider non-healthcare workforces.

3.9. Service Utilisation

It is through utilizing service that the healthcare delivery system achieves its impact on the place of death. Service utilization can be measured at area level by the number of admissions, lengths of stays, and bed occupancies in hospitals, hospices, and emergency units. Ecological level (e.g., national, area) statistics on health service use are routinely released to the public domain [47–50]. These data are often summarised by care settings though that which are specific to PEoLC are very limited. The National End of Life Care Intelligence Network of Public Health England (http://www.endoflifecare-intelligence.org.uk) has been set up to fill this information gap but is still well-behind other care settings. According to our framework, service utilization should be modelled as a mediating factor between service characteristics and place of death outcome [51].

3.10. Needs and Other Environmental Factors

The focus of this framework is the healthcare service input on the place of death. Therefore, we group all other non-health service variables that may influence place of death as needs and other environmental factors. Needs factors include the clinical and socio-demographic characteristics of individuals [7,52]. The provision of PEoLC was historically focused on patients with terminal cancer. However, the modern view is that PEoLC services should be provided on the basis of needs rather than the diagnosis. Patients with certain non-cancer conditions, frail older people, and patients with multiple morbidities may have PEoLC needs and can benefit from palliative care input [53]. One method of measuring service needs at the population level can be using underlying (e.g., cancer versus non-cancer) and contributory causes of deaths (e.g., the number of comorbidities) reported in routine death registry data [54].

Family and community support are crucial in enabling dying people to remain at home or in their usual residence. Marital status is often used as a proxy for family support. A national population-based study in cancer patients in England found patients who are single, divorced, or widowed were less likely to die at home, compared to those who are married [2]. At the population level, the percentage of individuals summarised according to their marital status is freely available through official statistics websites, e.g., the Office for National Statistics (ONS)'census portal [55]. Area-level spending on social care may serve as an indicator of the level of social care provision. There has not yet been a formal evaluation of the impact of social care provision on place of death, but social care (measured at the individual level) costs were negatively associated with inpatient care costs [56], suggesting social care may play a role in place of death. A recent Australian study provided further qualitative evidence that specially trained community care workers can effectively support patients and their families in home settings at the end of life [57], though none of them have quantified the effects of social care.

4. Discussion

We present a conceptual framework identifying service factors that may affect the place of death and how. To our knowledge, this is the first-of-its-kind for an important end of life care outcome—place of death. This model can be used to guide the evaluation of the population-based impact of service factors on place of death, from data collection to data analysis and interpretation. To date, the majority of published studies on the place of death has a focus on individual socio-demographic and clinical characteristics [2,16,58,59]. A large-scale observational study conducted in the UK found that only a quarter, or even less for certain diseases, of the geographical variation in place of death are explained by patient-level characteristics [3].

The framework notes the importance of various service components in determining where people die; they are positioned in the middle of a causal pathway. The chain of reaction starts from the national policy followed by service commissioning. They go on to affect service characteristics, which then influence service utilization and ultimately place of death. The framework can be used to guide population-based service planning and development. Service commissioners should take into consideration four aspects of service factors: type, capacity (facilities), location, and workforce. The relative contribution of the individual components to service utilization and place of death has not yet been quantified, but it is critical to help design programs and prioritize intervention. It is worth noting that the feedback loop between service utilization, place of death, and policies that will change service characteristics through planning and commissioning, highlighting intervention at any levels (e.g., policy, planning and commissioning, service), should be a dynamic rather than a one-off process of learning.

A patient's palliative care needs encompass four dimensions: physical, psychological, social, and spiritual. According to Maslow [60], these needs are in hierarchical structures with physical at the lowest and spiritual the highest level. It means that the higher needs may not be relevant until the lower ones are met. Therefore, unless we can provide high-quality end of life care to meet a patient's lower level (e.g., physical) needs across all available settings, the preferred place of care and death do not have a real meaning to patients and families. In fact, patients choose a hospital as their preferred setting for the end of life care because they feel that the hospital is safer than other care settings, e.g., their own home or usual residence [61]. In other words, patients do not always feel safe at home or that care need can be best met at home—this, per se, indicates service gaps.

The key challenge for population-based service evaluation is data availability. The data scoping exercise for the GUIDE_Care Services project identified large gaps in service data. There exists very limited national-level service data in palliative and end of life care. Even a master list of hospices was not available in the public domain with easy access options to researchers and stakeholders. This is in contrast to personal-level data, where the major challenge lies in accessibility issues related to information governance, confidentiality, and data protection [62]. Service data are collected at the aggregate level and do not require ethical approvals for access. Even for commissioning data, which is supposed to be open and transparent, there is no centralized data portal. In England, only an annual CCG spending of over 25 k on palliative and end of life care is available in the public domain; however, not all CCGs submit this data. Service data collection is not as well developed as that of person-level data; most of the service-level data collections take place at the local level and a few at a larger scale or national level. The methods for local data collection vary widely, and data reporting and capture are far from being a routine at all levels. These all hamper the effort to evaluate and understand the role of service factors in place of death. There is urgent need to develop systems for service data collection.

As service variables are collected at the aggregate level, the choice of analytical methods is dependent on the study unit. If it is at service level, then the data can be analyzed using conventional statistical methods, which assume the independence of units of analysis. For studies with patients as the unit of analysis and involving a mixture of service- and individual-level variables, more sophisticated analytical methods such as multilevel models or more appropriately causal modelling should be used to account for the hierarchical structure of the data and the complex relationship between the variables at various levels.

We did not include a quality aspect (e.g., the quality of service delivery) for it is hard to measure, particularly at the population level. Even in a research context, it is challenging to ensure that healthcare service is delivered as intended [63]. Therefore, when applying the framework, one should bear in mind that the service characteristics may not be fully reflected in the variables collected for analysis. One should also note that the major building blocks of our framework were drawn from robust theoretical models and comprehensive systematic reviews, based primarily on studies undertaken in the UK, western European countries and the USA, and therefore they may not be relevant to other healthcare systems. Finally, as the place of death reflects only the last moments of a person's life, it should be viewed in conjunction with the other end of life care outcome measures, for example, place of care and care transitions [24]. This will provide a more comprehensive perspective about how patients are cared for at the end of life.

Currently, there are a limited number of studies investigating the service characteristics that are most amenable to change. We hope our proposed framework will facilitate research efforts on the place of death to include more healthcare service factors.

5. Conclusions

We propose a framework which conceptualizes the impact of healthcare services on the place of death. The impact pathway is proceeding from the end of life care policies, which, in turn, influence service commissioning and shape healthcare service characteristics, including service type, capacity (facilities), location and workforce, through which service utilization and ultimately place of death are affected. Patient socio-demographics, disease-related variables, and social care and support related factors also influence place of death, but they are not the focus of this framework; they are therefore grouped as needs and other environmental factors. Information on service utilization together with place of death outcome create a loop feedback to inform policy and service commissioning. The framework can be used to guide the planning, analysis, and interpretation of the service-related factors that may influence place of death. It can also be used to potentially identify service factors that may be addressed to improve end of life care.

Author Contributions: W.G. and I.J.H. acquired the funding to support this study. S.H. and W.G. jointly developed an early draft of the manuscript. W.G. with significant input from M.M. contributed to the subsequent major revisions of the manuscript. All authors commented on, contributed to the final draft, and agreed with manuscript results and conclusions; all authors read and meet ICMJE criteria for authorship and approved this submission.

Funding: This study was funded by the National Institute for Health Research, Health Services and Delivery Research Programme (NIHR HS & DR, 14/19/22). This work is independent research partly supported by the National Institute for Health Research (NIHR) Collaboration for Leadership in Applied Health Research & Care (CLAHRC) South London. CLAHRC South London is part of the National Institute for Health Research (NIHR) and is a partnership between King's Health Partners, St. George's, University London, and St George's Healthcare NHS Trust.

Acknowledgments: Guide_Care Services project is a large-scale observational study investigating the role of service factors in place of death funded by the National Institute for Health Research, Health Services and Delivery Research Programme (NIHR HS & DR, 14/19/22), led by King's College London, Cicely Saunders Institute, Department of Palliative Care, Policy & Rehabilitation, UK. Guide_Care Services Investigators: Wei Gao (co-PI), Irene J Higginson (co-PI), Julia Verne, Emma Gordon and Giovanna Polato. Guide_Care Services Project Advisory Group members: Tony Bonser, Nicola Bowtell, Kate Heaps, Claire Henry, Jamie Jenkins, Katie Lindsey, Catherine Millington-Sanders, Rajiv Mitra, Myfanwy Morgan, Carolyn Morris, Robert Mulliss, Andy Pring, Sarah Russell, Jane Smith, Ros Taylor, Claudia Wells, Paula Young. Guide_Care Services Researchers: Emeka Chukwusa (Project Manager), Peihan Yu, Rebecca Wilson, Clare Pearson, Sumaya Huque. Administrative support: Halle Johnson, Daniel Gulliford, Sophie Watson, Zaynah Sheikh. The views expressed in this publication are those of the authors and not necessarily those of the National Health Service, the National Institute for Health Research, or the Department of Health.

Appendix A. Details of the Literature Search

Aim:

To identify the published conceptual framework on the determinants of place of death.

Search databases:

1.　Embase 1974 to 2018 Week 34

2.   Ovid MEDLINE(R) and Epub Ahead of Print, In-Process & Other Non-Indexed Citations and Daily 1946 to August 22, 2018

3.   PsycINFO 1806 to August Week 3 2018

Search strategy:

(Palliative care or end of life care or hospice care or terminal care or death or dying or terminally ill or palliative nursing) AND (conceptual framework or conceptual model or pragmatic framework or pragmatic model or theoretical model or theoretical framework) AND (site of death or place of death or home death or hospital death or hospice death or nursing home death or care home death) in all searchable fields in the three databases. Duplicated records were deleted.

Result:

Only one conceptual model (Gomes & Higginson, 2006) was identified.

References

1.   Higginson, I.J.; Astin, P.; Dolan, S. Where do cancer patients die? Ten-year trends in the place of death of cancer patients in England. *Palliat. Med.* **1998**, *12*, 353–363. [CrossRef] [PubMed]

2.   Gao, W.; Ho, Y.K.; Verne, J.; Glickman, M.; Higginson, I.J. GUIDE_Care project changing patterns in place of cancer death in England: A population-based study. *PLoS Med.* **2013**, *10*, e1001410. [CrossRef] [PubMed]

3.   Gao, W.; Ho, Y.K.; Verne, J.; Gordon, E.; Higginson, I.J. Geographical and temporal understanding in place of death in England (1984–2010): Analysis of trends and associated factors to improve end-of-life care (GUIDE_Care)—Primary research. *Health Serv. Deliv. Res.* **2014**, *2*, 1–104. [CrossRef] [PubMed]

4.   Department of Health. *End of Life Care Strategy*; Department of Health: London, UK, 2008; p. 171.

5.   Department of Health. Our Commitment to you for end of life care. In *The Government Response to the Review of Choice in End of Life Care*; Department of Health: London, UK, 2016.

6.   Reyniers, T.; Deliens, L.; Pasman, H.R.; Vander Stichele, R.; Sijnave, B.; Cohen, J.; Houttekier, D. Reasons for end-of-life hospital admissions: Results of a survey among family physicians. *J. Pain Symptom Manag.* **2016**, *52*, 498–506. [CrossRef] [PubMed]

7.   Gomes, B.; Higginson, I.J. Factors influencing death at home in terminally ill patients with cancer: Systematic review. *Br. Med. J.* **2006**, *332*, 515–518. [CrossRef] [PubMed]

8.   Costa, V. The determinants of place of death: An evidence-based analysis. *Ont. Health Technol. Assess. Ser.* **2014**, *14*, 1–78. [PubMed]

9.   Phillips, K.A.; Morrison, K.R.; Andersen, R.; Aday, L.A. Understanding the context of healthcare utilization: Assessing environmental and provider-related variables in the behavioral model of utilization. *Health Serv. Res.* **1998**, *33*, 571–596. [PubMed]

10.   Andersen, R.; Newman, J.F. Societal and individual determinants of medical care utilization in the United States. *Milbank Q.* **2005**, *83*, 1–28. [CrossRef]

11.   Levesque, J.-F.; Harris, M.F.; Russell, G. Patient-centred access to health care: Conceptualising access at the interface of health systems and populations. *Int. J. Equity Health* **2013**, *12*, 18. [CrossRef] [PubMed]

12.   Donabedian, A. The quality of care: How can it be assessed? *J. Am. Med. Assoc.* **1997**, *260*, 1743–1748. [CrossRef]

13.   Kindig, D.A.; Asada, Y.; Booske, B. A population health framework for setting national and state health goals. *JAMA* **2008**, *299*, 2081–2083. [CrossRef] [PubMed]

14.   Laguna, J.; Enguídanos, S.; Siciliano, M.; Coulourides-Kogan, A. Racial/ethnic minority access to end-of-life care: A conceptual framework. *Home Health Care Serv. Q.* **2012**, *31*, 60–83. [CrossRef] [PubMed]

15.   Appleby, J.; Lyscom, T.; Raleigh, V.; Frosini, F.; Bevan, G.; Gao, H. *Variations in Health Care*; King's Fund: London, UK, 2011; pp. 1–40.

16.   Higginson, I.J.; Reilly, C.C.; Bajwah, S.; Maddocks, M.; Costantini, M.; Gao, W. Which patients with advanced respiratory disease die in hospital? A 14-year population-based study of trends and associated factors. *BMC Med.* **2017**, *15*, 19. [CrossRef] [PubMed]

17.   Sleeman, K.E.; Ho, Y.K.; Verne, J.; Gao, W.; Higginson, I.J. Reversal of English trend towards hospital death in dementia: A population-based study of place of death and associated individual and regional factors, 2001-2010. *BMC Neurol.* **2014**, *14*, 59. [CrossRef] [PubMed]

18. Gao, W.; Verne, J.; Peacock, J.; Stiller, C.; Wells, C.; Greenough, A.; Higginson, I.J. Place of death in children and young people with cancer and implications for end of life care: A population-based study in England, 1993-2014. *BMC Cancer* **2016**, *16*, 727. [CrossRef] [PubMed]

19. Muramatsu, N.; Hoyem, R.L.; Yin, H.; Campbell, R.T. Place of death among older Americans: Does state spending on home- and community-based services promote home death? *Med. Care* **2008**, *46*, 829–838. [CrossRef] [PubMed]

20. Flory, J.; Yinong, Y.X.; Gurol, I.; Levinsky, N.; Ash, A.; Emanuel, E.; Young-Xu, Y.; Gurol, I.; Levinsky, N.; Ash, A.; et al. Place of death: U.S. trends since 1980. *Health Aff.* **2004**, *23*, 194–200. [CrossRef]

21. Feudtner, C.; Feinstein, J.A.; Satchell, M.; Zhao, H.; Kang, T.I. Shifting place of death among children with complex chronic conditions in the United States, 1989–2003. *JAMA* **2007**, *297*, 2725–2732. [CrossRef] [PubMed]

22. Wilson, D.M.; Truman, C.D.; Thomas, R.; Fainsinger, R.; Kovacs-Burns, K.; Froggatt, K.; Justice, C. The rapidly changing location of death in Canada, 1994–2004. *Soc. Sci. Med.* **2009**, *68*, 1752–1758. [CrossRef] [PubMed]

23. Houttekier, D.; Cohen, J.; Surkyn, J.; Deliens, L. Study of recent and future trends in place of death in Belgium using death certificate data: A shift from hospitals to care homes. *BMC Public Health* **2011**, *11*, 228. [CrossRef] [PubMed]

24. Teno, J.M.; Gozalo, P.L.; Bynum, J.P.; Leland, N.E.; Miller, S.C.; Morden, N.E.; Scupp, T.; Goodman, D.C.; Mor, V. Change in end-of-life care for Medicare beneficiaries: Site of death, place of care, and health care transitions in 2000, 2005, and 2009. *JAMA* **2013**, *309*, 470–477. [CrossRef] [PubMed]

25. Gruneir, A.; Mor, V.; Weitzen, S.; Truchil, R.; Teno, J.; Roy, J. Where people die: A multilevel approach to understanding influences on site of death in America. *Med. Care Res. Rev.* **2007**, *64*, 351–378. [CrossRef] [PubMed]

26. Chitnis, X.A.; Georghiou, T.; Steventon, A.; Bardsley, M.J. Effect of a home-based end-of-life nursing service on hospital use at the end of life and place of death: A study using administrative data and matched controls. *BMJ Support. Palliat. Care* **2013**, *3*, 422–430. [CrossRef] [PubMed]

27. Aabom, B.; Kragstrup, J.; Vondeling, H.; Bakketeig, L.S.; Stovring, H.; Støvring, H. Population-based study of place of death of patients with cancer: Implications for GPs. *Br. J. Gen. Pract.* **2005**, *55*, 684–689. [PubMed]

28. Lavergne, M.R.; Lethbridge, L.; Johnston, G.; Henderson, D.; D'Intino, A.F.; McIntyre, P. Examining palliative care program use and place of death in rural and urban contexts: A Canadian population-based study using linked data. *Rural Remote Health* **2015**, *15*, 3134. [PubMed]

29. Radbruch, L.; Payne, S. White Paper on standards and norms for hospice and palliative care in Europe: Part 2. *Eur. J. Cancer Care* **2010**, *17*, 12.

30. O'Dowd, E.L.; McKeever, T.M.; Baldwin, D.R.; Hubbard, R.B. Place of death in patients with lung cancer: A retrospective cohort study from 2004–2013. *PLoS ONE* **2016**, *11*, e0161399. [CrossRef] [PubMed]

31. Hare, T.S.; Barcus, H.R. Geographical accessibility and Kentucky's heart-related hospital services. *Appl. Geogr.* **2007**, *27*, 181–205. [CrossRef]

32. Aoun, N.; Matsuda, H.; Sekiyama, M. Geographical accessibility to healthcare and malnutrition in Rwanda. *Soc. Sci. Med.* **2015**, *130*, 135–145. [CrossRef] [PubMed]

33. Gatrell, A.C.; Harman, J.C.; Francis, B.J.; Thomas, C.; Morris, S.M.; McIllmurray, M. Place of death: Analysis of cancer deaths in part of North West England. *J. Public Health Med.* **2003**, *25*, 53–58. [CrossRef] [PubMed]

34. Pearson, C.; Verne, J.; Wells, C.; Polato, G.M.; Higginson, I.J.; Gao, W. Measuring geographical accessibility to palliative and end of life (PEoLC) related facilities: A comparative study in an area with well-developed specialist palliative care (SPC) provision. *BMC Palliat. Care* **2017**, *16*, 14. [CrossRef] [PubMed]

35. Delamater, P.L.; Messina, J.P.; Shortridge, A.; Grady, S.C. Measuring geographic access to health care: Raster and network methods. *Int. J. Health Geogr.* **2012**, *11*, 15. [CrossRef] [PubMed]

36. Rainsford, S.; MacLeod, R.D.; Glasgow, N.J. Place of death in rural palliative care: A systematic review. *Palliat. Med.* **2016**, *30*, 745–763. [CrossRef] [PubMed]

37. Goodridge, D.; Lawson, J.; Rennie, D.; Marciniuk, D. Rural/urban differences in health care utilization and place of death for persons with respiratory illness in the last year of life. *Rural Remote Health* **2010**, *10*, 1349. [PubMed]

38. England NHS. *England Five Year Forward View*; England NHS: London, UK, 2014.

39. Addicott, R.; Maguire, D.; Jabbal, J.; Honeyman, M. *Workforce Planning in the NHS*; The Kings Fund: London, UK, 2015; p. 43.

40. Neergaard, M.A.; Vedsted, P.; Olesen, F.; Sokolowski, I.; Jensen, A.B.; Sondergaard, J. Associations between home death and GP involvement in palliative cancer care. *Br. J. Gen. Pract.* **2009**, *59*, 671–677. [CrossRef] [PubMed]

41. Neergaard, M.A.; Vedsted, P.; Olesen, F.; Sokolowski, I.; Jensen, A.B.; Sondergaard, J. Associations between successful palliative trajectories, place of death and GP involvement. *Scand. J. Prim. Health Care* **2010**, *28*, 138–145. [CrossRef] [PubMed]

42. Spetz, J.; Donaldson, N.; Aydin, C.; Brown, D.S. Methods how many nurses per patient? Measurements of nurse staffing in health services research. *Health Serv. Res.* **2008**, *43*, 1674–1692. [CrossRef] [PubMed]

43. Nancarrow, S.A.; Booth, A.; Ariss, S.; Smith, T.; Enderby, P.; Roots, A. Ten principles of good interdisciplinary team work. *Hum. Resour. Health* **2013**, *11*, 19. [CrossRef] [PubMed]

44. Buchan, J.; Dal Poz, M.R. Skill mix in the health care workforce: Reviewing the evidence. *Bull. World Health Organ.* **2002**, *80*, 575–580. [PubMed]

45. National Institute for Health and Care Excellence. *End of Life Care for Adults: Quality Standard*; NICE: London, UK, 2011.

46. Radbruch, L.; Payne, S.; Bercovitch, M.; Caraceni, A.; De Vlieger, T.; Firth, P.; Hegedus, K.; Nabal, M.; Rhebergen, A.; Schmidlin, E.; et al. White Paper on standards and norms for hospice and palliative care in Europe: Part 1. *Eur. J. Palliat. Care* **2009**, *16*, 278–289.

47. NIH Library Financial or Service Utilization Data. Available online: https://www.nihlibrary.nih.gov/resources/subject-guides/health-data-resources/financial-or-service-utilization-data (accessed on 30 January 2018).

48. NHS Digital Indicator Portal. Available online: https://indicators.hscic.gov.uk/webview/ (accessed on 30 January 2018).

49. AHWI Health & Welfare Services. Available online: https://www.aihw.gov.au/reports-statistics/health-welfare-services (accessed on 30 January 2018).

50. Canadian Institute for Health Information Quick Stats. Available online: https://www.cihi.ca/en/quick-stats (accessed on 30 January 2018).

51. Roux, A.V.D. The study of group-level factors in epidemiology: Rethinking variables, study designs, and analytical approaches. *Epidemiol. Rev.* **2004**, *26*, 104–111. [CrossRef] [PubMed]

52. Costa, V.; Earle, C.C.; Esplen, M.J.; Fowler, R.; Goldman, R.; Grossman, D.; Levin, L.; Manuel, D.G.; Sharkey, S.; Tanuseputro, P.; et al. The determinants of home and nursing home death: A systematic review and meta-analysis. *BMC Palliat. Care* **2016**, *15*, 8. [CrossRef] [PubMed]

53. Campion, E.W.; Kelley, A.S.; Morrison, R.S. Palliative care for the seriously Ill. *N. Engl. J. Med.* **2015**, *373*, 747–755. [CrossRef]

54. Murtagh, F.E.M.; Bausewein, C.; Verne, J.; Groeneveld, E.I.; Kaloki, Y.E.; Higginson, I.J. How many people need palliative care? A study developing and comparing methods for population-based estimates. *Palliat. Med.* **2014**, *28*, 49–58. [CrossRef] [PubMed]

55. ONS Nomis—Official Labour Market Statistics. Available online: https://www.nomisweb.co.uk/ (accessed on 12 February 2018).

56. Bardsley, M.; Georghiou, T.; Dixon, J. *Social Care and Hospital Use at the End of Life*; The Nuffield Trust: London, UK, 2010.

57. Poulos, R.G.; Harkin, D.; Poulos, C.J.; Cole, A.; MacLeod, R. Can specially trained community care workers effectively support patients and their families in the home setting at the end of life? *Health Soc. Care Community* **2018**, *26*, e270–e279. [CrossRef] [PubMed]

58. Gill, A.; Laporte, A.; Coyte, P.C.; Peter, C. Predictors of home death in palliative care patients: A critical literature review. *J. Palliat. Care* **2013**, *29*, 113–118. [PubMed]

59. Cohen, J.; Bilsen, J.; Hooft, P.; Deboosere, P.; Van der Wal, G.; Deliens, L.; Van der Wal, G.; Deliens, L. Dying at home or in an institution: Using death certificates to explore the factors associated with place of death. *Health Policy* **2006**, *78*, 319–329. [CrossRef] [PubMed]

60. Maslow, A.H. A theory of human motivation. *Psychol. Rev.* **1943**, *50*, 370–396. [CrossRef]

61. Henson, L.A.; Higginson, I.J.; Daveson, B.A.; Ellis-Smith, C.; Koffman, J.; Morgan, M.; Gao, W. 'I'll be in a safe place': A qualitative study of the decisions taken by people with advanced cancer to seek emergency department care. *BMJ Open* **2016**, *6*, e012134. [CrossRef] [PubMed]

62. Davies, J.M.; Gao, W.; Sleeman, K.E.; Lindsey, K.; Murtagh, F.E.; Teno, J.M.; Deliens, L.; Wee, B.; Higginson, I.J.; Verne, J. Using routine data to improve palliative and end of life care. *BMJ Support. Palliat. Care* **2016**, *6*, 257–262. [CrossRef] [PubMed]

63. Ang, K.; Hepgul, N.; Gao, W.; Higginson, I.J. Strategies used in improving and assessing the level of reporting of implementation fidelity in randomised controlled trials of palliative care complex interventions: A systematic review. *Palliat. Med.* **2018**, *32*, 500–516. [CrossRef] [PubMed]

13

Improving Cardiovascular Disease Knowledge among Rural Participants: The Results of a Cluster Randomized Trial

Laurie S. Abbott [1],* [ORCID] and Elizabeth H. Slate [2]

1   College of Nursing, Florida State University, Tallahassee, FL 32306-4310, USA
2   Department of Statistics, Florida State University, Tallahassee, FL 32306-4310, USA; slate@stat.fsu.edu
*   Correspondence: labbott@fsu.edu

Abstract: Cardiovascular disease (CVD) is a major cause of death and disability, especially among people living in the rural, southern United States. Rural African Americans are often diagnosed with CVD earlier in life, and they bear a disproportionate burden of CVD risk factors, morbidity, and mortality. Health equity among historically underserved, rural populations can potentially be attained through culturally relevant interventions that teach people skills to stay well and avoid CVD-related risk and diagnoses. The purpose of this secondary analysis was to determine the effect of an evidence-based intervention on cardiovascular health knowledge and the stages of change toward the action and maintenance phases. The pre-test-post-test data were obtained during a cluster randomized trial involving twelve rural churches that were randomized to intervention ($n = 6$) and control ($n = 6$) groups. Participants ($n = 115$) in the intervention group received a cardiovascular health intervention, and those ($n = 114$) in the control group could receive the intervention following the study's completion. The data were analyzed using a linear mixed model to compare group differences from pre-test to post-test. The cardiovascular health promotion intervention significantly improved cardiovascular health knowledge and was associated with advancements in the stages of change toward the action and maintenance phases.

Keywords: community health; health promotion; rural health; cardiovascular disease

1. Introduction

Cardiovascular disease (CVD) is a public health problem that is a major cause of death and disability among people living in the United States [1]. The prevalence of CVD is expected to rise during the next decade because of the aging population and the increased pervasiveness of risk factors, such as too little physical activity, poor diet, uncontrolled hypertension, and diabetes—all of which are modifiable [2]. African Americans bear a disproportionate burden of CVD and an increased risk of hypertension and stroke, and these disparities are especially apparent among those living in the rural southern United States [2–6]. The national objectives listed by Healthy People 2020, a health initiative of the United States government, include improving the overall cardiovascular health among all American people, reducing CVD risk factors, and enhancing the awareness of stroke and heart attack symptoms to stimulate recognition and early medical intervention [7]. In general, African Americans are often diagnosed with CVD at earlier ages, and the early onset of CVD within this population has been attributed to a higher prevalence of CVD risk factors and related adverse health behaviors [8]. Bridging knowledge gaps of CVD through health education interventions is an important step toward achieving these goals and advancing health equity, especially among historically underserved groups [9].

People living in rural areas of the United States have reduced knowledge and awareness about cardiovascular health issues such as knowing the symptoms of a heart attack or a stroke [9,10]. They are also more likely to have low self-efficacy for reading food labels and cooking heart-healthy foods [11]. Limited knowledge and low health literacy about CVD risk factors and associated diagnoses such as heart disease, stroke, and heart failure can hinder CVD risk reduction and the prevention of chronic heart disease exacerbation at home [12–14]. Having limited cardiovascular health knowledge is associated with low perceived risk of cardiovascular disease and stroke. For example, African American women living in rural, southern areas of the United States typically understand the causal factors associated with CVD through a combination of learned medical factors and vicarious knowledge that is gained through the experiences of family members and friends that are diagnosed with heart disease [15]. However, having a family history of chronic disease, such as stroke, does not predict improved health knowledge and habits, such as a good diet and exercise [12].

Educational interventions that are designed to improve knowledge, heart health habits, and related skills are crucial for advancing cardiovascular health equity among people living in underserved areas in the rural, southern United States [5,12–14]. Research is needed to determine whether educational interventions increase the knowledge that is necessary to promote health behavior changes and to reduce the overall cardiovascular disease risk [12]. The purpose of this secondary analysis was to examine the effects of the culturally relevant With Every Heartbeat is Life intervention on cardiovascular health knowledge [16]. The Integrated Model of Behavioral Prediction was the theoretical framework that was used to guide the study [17]. This health behavior model explains the relationships among factors such as norms, attitudes, and self-efficacy in regard to intentions to adopt recommended health practices [17]. Health knowledge fosters essential health skills that are associated with progressing intentions toward active health behavior performance [17].

2. Materials and Methods

The current study is a secondary analysis that examined data that was collected during a cluster randomized trial among African American participants living in the rural, southeastern United States. The parent study had a pre-test-post-test strategy that observed the intervention effects of a health promotion program among the participants who were recruited from randomized churches that were located in two rural counties. Detailed information about the methods, recruitment strategies, and sample size calculations that were used during the parent study has been previously published in a manuscript that described the effect of the intervention on psycho-social aspects such as intentions, norms, attitudes, and self-efficacy [18]. The procedures and human ethics of this secondary data analysis that analyzed knowledge and stage of change variables were reviewed and approved by the institutional review board (IRB) of Florida State University.

2.1. Sample and Setting

The participants ($n = 229$) in the parent study were recruited from twelve rural churches that were randomized to intervention ($n = 6$) and control ($n = 6$) groups. Church settings have been found to be a cultural strength within an already established community that facilitates reaching African American groups and may influence participation in health behavior change interventions [8,11]. Of the total 229 participants, 115 people were in the intervention group and 114 participants were in the control group. Eligible participants were (a) men and women who self-identified as African American, (b) at least 24 years of age, and (c) able to read, write, and understand English. The informed consent forms were signed after all questions about the study were satisfactorily answered. The participants from churches that were randomized to the intervention group received the heart health curriculum from the same public health nurse. The pastors of the control group churches were given the option of having the intervention delivered in their churches following the completion of the study. A US $20 gift card incentive was issued to the participants in both the intervention and the control groups during the final data collection period.

2.2. Intervention

The participants in the churches who were randomized to the intervention group received the With Every Heartbeat is Life cardiovascular health promotion program [16]. The curriculum was developed and culturally tailored specifically for African American groups by the National Heart, Lung, and Blood Institute (NHLBI). Although it was designed to be implemented over ten, weekly sessions of approximately 45 min to an hour each, we adapted the program for delivery in six, weekly sessions, each lasting about ninety minutes to accommodate schedule logistics. Related topics were combined into one session, and the time frame for each session was lengthened to include the increased educational material and interactive activities. This adaptation was done in response to feedback from the church group representatives that the initially planned twelve-session intervention, including two additional days for pre-test and post-test data collection, was too lengthy and would result in reduced participation. The weekly topics addressed major CVD risk factors such as diabetes, hypertension, diet, elevated serum cholesterol, excessive weight, physical inactivity, and smoking.

2.3. Measures

The data used in the secondary analysis were collected during two time periods. Within the intervention group, data were collected at baseline and after the sixth week's session. Within the control group, the data were collected at baseline and six weeks later. The program-specific "My Health Knowledge" instrument had twenty-one items for measuring cardiovascular health knowledge [19]. There was one item that measured participant movement toward an action phase or stage of change.

Heart health knowledge. The "My Health Knowledge" instrument measured participant knowledge about cardiovascular health topics: heart disease risk, heart attack and stroke symptoms, diet including cholesterol, diabetes, weight management, smoking, and the effects of alcohol. Similar items within the measure were evaluated by adapting a method from a previous study using an earlier, yet similar version of the instrument that was published for use with the With Every Heartbeat is Life curriculum [20]. The categories are (a) Risk Factors, (b) Disease Symptoms, (c) Risk Reduction, and (d) Heart Health Facts. For example, the Risk Factors section includes questions about factors that influence cardiovascular disease risk. The Disease Symptoms area has items for measuring knowledge about the signs and symptoms of diabetes, heart attack, and stroke. The Risk Reduction category asks about strategies for reducing cardiovascular disease risk, and the Heart Health facts includes basic information about cardiovascular disease issues, such as the parameters for normal blood pressure, blood glucose, and blood cholesterol levels. The combined value of all of the items in the "My Health Knowledge" measure equaled 100 points, and the summed participant responses were indicative of the percentage of correctly answered items.

Stages of change. There was one item on the "My Health Knowledge" instrument that was titled, "A Day with the Harris Family" that measured the participants' readiness to make cardiovascular health habit changes. The item was based on the 5-stage continuum that was described by the Trans-Theoretical Model: precontemplation, contemplation, preparation, action, and maintenance [21]. A scenario was provided that described the situation, and the answer options included five fictitious people who represented one of the five stages of change. For example, choosing Ms. Diane, "I am taking action.", signified the action stage. Using the classification method which was adapted from a previous publication by Hurtado et al., the 5-point measure was dichotomized by combining the first three stages (precontemplation, contemplation, and preparation) and the last two stages (action and maintenance) [20].

2.4. Data Analysis

The socio-demographic characteristics of the participants were described using frequencies, averages, and standard deviations. The statistical procedure that was used to assess group differences from pre-test to post-test was the significance of the interaction between time and group assignment in a repeated measures linear mixed model (LMM) using the mixed procedure. The model included fixed effects for study group assignment, time, and the time-by-group interaction, together with a random effect for church—the last of which accommodated the within-cluster correlation among the responses. All of the analyses used the intention-to-treat paradigm in which all participants were included in the group to which their church was randomized. Missing post-test responses ($n = 12$ and $n = 4$ in the intervention and control groups, respectively) were handled via a maximum likelihood estimation of the LMM. Results are presented as point estimates and confidence intervals for the time-by-group interaction effect and the changes from pre-test to post-test for the two groups. No multiplicity adjustment was used. Analyses were performed using the mixed procedure in IBM SPSS Statistics, version 22 (IBM, Armonk, NY, USA).

3. Results

There were no substantial group differences regarding socio-demographic characteristics such as gender, age, educational attainment, and employment levels (Table 1). The results of the secondary analysis indicated that participation in the intervention was associated with cardiovascular health knowledge improvements. Compared with the control group, the intervention group had statistically significant overall differences ($p < 0.001$) from pre-test to post-test (Table 2). The results for the overall test were summed from the individual items, with 100 being the best possible score. The mean (M) baseline or pre-test scores for both the intervention ($M = 78.03$) and control ($M = 78.86$) groups were similar. However, the mean post-test score for the intervention group ($M = 94.52$) was substantially higher than the mean post-test score ($M = 80.86$) for the control group. The findings for each classification are listed with detailed descriptions about the items that were included within each of the categorical headings.

Table 1. Sociodemographic characteristics of the sample.

Demographic Variable	Intervention Group ($n = 115$)				Control Group ($n = 114$)			
	n	%	M	SD	n	%	M	SD
Age (years)			59.03	12.91			56.56	13.49
Race								
African American	115	100			114	100		
Gender								
Male	31	27.0			35	30.7		
Female	84	73.0			79	69.3		
Educational level								
Did not finish high school	21	18.3			22	19.3		
Graduated from high school/General Education Diploma (GED)	28	24.3			45	39.5		
Attended some college	32	27.8			23	20.0		
Graduated from college	23	20.0			14	12.3		
Earned a graduate/professional degree	11	9.6			10	8.8		
Employment Status								
Employed (Full-time or Part-time)	53	46.1			59	51.8		
Not Employed (Retired/Homemaker or Unemployed)	62	54			55	48.2		

Note: The entries provided are counts (n) and percentages (%) except for age (M = average, SD = standard deviation).

3.1. Knowledge of Risk Factors

The results of the overall score for the Risk Factors knowledge category showed statistically significant ($p < 0.001$) group differences (Table 2). Within this category, five of the six individual items about risk factor topics that had statistically significant results were (a) general heart disease risk ($p = 0.005$), (b) cholesterol levels ($p = 0.044$), (c) risk for diabetes ($p = 0.004$), (d) smoking as a chronic disease risk factor ($p < 0.001$), and e) blood pressure increased by alcohol consumption ($p < 0.001$).

There was one item within this topic grouping about second-hand smoke as a risk factor for heart and lung disease that showed no significant knowledge improvement ($p = 0.117$).

Table 2. A comparison of study outcomes for the intervention and control groups.

Variable	Control Group *		Intervention Group +		Intervention Effect ±		
	Δ_C	95% CI	Δ_I	95% CI	b	95% CI	p
My Health Knowledge (MHK), Overall	2.00	(−1.57, 5.58)	15.50	(12.84, 20.16)	14.49	(9.38, 19.61)	0.000
Risk Factors (RF)							
RF, Overall	1.043	(−0.343, 2.429)	5.395	(3.978, 6.811)	4.352	(2.370, 6.333)	0.000
HDRisk1	0.412	(−0.157, 0.982)	1.580	(0.998, 2.160)	1.17	(0.353, 1.98)	0.005
Cholest2	0.300	(−0.034, 0.634)	0.790	(0.449, 1.131)	0.490	(0.013, 0.967)	0.044
DiaRisk3	0.423	(−0.013, 0.859)	1.335	(0.891, 1.780)	0.913	(0.289, 1.536)	0.004
SmRisk9	−0.159	(−0.643, 0.324)	1.318	(0.825, 1.811)	1.477	(0.787, 2.168)	0.000
Alcoh19	0.063	(−0.031, 0.156)	0.343	(0.248, 0.439)	0.280	(0.147, 0.414)	0.000
Smok20	0.005	(−0.043, 0.054)	0.061	(0.011, 0.110)	0.055	(0.014, 0.125)	0.117
Disease Symptoms (DS)							
DS, Overall	0.709	(−0.527, 1.946)	4.605	(3.342, 5.868)	3.900	(2.129, 5.663)	0.000
DiaSym4	0.238	(−0.167, 0.642)	1.053	(0.640, 1.466)	0.815	(0.237, 1.393)	0.006
StrSigns5	0.145	(−0.444, 0.734)	1.862	(1.260, 2.463)	1.716	(0.874, 2.558)	0.000
HASigns6	0.324	(−0.186, 0.834)	1.700	(1.179, 2.220)	1.375	(0.647, 2.104)	0.000
Risk Reduction (RR)							
RR, Overall	0.235	(−0.963, 1.433)	2.535	(1.313, 3.757)	2.300	(0.588, 4.011)	0.009
HDRiskRed8	0.185	(−0.308, 0.678)	1.095	(0.591, 1.600)	0.910	(0.205, 1.615)	0.012
WeiLoss10	0.026	(−0.428, 0.481)	0.728	(0.266, 1.190)	0.702	(0.053, 1.350)	0.034
Exerc11	0.026	(−0.428, 0.481)	0.728	(0.266, 1.190)	0.702	(0.053, 1.350)	0.034
MinEx15	−0.019	(−0.111, 0.073)	0.123	(0.029, 0.216)	0.142	(0.011, 0.273)	0.034
Heart Health Facts (HHF)							
HHF, Overall	−0.042	(−0.472, 0.388)	2.645	(2.207, 3.084)	2.687	(2.073, 3.301)	0.000
HAFacts7	0.061	(−0.328, 0.450)	1.416	(1.020, 1.813)	1.356	(0.800, 1.911)	0.000
VeServ12	0.000	(−0.106, 0.106)	0.290	(0.182, 0.398)	0.290	(0.139, 0.441)	0.000
WomWai13	0.081	(−0.019, 0.180)	0.325	(0.224, 0.427)	0.245	(0.102, 0.387)	0.001
MenWai14	0.010	(−0.092, 0.113)	0.485	(0.380, 0.589)	0.474	(0.328, 0.621)	0.000
BP16	−0.076	(−0.185, 0.032)	0.163	(0.052, 0.274)	0.240	(0.275, 0.936)	0.003
Chol17	−0.030	(−0.261, 0.202)	0.576	(0.341, 0.812)	0.606	(−0.055, 0.338)	0.000
BlGlu18	−0.047	(−0.218, 0.124)	0.726	(0.552, 0.900)	0.773	(0.529, 1.017)	0.000
BP21	0.016	(−0.040, 0.071)	0.070	(0.013, 0.126)	0.054	(−0.025, 0.133)	0.182
Stage of Change (SC)							
SC	0.022	(−0.246, 0.203)	0.651	(0.422, 0.881)	0.673	(0.352, 0.994)	0.000

* Δ_C is the pre-test to post-test change for the control group, as estimated from the LMM. + Δ_I is the pre-test to post-test change for the intervention group, as estimated from the LMM. ± b is the estimate of the effect of the intervention, i.e., the estimate of the coefficient for the interaction between time (pre-test to post-test) and study group in the LMM (also, $b = \Delta_I − \Delta_C$).

3.2. Disease Symptoms

There were statistically significant group differences ($p < 0.001$) for the overall score in the Disease Symptoms category. All of the individual items within this classification had statistically significant results including (a) diabetes symptoms ($p = 0.006$), (b) stroke signs ($p < 0.001$), and (c) heart attack signs ($p < 0.001$).

3.3. Risk Reduction

There were statistically significant findings ($p = 0.009$) for the overall score in the Risk Reduction category. All of the individual items that were grouped in this category had significant results, and these were (a) heart disease risk reduction ($p = 0.012$), (b) weight loss ($p = 0.034$), (c) exercise ($p = 0.034$), and (d) minimal time each day that should be spent exercising ($p = 0.034$).

3.4. Heart Health Facts

There were statistically significant results ($p < 0.001$) for the overall score in the Heart Health Facts category. The statistically significant individual items within this grouping were general facts about heart health, such as (a) heart attack facts ($p < 0.001$), (b) vegetable servings per day ($p < 0.001$), (c) women's waist measurement ($p = 0.001$), (d) men's waist measurement ($p < 0.001$), (e) blood pressure reading ($p = 0.003$), (f) cholesterol levels ($p < 0.001$), and (g) blood glucose levels ($p < 0.001$). The one item that was not statistically significant between groups was about blood pressure being a silent killer ($p = 0.182$).

3.5. Stage of Change

The one item within the Stage of Change category indicated that there were statistically significant changes from baseline ($p < 0.001$) between the groups. For Stage of Change, the proportion of participants either taking action or maintaining a healthy path was similar at pre-test for the control and the intervention groups at 53.5% and 50.4%, respectively. At post-test, these proportions increased to 59.1% and 80.6%, respectively.

4. Discussion

The results of this secondary analysis indicate that the educational intervention in a rural community setting was useful for improving cardiovascular knowledge and may promote healthier lifestyle choices and behaviors. Compared with the control group, the participants in the intervention group had significantly improved knowledge associated with CVD, risk reduction strategies, and recognizing the signs and symptoms of cardiovascular events such as heart attack and stroke. For the people in the intervention group, participation in the intervention significantly influenced stage of change toward the action and maintenance phases. Theoretically, movement toward the action phase indicates active performance of a recommended health behavior, and the maintenance phase involves sustained behavior over time [21]. Having increased knowledge about CVD pathophysiology, related CVD risk factors, and prevention strategies using understandable language, culturally relevant examples, and skill-building activities such as role-plays and label-reading exercises may have influenced the intervention group participants and motivated them to actively engage in the recommended cardiovascular health behaviors.

There were two items that did not demonstrate statistically significant changes in participant knowledge from baseline to post-test. The items that measured knowledge about the dangers of second-hand smoke exposure ($p = 0.117$) and blood pressure ($p = 0.182$) had no significant between-group post-test differences. An influencing factor may have been that the two questions asked about topics that are considered simple knowledge, meaning the participants had high scores at baseline, leaving little room for improvement. The smoking question asked whether second-hand smoke was associated with increased heart and lung disease, and the question about blood pressure asked whether hypertension was considered a "silent killer" because people do not recognize the symptoms. Further, both questions had "Yes", "No", or "Don't Know" answer options which made guessing the correct answer easier.

The findings of other studies indicate that evidence-based guidelines that incorporate cultural preferences and attitudes can positively influence health behavior modifications among African American populations [8]. Educational health programs have typically been effective strategies for improving knowledge about CVD, which is necessary for making heart healthy choices and reducing modifiable CVD risk factors [22]. Such interventions are crucial for bridging knowledge gaps among people at increased risk for adverse cardiovascular outcomes [9]. For example, the outcomes of a nutritional intervention study included improvements on weight and blood pressure parameters, increased produce consumption, and reduced intake of overly processed foods with a high sodium content [23]. A different intervention showed that an educational intervention and access to produce in a community garden had greater improvements in produce consumption than access to the community garden alone [24]. Educational interventions can empower participants to better care for themselves and make healthier lifestyle choices that are associated with decreased risk reduction [11]. The outcomes of an educational intervention among minority women increased their knowledge about heart disease and stroke, CVD risk factors, and taking appropriate action for symptom presentation [9]. A stroke prevention program implemented among African American participants in rural churches had the positive effects of increasing CVD knowledge and reducing blood pressure measures [25]. Another intervention in rural African American church settings successfully improved awareness about CVD and the need for eating a heart-healthy diet and increasing physical activity levels [26].

A limitation of the study is the narrow geographical location from which the participants were recruited, meaning that the results may not be generalizable to other areas. The implementation of the study in two neighboring rural counties could have increased the possibility of cross-contamination between the two study groups. Additionally, the aim of the study design was to analyze the intervention effect on knowledge from pre-test to post-test, however it did not evaluate whether knowledge predicted health behavior changes. Another limitation was that the study did not address whether the knowledge was retained over longer lengths of time. Future research efforts could determine the long-term effects of increased cardiovascular knowledge on lifestyle choices and improvements in biological parameters such as weight, blood pressure, and plasma cholesterol levels.

5. Conclusions

A culturally relevant health education intervention designed to improve CVD knowledge can potentially advance health equity and improve cardiovascular health outcomes among underserved populations. African Americans living in the rural, southern United States are disproportionately burdened by CVD and related chronic diseases and have been historically difficult to engage in health promotion research efforts. The positive results of this study support future efforts targeting CVD risk reduction and health knowledge improvement efforts within rural communities. Public health nurses are particularly well-suited to implement evidence-based health promotion programs in remote community settings and to participate in health disparity research efforts.

Author Contributions: For research articles with several authors, a short paragraph specifying their individual contributions must be provided. The following statements should be used "Conceptualization, L.S.A. and E.H.S.; Methodology, L.S.A. and E.H.S.; Software, L.S.A. and E.H.S.; Formal Analysis, L.S.A. and E.H.S.; Investigation, L.S.A. and E.H.S.; Resources, L.S.A.; Data Curation, L.S.A.; Writing-Original Draft Preparation, L.S.A.; Writing-Review & Editing, L.S.A. and E.H.S.; Visualization, L.S.A.; Supervision, E.H.S.; Project Administration, L.S.A. and E.H.S.; Funding Acquisition, N/A", please turn to the CRediT taxonomy for the term explanation. Authorship must be limited to those who have contributed substantially to the work reported.

Funding: This research received no external funding.

References

1.   Benjamin, E.J.; Virani, S.S.; Callaway, C.W.; Chang, A.R.; Cheng, S.; Chiuve, S.E.; Cushman, M.; Delling, F.N.; Deo, R.; de Ferranti, S.; et al. Heart Disease and Stroke Statistics-2018 Update: A Report from the American Heart Association. *Circulation* **2018**, *137*. [CrossRef] [PubMed]

2.   Havranek, E.P.; Mujahid, M.S.; Barr, D.A.; Blair, I.V.; Cohen, M.S.; Cruz-Flores, S.; Davey-Smith, G.; Dennison-Himmelfarb, C.R.; Lauer, M.S.; Lockwood, D.W.; et al. Social determinants of risk and outcomes for cardiovascular disease A scientific statement From the American Heart Association. *Circulation* **2015**, *132*, 1–26. [CrossRef] [PubMed]

3.   Howard, G.; Kleindorfer, D.; Cushman, M.; Long, D.L.; Jasne, A.; Judd, S.E.; Higginbotham, J.C.; Howard, V.J. Contributors to the excess stroke mortality in rural areas in the United States. *Stroke* **2017**, *48*, 1773–1778. [CrossRef] [PubMed]

4. Kulshreshtha, A.; Goyal, A.; Dabhadkar, K.; Veledar, E.; Vaccarino, V. Urban-rural differences in coronary heart disease mortality in the United States: 1999–2009. *Public Health Rep.* **2014**, *129*, 19–29. [CrossRef] [PubMed]

5. Limdi, N.; Howard, V.; Higginbotham, J.; Parton, J.; Safford, M.; Howard, G. US Mortality: Influence of race, geography and cardiovascular risk among participants in the population-based REGARDS cohort. *J. Racial Ethnic Health Disparities* **2016**, *3*, 599–607. [CrossRef] [PubMed]

6. Singh, G.K.; Daus, G.P.; Allender, M.; Ramey, C.T.; Martin, E.K.; Perry, C.; de Los Reyes, A.; Vedamuthu, I.P. Social determinants of health in the United States: Addressing major health inequality trends for the nation, 1935–2016. *IJMA* **2017**, *6*, 139–164. [CrossRef] [PubMed]

7. Healthy People 2020. Heart Disease and Stroke: Goal. 2018. Available online: https://www.healthypeople.gov/2020/topics-objectives/topic/heart-disease-and-stroke (accessed on 22 February 2018).

8. Carnethon, M.; Pu, J.; Howard, G.; Albert, M.A.; Anderson, C.A.; Bertoni, A.G.; Mujahid, M.S.; Palaniappan, L.; Taylor, H.A.; Willis, M.; et al. Cardiovascular health in African Americans: A scientific statement from the American Heart Association. *Circulation* **2017**, *136*, E393–E423. [CrossRef] [PubMed]

9. Villablanca, A.C.; Slee, C.; Lianov, L.; Tancredi, D. Outcomes of a clinic-based educational intervention for cardiovascular disease prevention by race, ethnicity, and urban/rural status. *J. Womens Health* **2016**, *25*, 1174–1186. [CrossRef] [PubMed]

10. Swanoski, M.T.; Lutfiyya, M.N.; Amaro, M.L.; Akers, M.F.; Huot, K.L. Knowledge of heart attack and stroke symptomology: A cross-sectional comparison of rural and non-rural US adults. *BMC Public Health* **2012**, *12*, 283–290. [CrossRef] [PubMed]

11. Martinez, D.J.; Turner, M.M.; Pratt-Chapman, M.; Kashima, K.; Hargreaves, M.K.; Dignan, M.B.; Hébert, J. The effect of changes in health beliefs among African-American and rural White church congregants enrolled in an obesity intervention: A qualitative evaluation. *J. Community Health* **2016**, *41*, 518–525. [CrossRef] [PubMed]

12. Aycock, D.; Clark, P.; Kirkendoll, K.; Coleman, K.; Alexandrov, A.; Albright, K. Family history of stroke among African Americans and its association with risk factors, knowledge, perceptions, and exercise. *J. Cardiovasc. Nurs.* **2015**, *30*, E1–E6. [CrossRef] [PubMed]

13. Davis, S.K.; Gebreab, S.; Quarells, R.; Gibbons, G. Social determinants of cardiovascular health among Black and White women residing in stroke belt and buckle regions of the south. *Ethn. Dis.* **2014**, *24*, 133–143. [PubMed]

14. Dracup, K.; Moser, D.; Pelter, M.M.; Nesbitt, T.; Southard, J.; Paul, S.M.; Robinson, S.; Hemsey, J.Z.; Cooper, L. Rural patients' knowledge about heart failure. *J. Cardiovasc. Nurs.* **2014**, *29*, 423–428. [CrossRef] [PubMed]

15. Evans, L.K. Because we don't take better care of ourselves: Rural Black women's explanatory models of heart disease. *J. Women Aging* **2010**, *22*, 94–108. [CrossRef] [PubMed]

16. National Institutes of Health. With Every Heartbeat Is Life: A Community Health Worker's Manual for African Americans. 2007. Available online: http://www.nhlbi.nih.gov/files/docs/resources/heart/aa_manual.pdf (accessed on 15 January 2018).

17. Fishbein, M.; Yzer, M.C. Using theory to design effective health behavior interventions. *Commun. Theory* **2003**, *13*, 164–183. [CrossRef]

18. Abbott, L.S.; Williams, C.; Slate, E.H.; Gropper, S. Promoting heart health among rural African Americans. *J. Cardiovasc. Nurs.* **2018**, *33*, E8–E14. [CrossRef] [PubMed]

19. National Heart, Lung, and Blood Institute (NHLBI). My Health Knowledge. 2012. Available online: https://www.nhlbi.nih.gov/health/educational/healthdisp/pdf/resources/CHWI_MyHealthHabits_Pre_EN.pdf (accessed on 15 January 2018).

20. Hurtado, M.; Spinner, J.R.; Yang, M.; Evensen, C.; Windham, A.; Ortiz, G.; Tracy, R.; Ivy, E.D. Knowledge and behavioral effects in cardiovascular health: Community health worker health disparities initiative, 2007–2010. *Prev. Chronic Dis.* **2014**, *11*, 1–9. [CrossRef] [PubMed]

21. Prochaska, J.O.; Velicer, W.F. The transtheoretical model of health behavior change. *Am. J. Health Promot.* **1997**, *12*, 38–48. [CrossRef] [PubMed]

22. Scarinci, I.; Moore, A.; Wynn-Wallace, T.; Cherrington, A.; Fouad, M.; Li, Y. A community-based, culturally relevant intervention to promote healthy eating and physical activity among middle-aged African American women in rural Alabama: Findings from a group randomized controlled trial. *Prev. Med.* **2014**, *69*, 13–20. [CrossRef] [PubMed]

23. Baker, E.A.; Barnidge, E.K.; Schootman, M.; Sawicki, M.; Motton-Kershaw, F.L. Adaptation of a modified DASH diet to a rural African American community setting. *Am. J. Prev. Med.* **2016**, *51*, 967–974. [CrossRef] [PubMed]

24. Barnidge, E.K.; Baker, E.A.; Schootman, M.; Motton, F.; Sawicki, M.; Rose, F. The effect of education plus access on perceived fruit and vegetable consumption in a rural African American community intervention. *Health Educ. Res.* **2015**, *30*, 773–785. [CrossRef] [PubMed]

25. Williams, L.B.; Franklin, B.; Evans, M.B.; Jackson, C.; Hill, A.; Minor, M. Turn the beat around: A stroke prevention program for African American churches. *Public Health Nurs.* **2016**, *33*, 11–20. [CrossRef] [PubMed]

26. Williamson, W.; Kautz, D.D. "Let's get moving: Let's get praising": Promoting health and hope in an African American church. *ABNF J.* **2009**, *20*, 102–105. [PubMed]

14

The Delivery of Health Promotion and Environmental Health Services; Public Health or Primary Care Settings?

Lene Bjørn Jensen [1], Irena Lukic [2] and Gabriel Gulis [2],* (iD)

[1] Public Health Consultant, Haderslev Municipality, Noerregade 41, 6100 Haderslev, Denmark; lbjj@haderslev.dk
[2] Unit for Health Promotion Research, University of Southern Denmark, 6700 Esbjerg, Denmark; irenalukic@hotmail.com
* Correspondence: ggulis@health.sdu.dk

Abstract: The WHO Regional Office for Europe developed a set of public health functions resulting in the ten Essential Public Health Operations (EPHO). Public health or primary care settings seem to be favorable to embrace all actions included into EPHOs. The presented paper aims to guide readers on how to assign individual health promotion and environmental health services to public health or primary care settings. Survey tools were developed based on EPHO 2, 3 and 4; there were six key informant surveys out of 18 contacted completed via e-mails by informants working in Denmark on health promotion and five face-to-face interviews were conducted in Australia (Melbourne and Victoria state) with experts from environmental health, public health and a physician. Based on interviews, we developed a set of indicators to support the assignment process. Population or individual focus, a system approach or one-to-one approach, dealing with hazards or dealing with effects, being proactive or reactive were identified as main element of the decision tool. Assignment of public health services to one of two settings proved to be possible in some cases, whereas in many there is no clear distinction between the two settings. National context might be the one which guides delivery of public health services.

Keywords: public health operations; settings; decision tools; primary care

1. Introduction

To identify the most important public health services and activities, several "essential public health functions" have been suggested over the years. In 1997, an international Delphi study produced a set of essential public health functions [1], which were modified by the Pan American Health Organization and the WHO Regional Office for the Western Pacific [2]. Adjustments to these essential public health functions have been developed by the WHO Regional Office for Europe (WHO EURO) and resulted in the ten Essential Public Health Operations (EPHO) [3], as follows:

1. Surveillance of population health and well-being.
2. Monitoring and response to health hazards and emergencies.
3. Health protection, including environmental, occupational, food safety, and others.
4. Health promotion, including action to address social determinants and health inequity.
5. Disease prevention, including early detection of illness.
6. Ensuring governance for health and well-being.
7. Ensuring a sufficient and competent public health workforce.

8.   Ensuring sustainable organizational structures and financing.
9.   Advocacy, communication and social mobilization for health.
10.   Advancing public health research to inform policy and practice.

To each EPHO, a set of individual actions has been pre-defined by WHO EURO leading to question in which setting should those actions be conducted? Public health or primary care settings seem to be favorable to embrace all actions included into EPHOs, yet a recommendation on which action should be conducted where is not a simple task.

The focus of public health lies in the health of populations and is concerned with all factors, which have an influence on the health of both groups of people and individuals [4]. Public health was defined by Acheson in 1988 as "the art and science of preventing disease, prolonging life and promoting health through the organized efforts of society" [5]. Natural disasters and the newly emerging infections have underlined the global responsibility of early coordinated responses [6] and with the beginning of the 21st century the importance of public health services and approaches has increased. The understanding of tasks and limits of public health services differ among European countries, as well as the extent to which public health is featured on national agendas. Despite the differences across countries, the focus in Europe has evolved in recent decades from sanitary provision and communicable disease control to the new public health which include health promotion, disease prevention and intersectional action.

The concepts of primary care and primary health care have often been used instinctively in the literature, although they derive from different contexts. Historically, primary care is dated back to the United Kingdom (UK) in 1920, where it was intended for the regionalization of health services. Since then the concept has evolved and reached its potential with the establishment of UK National Health Services and the British model of general practice after World War II. These changes in the UK transcended into health systems throughout the industrialized countries and transformed into great variation [7]. The variety of notions used about primary care often refers to the level of health care services closest to communities or health care provided by health professionals at a person's first point of entry into the health care system. For the public, at large in the industrialized world, primary care is mostly associated with medical care because the physician is their first point of entry to the health care system [7]. Primary care can be formally defined as "a multidimensional system structured by primary care governance, economic conditions, and a primary care development, facilitating access to a wide range of primary care services in a coordinated way, and on a continuous basis, by applying resources efficiently to provide high quality care, contributing to the distribution of health in the population" [8]. Primary care is profession centered and often only implies clinical contact [9].

Public health and primary care should be part of one health system [10]. The presented paper aims to guide readers on how to assign individual public health services to either public health or primary care settings. It covers health promotion and environmental health related services only, but generalizes findings in the discussion and conclusion part.

2. Materials and Methods

A pilot study design was employed to develop the guidance to assign individual public health services to both or one of target settings. Denmark and Australia (Victoria state) were selected as study areas with interest to test the process in different health system settings.

To select individual EPHOs and services enlisted under them we used the "Self-assessment tool for evaluation of essential public health operations in the WHO European Region (2015)" [11]. EPHO 4 "Health promotion" was selected direct as individual EPHO and services were edited with aim to shorten the survey tool. Environmental health services were gathered into one set from three EPHOs; EPHO 2, 3 and 4 and created a survey tool. The survey tools were discussed among authors and with an expert from clinical medicine who served as co-supervisor on health promotion services related analyses, but were not pretested.

For health promotion services, there were 6 key informant surveys out of 18 contacted completed via e-mails by informants working in Denmark. On environmental health five face-to-face interviews were conducted in Australia (Melbourne and Victoria state) with experts from environmental health, public health and a physician. Respondents were asked to categorize individual services either to one of key potential provider settings or to both and justify their choice.

3. Results

3.1. Health Promotion Services

The health promotion services that could be provided in agreement of respondents in primary care constituted of nine services. The major characteristic of these public health services is mostly related to services that are provided directly through patient contact. Most of the services require authorized health care professionals to be provided. These services are summarized in Table 1.

Table 1. Health promotion services provided in a primary care setting [11].

Provision of early childhood care, including regular check-ups, preventive services and healthy child development services
Screening and treatment of sexually transmitted infections
Access to fertility treatments
Access to safe medical and surgical abortion
Breastfeeding counselling and support in special-needs situations
Nutritional care and support for children living with HIV
Nutrition for children in an emergency context
Iron supplementation
Folic acid supplementation

The health promotion services that could be provided in public health settings according to respondents are constituted by 22 services. The major characteristic of these public health services is mostly related to community work, inter-sectoral collaboration and information systems. These services are summarized in Table 2.

Table 2. Health promotion services provided in a public health setting [11].

Empowerment of communities through local capacity-building, education, training and community mobilization
Community-based initiatives and partnerships
Establishment of information system, defining responsibilities and methodologies for data collection, analysis and use
Coherence of nutrition strategy with other policies related to health, agriculture, food safety, food industry, etc., information systems, monitoring and evaluation
Health promotion programs in community settings, including schools and workplaces
"Active transport" and urban development policies to promote walking and cycling, at the local and national levels
Efforts at a municipal or national level to ensure access to green space in urban environments
Communication campaigns to reduce obesity, including elements of diet and physical activity
Community-based strategies in sexual health education, including for vulnerable populations
Culturally sensitive communication campaigns to positively change social norms (on HIV, homosexuality, etc.)
Engagement with cultural and religious leaders to positively influence attitudes on sexual health
Quality of childbirth facilities, services and professionals
Information campaigns for the prevention of substance abuse, information systems, monitoring and evaluation
Performance of needs assessment research; generation of policy reports to obtain a comprehensive picture of mental health needs in the country
List of mental health services available within public health care system
Linkage with health and social services for prevention, detection, promotion and rehabilitation (including screening and prevention programmes for suicide and suicide risk)

Table 2. *Cont.*

Context-specific research on the causes of violence and effective prevention/protection strategies
Policies and programmes related to injury prevention, indicators and monitoring
Policies adapted to local conditions (urban versus rural, ethnic mix, gender issues, etc.) and developed in cooperation with local community leaders)
Strategy based on a critical analysis of the underlying causes for health inequities and identification of areas amenable to assessment
Development of information systems to track relevant target-based indicators, including income inequality, educational quality, access to healthy environments, employment opportunities, etc.
Measures aimed at building community support for health equity (e.g., through communication campaigns and awareness raising)

The public health services that could be provided in both a public health setting and primary care setting are constituted by 23 services according to respondents. This group contains both services where the public health setting does not apply, e.g., "management of moderate and severe acute malnutrition in infants and young children" and "intermittent supplementation of folic acid and iron for women in reproductive age", and services where the primary care setting does not apply, e.g., "nutrition education, including food safety and physical activity, included in curriculum" and "Safe school environment for girls; skills-based education covering gender issues; promotion of girls' education and empowerment". Decision upon setting could be context based in different countries. Compared to agreement level on previous two categories (primary care or public health), the agreement level with these services was low. Summary of services is in Table 3.

Table 3. Health promotion services to be provided both in primary care or public health settings [11].

Youth-friendly sexual health services Ensuring broad access to information on the harm done by tobacco consumption, exposure to second-hand smoke and the benefits of quitting
Provision of direct support to smokers wishing to quit within the health care system, both in primary care and in specialized services
Increased capacity for prevention, treatment and care for all individuals and families affected by harmful use of alcohol
Specific programmes targeted to vulnerable groups Dissuasive warnings on consumption of illicit alcohol to public Facility- and community-level breastfeeding programmes/support Maternity protection Management of moderate and severe acute malnutrition in infants and young children Intermittent supplementation of folic acid and iron for women in reproductive age Nutritional support during emergencies for pregnant women Nutrition education, including food safety and physical activity, included in curriculum
Specific food programmes for vulnerable populations (e.g., school lunch programme, food subsidies, etc.)
Programmes aimed at increasing intake of fruit and vegetables
Communication and educational programmes in community settings (health centres, workplaces, etc.)
Measures to identify and address malnutrition in adult and elderly populations Family planning services
Linkage with health and social services for prevention, detection, promotion and rehabilitation (including screening and prevention programmes for suicide and suicide risk), monitoring and evaluation
Safe school environment for girls; skills-based education covering gender issues; promotion of girls' education and empowerment
Use of reproductive/family planning services as entry points to support for victims Research, analysis and dissemination
Defined roles in health and other sectors for a range of injuries and violence (poisoning, fires, drowning, falls, road traffic accidents, violence, etc.)
Public health approach followed (1) surveillance, (2) identification of risk factors, (3) development and evaluation, (4) implementation

3.2. Environmental Health Services

Table 4 summarizes categorization of service delivery places for environmental health services.

Table 4. Division of environmental health services.

Primary Care	None
Public Health	• Reducing air pollution • Sanitation and drinking water • Sanitation of swimming pools and public lakes • Dust storms • Bushfires, heatwaves and floods • Indoor air quality • Alert systems
Uncertain/either/or	• Preparing for adaptation to impacts of climate change • Land contamination • Radiation inside and outside of hospital • Reducing noise • Indoor air pollutants • Food safety both public and private spaces • Investigation of disease clusters

In fact, only those broad services are assigned to public health where the five interviewees reached agreement. In those in "uncertain" they did not reached agreement, yet with exception of radiation control they categorized public health or either/or as delivery place. The services on radiation control are the only one where primary care has been mentioned by one interviewee direct.

3.3. Indicators

Even more interesting as direct categorization of delivery places for individual health promotion or environmental health services are the indicators employed by respondents and interviewees to assign a delivery place. Summary of those decision tools is in Table 5.

Table 5. Decision tools.

Public Health		Primary Care
Population-based	⟵⟶	Individual perspective
System dimension	⟵⟶	One-on-one relationship
Dealing with hazard	⟵⟶	Dealing with the effects
Proactive	⟵⟶	Reactive
Large scale/area/living environment/a whole community		Reporting system
Research		Monitoring of individuals
The bigger picture		Ill health
Prevention		
Monitoring		
Regulations		
Public spaces		
Creating and implementing guidelines		

The arrows signalize that the indicators were used with regard both settings, though in some case more often for primary care as for public health, or equally.

4. Discussion

Looking at formal definitions of primary care and public health, there is a clear distinction. However, the distinction become less clear when looking deeper into what literature is explaining especially in terms of areas of responsibility and into practical routine work. Brown, Upshur and Sullivan [10] put the question "Public Health and Primary Care: Competition or Collaboration?" direct as title of their editorial. They conclude that public health and primary care should be two integrated parts of the same health system. The integration can for example be seen in the explanation of strong primary care, presenting preventive programs as part of strong primary care [12]. Literature also creates confusion in the differentiation of the terms primary care and primary health care. Primary health care includes both public health and primary care in its framework, placing primary care as the main setting, building the health care system around the primary care to create the health system that meets the need of all [13].

Even though the Health 2020 report in many ways is focused on strengthening public health, it recognizes primary health care as the center of service delivery [14]. In one instance, primary health care puts public health as the main actor, which is when focusing on public policies [13].

A major limitation of our study is the sample size and selection of two remote countries as study settings. The sample size is too small in both surveys to be able to make conclusions based on the results. One of the key barriers to get a larger sample size was the length of survey tool due to substantial listing of services. This also means that the results cannot be generalized, though it is a general question whether any results on the issue of public health—primary care can be generalized due to the significant role of national contexts. The results also must be seen in the light of the possibility of professional bias. To control for it, we tried to provide precise definitions of the public health setting and the primary care setting, but it seems like the respondents have not made sufficient use of the definitions. Respondents were likely to respond and categorize services according to their own professional background. In future research, noting the professional background of respondents and aiming to increase a balanced and most importantly larger sample size can lead to improved validity of results.

However, the most important product of this research is the listing of indicators used by respondents to decide whether a service delivery is closer to a public health or primary care setting. Both the Danish survey respondents and the Australian interviewees used the same categories proving global generalizability of the presented categories. They can be of help also to national health policy makers while designing strategies and legislation on public health.

Despite all limitations of our pilot study, we believe that our findings place the EPHOs in slightly other perspective highlighting more the collaboration between public health and primary care. The EPHOs in addition to their original purpose to define essential public health services can be used also as an integration framework for settings providing the individual services in a specific governance and administration context.

5. Conclusions

The presented research aimed to categorize health promotion and environmental health services of public health according to delivery setting, which was set as both or either a public health or a primary care setting. This proved to be possible in some cases, whereas in many there is no clear distinction between the two settings. Obviously, public health and primary care are both part of a health system and one of the key messages is, therefore, a need to coordinate the work of two settings rather then look for differences. National context is likely the one that guides delivery of public health services in a close collaboration with primary care.

An important product of the research is a set of indicators, which can serve as decision tools while designing policies to provide all public health services. More research is needed on these indicators under specific national health system settings.

In addition, and integrative perspective of EPHOs was identified as well. Despite being oriented on public health, a detailed analysis of services with focus on providing settings can identify different institutions inside and beyond a traditional health system. Future research should therefore include settings outside heath sector like for example municipalities, environmental directorates and other settings.

Author Contributions: L.B.J. did the part of environmental health related EPHO analysis, I.L. conducted the study on health promotion EPHO and G.G. designed the study and wrote the initial draft of the manuscript. All authors read and approved the final draft of the manuscript.

Funding: This research received no external funding.

Acknowledgments: Not applicable; all work was done as master thesis at a study program on public health research.

References

1. Bettcher, D.W.; Sapirie, S.; Goon, E.H. Essential public health functions: Results of the international Delphi study. *World Health Stat. Q.* **1998**, *51*, 44–54. [PubMed]
2. PAHO. *PAHO Resolution CD 42.R14*; PAHO: Washington, DC, USA, 2000.
3. World Health Organization. *Review of Public Health Capacities and Services in the European Region*; World Health Organization: København, Denmark, 2012.
4. Ashton, J. Public health and primary care: Towards a common agenda. *Public Health* **1990**, *104*, 387–398. [CrossRef]
5. Rechel, B.; McKee, M. *Facets of Public Health in Europe. European Observatory on Health Systems and Policies Series*; Open University Press: Maidenhead, UK, 2014.
6. Hill, A.P.; Griffiths, S.; Gillam, S. *Public Health and Primary Care: Partners in Population Health*; Oxford University Press: Oxford, NY, USA, 2007.
7. Felix-Bortolotti, M. Part 1—Unravelling primary health care conceptual predicaments through the lenses of complexity and political economy: A position paper for progressive transformation. *J. Eval. Clin. Pract.* **2009**, *15*, 861–867. [CrossRef] [PubMed]
8. Kringos, D.S.; Boerma, W.G.; Hutchinson, A.; van der Zee, J.; Groenewegen, P.P. The breadth of primary care: A systematic literature review of its core dimensions. *BMC Health Serv. Res.* **2010**, *10*, 65. [CrossRef] [PubMed]
9. White, F. Primary health care and public health: Foundations of universal health systems. *Med. Princ. Pract.* **2015**, *24*, 103–116. [CrossRef] [PubMed]
10. Brown, A.D.; Upshur, R.; Sullivan, T.J. Public Health and Primary Care: Competition or Collaboration? *Healthc. Pap.* **2013**, *13*, 4–8. [CrossRef] [PubMed]
11. WHO. Self-Assessment Tool for Evaluation of Essential Public Health Operations in the WHO European Region 2015. Available online: http://www.euro.who.int/en/health-topics/Health-systems/public-health-services/publications/2015/self-assessment-tool-for-the-evaluation-of-essential-public-health-operations-in-the-who-european-region-2015 (accessed on 11 April 2018).
12. Kringos, D.S.; Boerma, W.G.W.; Hutchinson, A.; Saltman, R.B. Building Primary Care in a Changing Europe. World Health Organization European Observatory on Health Systems and Policies. 2015. Available online: http://www.euro.who.int/en/publications/abstracts/building-primary-care-in-a-changing-europe (accessed on 28 April 2016).
13. Lerberghe, W.V.; World Health Organization. *The World Health Report 2008: Primary Health Care Now More Than Ever*; World Health Organization: Geneva, Switzerland, 2008; Available online: http://www.who.int/whr/2008/en/ (accessed on 3 March 2016).
14. World Health Organization Regional Office for Europe. Health 2020 A European Policy Framework and Strategy for the 21st Century. WHO Regional Office of Europe 2013. Available online: http://www.euro.who.int/en/health-topics/health-policy/health-2020-the-european-policy-for-health-and-well-being/about-health-2020 (accessed on 17 March 2016).

15

Veteran Treatments: PTSD Interventions

Steven G. Koven

Urban Studies Institute, University of Louisville, 426 West Bloom Street, Louisville, KY 40208, USA; steven.koven@louisville.edu

Abstract: Post-traumatic stress disorder (PTSD) has resulted in high social costs in terms of the lingering inability of veterans to adapt to societal norms. These costs accrue to individual veterans, their families, friends, and others. In addition, society suffers from the lost productivity of veterans. There is a need to pay greater attention to the extant literature regarding the effectiveness or ineffectiveness of various interventions. This study reviews the most relevant research regarding PTSD, veterans, interventions, treatment, counseling, job training and medication. Increasing awareness of the existing state of knowledge can lead to better targeting of resources and better health outcomes.

Keywords: post-traumatic stress disorder; meta-analysis; veterans; treatment; interventions

---

1. Introduction

Many veterans who are devoid of visible disabilities have acquired invisible scars that negatively affect them throughout their lifetimes. Both visible and invisible scars have severe repercussions for families, friends, communities and the collective society. Mental health disorders, divorce, alcoholism, drug abuse, homelessness, depression, unemployment, underemployment, and criminal activity represent some of the negative side effects of traumatic stress. Suicides and post-traumatic stress disorder (PTSD) are tangible indicators of the invisible wounds of military service [1–3].

Payments for PTSD have escalated in recent years. Some trace the escalation to a 2010 rule change by the U.S. Veterans Administration that is associated with an increase in the approval of PTSD claims. The 2010 rule dispenses with the need to corroborate that hostile military action produces stress disorder (Office of Public and Intergovernmental Affairs, 2010). Ambiguities and inconsistencies in diagnoses also contributed to rising costs. In a 2005 report, the Department of Veterans Affairs, Office of Inspector General concluded that in 25% of the PTSD cases reviewed, inconsistencies occurred in rating methods as well as the process of verifying evidence. Error rates ranged from a high of 40.7% (Maine) to a low of 11% (Oregon). Over the lifetimes of the veterans, the questionable payments approximated many billions of dollars [3].

PTSD claims increased rapidly between 1999 and 2004. According to a 2005 Veterans Affairs report, between 1999 and 2004 the number of total veterans receiving disability compensation grew by less than 15% while the number of PTSD cases in this time-period grew by almost 80%. Veteran compensation for PTSD expanded to represent more than 20% of all compensation payments [4].

The monetary payments that veterans receive are not the only costs that are associated with PTSD. Other costs include marital problems, family violence, raising children with behavioral difficulties, problems of trust, closeness, communication, drinking, intimacy, friendships, physical violence and drug abuse [3,5,6]. The social costs of PTSD are high. Given the high costs, it is useful to gain a greater understanding of the academic literature addressing PTSD. Such a review of existing literature provides a fuller understanding of what we know and do not know about PTSD.

This study describes the most relevant academic research according to Google Scholar criteria. Identified articles are indicative of currency and interest among scholars and the wider Internet audience. Some high-quality research may not be included in the identified articles because they do not comport with the Google Scholar criteria. Descriptions of veteran PTSD research included in this study, therefore, are not all inclusive of PTSD research. Identification prioritizes prevalence and circulation among other factors.

2. Methods

This study describes highly accessed PTSD research. This strategy is similar but not identical to meta-analysis in the sense that it pools various studies in an effort to make inferences. The medical definition of meta-analysis refers to a quantitative statistical analysis that is applied to separate but similar experiments of different and usually independent researchers and that involves pooling the data and using the pooled data to test the effectiveness of the results. More generally, researchers have applied the term meta-analysis to the analysis of prior analyses [7]. Researchers regard meta-analysis highly. Meta-analysis ranks at the top in the hierarchy of clinical evidence according to its freedom from various biases [8]. This study also employs content analysis. Content analysis refers to a method for studying documents and means of communication, which might be texts, pictures, audio or video. One of the key advantages of using content analysis is its non-invasive nature, in contrast to simulating social experiences or conducting surveys. Practices and philosophies of content analysis vary between academic disciplines. However, all content analysis studies involve systematic reading or observation of texts or artifacts that researchers assign labels to indicate the presence of meaningful pieces of content [9].

This paper combines aspects of content analysis and meta-analysis; it uses the google research tool for the selection of relevant studies. The criteria for the selection of the 20 articles (10 each for each of the two areas of investigation) includes a search of scholarly work using key words, a sorting based on relevance, and selection of the 10 most relevant scholarly articles for each avenue of inquiry. Google Scholar ranks relevance by multiple criteria. These criteria include weighing the full text of each document, where it was published, whom it was written by, as well as how often and how recently it has been cited in other scholarly literature. A previous study uses similar criteria in choosing research for meta-analysis [10]. This study ranks the most relevant manuscripts considering two foci of analysis. The first area of inquiry uses a search of the keywords PTSD, veterans, interventions and treatment. The second uses the keywords PTSD, veterans, counseling, job training and medication. The first search focuses on general veteran PTSD research. The second focuses more specifically on the type of treatments. Books are not included in the relevance rankings. Both groups of publications use PTSD and veterans in the content search. However, the distinction between the more general interventions used to identify the first group and the more specific terminology of counseling, job training and medication used to identify the second group was sufficiently distinctive to produce two entirely different cohorts. None of the identified articles appears in both groups.

Previous studies delineate methodologies for identifying prior research [11,12]. This study adds to the body of research that leverages electronic media for identifying relevant research. The study utilizes key terms PTSD, veterans, interventions, and treatment for identifying research based on criteria developed by Google Scholar, a highly visible source of data in the electronic age. In contrast, the study utilizes the terms counseling, job training and medication in an effort to target the specific type of intervention for veterans with PTSD. The goal of the search is to make inferences about the prevalence of obvious types of treatment.

3. Results

Table 1 delineates the 10 most relevant manuscripts for the keywords PTSD, veterans, intervention and treatment. The table identifies relevance, year published, authors, titles and publisher of these scholarly works.

Table 1. General treatment and intervention studies.

Relevance	Year	Author	Title	Journal
1	1996	Bremner Southwick Darnell Charney	Chronic PTSD in Vietnam Combat Veterans [13]	American Journal of Psychiatry
2	2004	Galovsky Lyons	Psychological Sequelae of Combat Violence [14]	Aggression and Violent Behavior
3	2011	Ulmer Edinger Calhoun	A Multi-Component Cognitive-Behavioral Intervention for Sleep Disturbance in Veterans with PTSD [15]	Journal of Clinical Sleep Medicine
4	2009	Bisson Mathews Pilling	Psychological treatments for chronic post-traumatic stress disorder [16]	British Journal of Psychiatry
5	2009	Murphy Thompson Murray Rainey Uddo	Effect of a Motivation Enhancement Intervention [17]	Psychological Services
6	2009	Monson Taft Fredman	Military-related PTSD and intimate relationships [18]	Clinical Psychology Review
7	2009	Cukor Spitalnik Difede Rizzo Rothbaum	Emerging Treatments for PTSD [19]	Clinical Psychology Review
8	2005	Drescher Rosen Burling Foy	Causes of Death among Male Veterans Who Receive Residential Treatment for PTSD [20]	Journal of Traumatic Stress
9	2013	Vujanovic Niles Pietrefesa Schmertz Potter	Mindfulness in the Treatment of Posttraumatic Stress Disorder Among Military Veterans [21]	Spirituality in Clinical Practice
10	2006	Southwick Gilmartin McDonough Morrissey	Logotherapy an Adjunctive Treatment for Chronic Combat-related PTSD [22]	American Journal of Psychotherapy

As a whole, the studies delineated in Table 1 identify a wide variety of authors and publication outlets. Steven Southwick assists in two of the manuscripts. Articles appear in an array of journals; two manuscripts appear in the journal *Clinical Psychology Review*. Psychology journals are the major outlets for publication. With regard to the question of general treatment and intervention, two foci exist: (1) a treatment focus and (2) a problem focus.

Three of the 10 general treatment and intervention studies deal with meta-analysis [16] or controlled experiments [15,17]. Murphy, et al. (2009) study the awareness of the need to change among patients [17]. The authors find that poor response to PTSD treatment may be due not to inadequate interventions or biologically driven symptoms but from ambivalence or lack of awareness about the need to change. They posit that traumatized combat veterans may not see coping styles (e.g., social isolation, mistrust of others) as psychiatric symptoms but as functional strategies. The authors conclude that there is a need to focus on readiness to change. Ulmer, et al. (2011) found that newly developed interventions can address nightmare problems but do not fully remove all aspects of PTSD-related sleep difficulties [15].

Three articles describe innovative treatments/therapy for PTSD. Vujanovic et al. (2013) focuses on the application of meditation to trauma-related mental health struggles [21]. They note that as the utilization of "mindfulness-based" interventions increases, more research is necessary to determine how the intervention might alleviate psychological problems. Cukor et al. (2009) reviews emerging psychotherapeutic and pharmacologic interventions (including propranolol, ketamin, prazosin, and methylendioxymethaphetamine) for the treatment of PTSD [19]. Their paper states that the high rate of treatment failures for PTSD calls for the innovation and dissemination of alternative treatments. The authors review emerging interventions for the treatment of PTSD. They examine the evidence for a range of interventions, from social and family-based treatments to technological-based treatments and describe recent findings regarding novel pharmacologic approaches. The article gives special emphasis to virtual reality as a treatment.

Southwick et al. (2006) present "logotherapy" (healing through meaning) as an innovative adjunctive treatment for PTSD [22]. Logotherapy is future-oriented, focuses on personal strengths and places responsibility for change on the patient. The main tenets of logotherapy include "tragic optimism" or optimism in the face of human suffering guilt and certain death. Tragic optimism encompasses the human potential to transform suffering into human achievement and guilt into meaningful action. The authors view logotherapy as an adjunctive therapy, enhancing rather than supplanting other treatment approaches. They demonstrate how providers can apply logotherapy to the treatment of veterans with PTSD in a variety of therapeutic settings. The study concludes that through a variety of means, including Socratic dialogue, topical discussion using quotations, volunteerism, collective service projects, and group process, veterans can rediscover meaning in their lives. Veterans can see post-traumatic stress as a "heavy gift" and see themselves stronger because of their symptoms.

The final four general articles delineated in Table 1 link PTSD with specific problems that emanate from stress disorder. Bremner et al. (1996) address the effects of alcohol and substance abuse on PTSD patients [13]. They note that an increase in alcohol and substance abuse typically parallels the increase in symptoms of PTSD. Family and relationship problems are the focus of attention in two articles [14,18]. These studies describe numbing, anger, divorce, and severe relationship problems as aspects of PTSD. The final article explores cause of death among male veterans who receive treatment for PTSD. Authors find that behavioral causes (e.g., accidents, substance abuse, suicide, homicide or shooting by police) reduce the life expectancy of PTSD patients [19].

Table 2 describes the most relevant research inserting the key words PTSD, veterans, counseling, job training and medication. A variety of researchers publish in this area; however, the scholarship of Edna Foa is most prominent. Scholarship appears in multiple journals; the publication outlet *Journal of Traumatic Stress* is most prominent for the articles identified in Table 2.

Table 2. Specific PTSD treatment and intervention studies.

Relevance	Year	Author	Title	Journal
1	2010	Karlin Ruzek Chard Eftekhari Monson Hembree Resick Foa	Dissemination of evidence-based psychological treatments for posttraumatic stress disorder in the Veterans Health Administration [23]	Journal of Traumatic Stress
2	1996	Hyler Boyd Scurfield Smith Burke	Effects of Outward Bound Experience as an adjunct to inpatient PTSD treatment of war veterans [24]	Journal of Clinical Psychology

Table 2. *Cont.*

Relevance	Year	Author	Title	Journal
3	2009	Rauch Defever Favorite Duroe Garrity Matis Leberzon	Prolonged exposure for PTSD in a Veterans Health Administration PTSD clinic [25]	Journal of Traumatic Stress
4	1995	Silver Brooks Obenchain	Treatment of Vietnam War Veterans with PTSD [26]	Journal of Traumatic Studies
5	2002	Rothbaum Schwartz	Exposure to therapy for posttraumatic stress disorder [27]	American Journal of Psychotherapy
6	2009	Burke Degeneffe Olney	A New Disability for Rehabilitation Counselors [28]	Journal of Rehabilitation
7	1991	Foa Rothbaum Riggs Murdock	Treatment of Posttraumatic Stress Disorder in Rape Victims [29]	Journal of Consulting and Clinical Psychology
8	2005	Foa Hembree Cahill Rauch Riggs Feeney Elna	Randomized Trial of Prolonged Exposure for Posttraumatic Stress Disorder with and without Cognitive Restructuring [30]	Journal of Consulting and Clinical Psychology
9	2011	Kearney McDermott Malte Martinez Simpson	Association of participation in a mindfulness program with measures of PTSD, depression and quality of life in a veteran sample [31]	Journal of Clinical Psychology
10	2007	McNally	Mechanisms of exposure therapy: How neuroscience can improve psychological treatments for anxiety disorders [32]	Clinical Psychology Review

Articles describe numerous treatment options. Hyer et al. (1996) discuss the effect of placing people in a novel setting, such as a wilderness [24]. The authors test whether an "Outward Bound Experience" of 5 days in a novel setting has positive effects on PTSD patients. They conclude that the "Outward Bound Experience" did not outperform inpatient programs although many veterans rated the experience positively. Another study (relevance 4) examine Eye Movement Desensitization and Reprocessing (EMDR) Therapy concluding that EMDR can produce significant improvements in reducing anxiety, anger, depression, isolation, intrusive thoughts, flashbacks, nightmares and relationship problems [26]. EMDR asks patients to recall distressing images while conducting actions such as side-to-side eye movements or hand tapping. The paper suggests that EMDR training is a more effective treatment for PTSD than those traditionally provided in an in-patient PTSD-specific program. A third study (relevance 9) explores the effectiveness of mindfulness-based stress reduction (MBSR) programs. MBSR uses a combination of meditation, body awareness, and yoga [31]. The authors conclude that MBSR can achieve significant improvements in PTSD symptoms.

In addition to these studies of various treatments, one manuscript (relevance 7) addresses prolonged exposure and three other types of treatments in rape victims [29]. The authors conclude that prolonged exposure (re-experiencing the traumatic event through remembering it and engaging with, rather than avoiding it) produces better outcomes on reducing PTSD symptoms than other techniques. Only one article (relevance 6) addresses the needs of veterans for vocational rehabilitation, independent living, and family support [28]. Authors provide a comprehensive listing of resources for veterans with traumatic brain injury and post-traumatic stress disorder.

The final five articles found in Table 2 (relevance 1,3,5,8,10) address Prolonged Exposure (PE) therapy in one manner or another [23,25,27,30,32]. Foa et al. (2005) specifically explored the impact of Prolonged Exposure therapy on female assault survivors [30]. The plethora of research on this treatment is testament to its currency and relevance. A consensus view is that Prolonged Exposure is effective in reducing the symptoms of PTSD in veterans who receive care in clinics. Studies indicate that prolonged exposure therapy has yielded gains infrequently or never seen in the past with PTSD patients [23], which is one of the success stories of clinical psychology and psychiatry [32] and has proven its effectiveness in the treatment of PTSD [25]. In addition, research finds that PE can effectively treat rape survivors [29,30] and is a well-established treatment for PTSD [27].

4. Discussion

A review of the general treatment and intervention studies (Table 1) reveals two basic streams of research. One describes treatments for PTSD; another describes the problems associated with PTSD. Relevant articles describe innovative approaches and techniques such as logotherapy, "mindfulness" and novel drugs. Recent research offers insights into how to mitigate the effects of PTSD. Keynan et al. (2016) argue that excluding veterans with combat PTSD (CPTSD) from eligibility for special recognition (such as the Purple Heart) strengthens their stigma and has detrimental implications for their wellbeing [33]. The authors contend that reclassifying PTSD to PTSI (posttraumatic stress injury) may mitigate the stigma of their wounds, increase their willingness to seek aid, and improve their chance to heal. Steenkamp et al. (2015) reviewed evidence from clinical trials of psychotherapies for PTSD in military and veteran populations. They found that two trauma therapies (cognitive processing therapy and prolonged exposure) are most frequently studied [34]. These treatments attained clinically meaningful symptom improvements; however, large proportions of patients retained their PTSD diagnosis after treatment.

A review of the more specific treatment and intervention literature (Table 2) focuses upon Prolonged Exposure (PE) as an effective treatment for PTSD. Some of the literature addresses relatively novel approaches such as mindfulness and Eye Movement Desensitization Reprogramming (EMDR). It is worth noting that despite keyword searches that utilize "counseling" and "job training", only one article [28] has a focus on rehabilitation and offers practical recommendations for counseling professionals. A dearth of attention to the practical problems of veteran reintegration into society through employment or education seems to represent a deficiency in the literature. Poor employment prospects of PTSD patients may contribute to this relative lack of attention. The literature, however, is not completely devoid of employment-related studies. Ellison et al. (2018) found that veteran peer interventions can have positive effects with veterans subsequently spending greater amounts of time on education activities [35]. Amara et al. (2018) discovered that an array of factors such as severity of traumatic brain injury, drug abuse, age, education, and marital status were related to employment status of male and female post-9/11 veterans. Unemployment rates were similar for male and female veterans evaluated in the Veterans Health Administration for traumatic brain injury [36].

5. Conclusions

PTSD among veterans represents a significant problem for society, for families and individuals. Meta-analysis of relevant literature indicates that psychology and psychiatry academic journals are most prominent in pushing the boundaries of knowledge concerning PTSD treatments. The meta-analysis indicates some consensus on the viability of Prolonged Exposure therapy compared to other treatments. Given the high societal costs of PTSD, it is incumbent upon medical researchers to continue to explore treatment options. It is distressing, however, that the most relevant extant research does not assign greater attention to issues of job training, job placement, and social integration. Researchers should recognize that PTSD is a health issue but that job training, education, and job placement can also play an important role in veteran rehabilitation.

Funding: The research received no external funding.

References

1.   Milliken, C.S.; Auchterlonie, J.L.; Hoge, C.W. Longitudinal assessment of mental health problems among active and reserve component soldiers returning from the Iraq war. *J. Am. Med. Assoc.* **2007**, *298*, 2141–2148. [CrossRef] [PubMed]

2.   Tanielian, T.; Jaycox, L. *Invisible Wounds of War: Psychological and Cognitive Injuries, their Consequences, and Services to Assist Recovery*; RAND Corporation: Santa Monica, CA, USA, 2008.

3.   U.S. Department of Veterans Affairs. PTSD: National Center for PTSD, Relationships and PTSD. Available online: http://www.ptsd.va.gov/public/family/ptsd-and-relationships.asp (accessed on 2 August 2018).

4.   Department of Veterans Affairs: Office of Inspector General. Review of State Variances in VA Disability Compensation Payments. Available online: http://www.va.gov/oig/52/reports/2005/VAOIG-05-00765-137.pdf (accessed on 2 August 2018).

5.   Calhoun, P.S.; Beckham, J.C. Caregiver burden and psychological distress in partners of veterans with chronic posttraumatic stress disorder. *J. Trauma. Stress* **2002**, *15*, 205–212. [CrossRef] [PubMed]

6.   Liss, M.; Willer, B. Traumatic brain injury and marital relationships: A literature review. *Int. J. Rehabil. Res.* **1990**, *13*, 309–320. [CrossRef] [PubMed]

7.   Glass, G.V. Primary, secondary, and meta-analysis of research. *Educ. Res.* **1976**, *5*, 3–8. [CrossRef]

8.   Haidich, A.B. Meta-analysis in medical research. *Hippokratia* **2010**, *14*, 29–37. [PubMed]

9.   Hodder, I. *The Interpretation of Documents and Material Culture*; Sage: Thousand Oaks, CA, USA, 1994.

10.   Koven, S.G. PTSD and suicides among veterans: Recent findings. *Public Integr.* **2016**, *19*, 500–512. [CrossRef]

11.   Bolton, A.J.; Dorstyn, D.S. Telepsychology for posttraumatic stress disorder: A systematic review. *J. Telemed. Telecare* **2015**, *21*, 254–267. [CrossRef] [PubMed]

12.   Simblett, S.; Birch, J.; Matcham, F.; Yaquez, L.; Morris, R. A systematic review and meta-analysis of e-mental health interventions to treat symptoms of posttraumatic stress. *J. Med. Internet Res.* **2017**, *4*, e14. [CrossRef] [PubMed]

13.   Bremner, J.D.; Soutwick, S.H.; Darnell, A.C.; Charney, D.S. Chronic PTSD in Vietnam combat veterans: Course of illness and substance abuse. *Am. J. Psychiatry* **1996**, *153*, 369–375. [PubMed]

14.   Galovsky, T.; Lyons, J. Psychological sequelae of combat violence: A review of the impact of PTSD on the veteran's family and possible interventions. *Aggress. Violent Behav.* **2004**, *9*, 477–501. [CrossRef]

15.   Ulmer, C.S.; Edinger, J.D.; Calhoun, P.S. A Multi-component cognitive-behavioral intervention for sleep disturbance in veterans with PTSD: A pilot study. *J. Clin. Sleep Med.* **2011**, *7*, 57–68. [PubMed]

16.   Bisson, J.A.; Matthews, R.; Pilling, S.; Richards, D.; Turner, S. Psychological treatments for chronic post-traumatic stress disorder: Systematic review and meta-analysis. *Br. J. Psychiatry* **2007**, *190*, 97–104. [CrossRef] [PubMed]

17.   Murphy, R.T.; Thompson, K.E.; Murray, M.; Rainey, Q.; Uddo, M.M. Effect of a motivation enhancement intervention on veterans' engagement in PTSD treatment. *Psychol. Serv.* **2009**, *6*, 264–278. [CrossRef]

18.   Monson, C.M.; Taft, C.T.; Fredman, S.J. Military-related PTSD and intimate relationships: From description to theory-driven research and intervention development. *Clin. Psychol. Rev.* **2009**, *29*, 707–714. [CrossRef] [PubMed]

19.   Cukor, J.; Spitolnik, J.; Difede, J.; Rizzo, A.; Rothbaum, B. Emerging treatments for PTSD. *Clin. Psychol. Rev.* **2009**, *29*, 715–726. [CrossRef] [PubMed]

20.   Drescher, K.D.; Rosen, C.S.; Burling, T.A.; Foy, D.W. Causes of death among male veterans who received residential treatment for PTSD. *J. Trauma. Stress* **2005**, *16*, 535–543. [CrossRef] [PubMed]

21. Vujanovic, A.A.; Niles, B.; Pietrefesa, A.; Schmertz, S.K.; Potter, C.M. Mindfulness in the treatment of posttraumatic stress disorder among military veterans. *Spiritual. Clin. Pract.* **2013**, *1*, 15–25. [CrossRef]

22. Southwick, S.M.; Gilmartin, R.; McDonough, P.; Morrissey, P. Logotherapy as an adjunctive treatment for chronic combat-related PTSD: A meaning-based intervention. *Am. J. Psychother.* **2006**, *60*, 161–174. [CrossRef] [PubMed]

23. Karlin, B.; Ruzek, J.; Chard, K.; Eftekhari, A.; Monson, C.; Hembree, E.; Resick, P.; Foa, E. Dissemination of evidence-based psychological treatments for posttraumatic stress disorder in the Veterans Health Administration. *J. Trauma. Stress* **2010**, *23*, 663–673. [CrossRef] [PubMed]

24. Hyler, L.; Boyd, S.; Scurfield, R.; Smith, D.; Burke, J. Effects of outward bound experience as an adjunct to inpatient PTSD treatment of war veterans. *J. Clin. Psychol.* **1996**, *52*, 263–278.

25. Rauch, S.; Defever, E.; Favorite, T.; Duroe, A.; Garrity, C.; Matis, B.; Leberzon, I. Prolonged exposure for PTSD in a Veterans Health Administration PTSD clinic. *J. Trauma. Stress* **2009**, *22*, 60–64. [CrossRef] [PubMed]

26. Silver, S.M.; Brooks, A.; Obenchain, J. Treatment of Vietnam War veterans with PTSD: A comparison of eye movement desensitization and reprocessing, biofeedback and relaxation training. *J. Trauma. Stud.* **1995**, *8*, 337–341. [CrossRef]

27. Rothbaum, B.O.; Schwartz, A.C. Exposure therapy for posttraumatic stress disorder. *Am. J. Psychother.* **2002**, *56*, 59–76. [CrossRef] [PubMed]

28. Burke, H.S.; Degeneffe, C.E.; Olney, M.E. A new disability for rehabilitation counselors: Iraq War veterans with traumatic brain injury and post-traumatic stress disorder. *J. Rehabil.* **2009**, *75*, 5–14.

29. Foa, E.B.; Rothbaum, B.O.; Riggs, D.S.; Murdock, T.B. Treatment of posttraumatic stress disorder in rape victims: A comparison between cognitive-behavioral procedures and counseling. *J. Consult. Clin. Psychol.* **1991**, *59*, 715–723. [CrossRef] [PubMed]

30. Foa, E.B.; Hembree, E.A.; Cahill, S.P.; Rauch, S.A.; Riggs, D.S.; Feeny, N.C.; Elna, Y. Randomized trial of prolonged exposure for posttraumatic stress disorder with and without cognitive restructuring: Outcome at academic and community clinics. *J. Consult. Clin. Psychol.* **2005**, *73*, 953–964. [CrossRef] [PubMed]

31. Kearney, D.J.; McDermott, K.; Malte, C.; Martinez, M.; Simpson, T. Association of participation in a mindfulness program with measures of PTSD, depression and quality of life in a veteran sample. *J. Clin. Psychol.* **2011**, *68*, 101–116. [CrossRef] [PubMed]

32. McNally, R.J. Mechanism of exposure therapy: How neuroscience can improve psychological treatments for anxiety disorders. *Clin. Psychol. Rev.* **2007**, *27*, 750–759. [CrossRef] [PubMed]

33. Keynan, I.; Keynan, J. War trauma, politics of recognition and purple heart: PTSD or PTSI? *Soc. Sci.* **2016**, *5*, 57. [CrossRef]

34. Steenkamp, M.; Litz, B.; Hoge, C.; Marmar, C. Psychotherapy for military-related PTSD: A review of randomized clinical trials. *J. Am. Med. Assoc.* **2015**, *314*, 489–500. [CrossRef] [PubMed]

35. Ellison, M.; Reilly, E.; Mueller, L.; Schultz, M.; Drebing, C. A supported education service pilot for returning veterans with posttraumatic stress disorder. *Psychol. Serv.* **2018**, *15*, 200–207. [CrossRef] [PubMed]

36. Amara, J.H.; Stolzmann, K.L.; Iverson, K.M.; Pogoda, T.K. Predictors of employment status in male and female post-9/11 veterans evaluated for traumatic brain injury. *J. Head Trauma Rehabil.* **2018**. [CrossRef] [PubMed]

16

Health Disparities Score Composite of Youth and Parent Dyads from an Obesity Prevention Intervention: iCook 4-H

Melissa D. Olfert [1],* [ID], Makenzie L. Barr [1], Rebecca L. Hagedorn [1] [ID], Lisa Franzen-Castle [2], Sarah E. Colby [3], Kendra K. Kattelmann [4] and Adrienne A. White [5]

[1] Davis College of Agriculture, Natural Resources & Design, Division of Animal and Nutritional Sciences, West Virginia University, G016 Agricultural Science Building, Morgantown, WV 26506, USA; mbarr6@mix.wvu.edu (M.L.B.); rlhagedorn@mix.wvu.edu (R.L.H.)

[2] Nutrition and Health Sciences Department, University of Nebraska-Lincoln, 110 Ruth Leverton Hall, Lincoln, NE 68583-0806, USA; lfranzen2@unl.edu

[3] Department of Nutrition, University of Tennessee, 1215 W. Cumberland Avenue, 229 Jessie Harris Building, Knoxville, TN 37996-1920, USA; scolby1@utk.edu

[4] Department of Health and Nutritional Sciences, South Dakota State University, Box 2275A, SWG 425, Brookings, SD 57007, USA; Kendra.Kattelmann@sdstate.edu

[5] School of Food and Agriculture, University of Maine, 5735 Hitchner Hall, Orono, ME 04469, USA; awhite@maine.edu

* Correspondence: Melissa.olfert@mail.wvu.edu

Abstract: iCook 4-H is a lifestyle intervention to improve diet, physical activity and mealtime behavior. Control and treatment dyads (adult primary meal preparer and a 9–10-year-old youth) completed surveys at baseline and 4, 12, and 24 months. A Health Disparity (HD) score composite was developed utilizing a series of 12 questions (maximum score = 12 with a higher score indicating a more severe health disparity). Questions came from the USDA short form U.S. Household Food Security Survey (5), participation in food assistance programs (1), food behavior (2), level of adult education completed (1), marital status (1), and race (1 adult and 1 child). There were 228 dyads (control n = 77; treatment n = 151) enrolled in the iCook 4-H study. Baseline HD scores were 3.00 ± 2.56 among control dyads and 2.97 ± 2.91 among treatment dyads, p = 0.6632. There was a significant decline in the HD score of the treatment group from baseline to 12 months (p = 0.0047) and baseline to 24 months (p = 0.0354). A treatment by 12-month time interaction was found (baseline mean 2.97 ± 2.91 vs. 12-month mean 1.78 ± 2.31; p = 0.0406). This study shows that behavioral change interventions for youth and adults can help improve factors that impact health equity; although, further research is needed to validate this HD score as a measure of health disparities across time.

Keywords: behavior; health disparities; nutrition; physical activity; family mealtime

---

1. Introduction

While there are many variations in how "Health Disparities" is defined [1–3], Braveman et al. (2014) defined health disparities as "worse health among socially disadvantaged individuals, specifically those of disadvantaged racial/ethnic groups" [4,5]. Although a clear classification system to identify individuals with health disparities has not yet been established, the idea that health disparities need to be eliminated, or at least mitigated, is widely accepted both nationally and internationally [6]. Health disparities adversely affect groups of people who have systematically experienced greater social and/or economic obstacles to being healthy, based on their racial or ethnic group, religion, socioeconomic status, gender, age, mental health (cognitive, sensory, or physical disability), sexual orientation or gender identity, geographic location, and other characteristics historically linked to discrimination or exclusion [1].

The United States (U.S.) Government has committed itself to the elimination of health disparities [1]. Every ten years, the U.S. Department of Health and Human Services publishes national objectives for improving the health of all Americans through health promotion and disease prevention [1,7]. Specifically, in Healthy People 2020, reducing health disparities was a primary objective with goals to "achieve health equity, eliminate disparities and improve the health of all groups". The Centers for Population Health and Health Disparities (CPHHD) Program, through the National Institutes of Health (NIH), has called for a new direction in health disparity research, with renewed focus on addressing disparities at the individual and community levels, by utilizing interventions that improve health behavior choices [8].

Efforts to reduce and prevent health disparities may be especially important with youth populations because health at a young age sets the stage for health across the lifespan [9]. Schreier et al. examined health disparities as they impact adolescents [10]. They identified that adolescents growing up in a low socioeconomic status (SES), or "health disparate" environments, were more likely to experience negative health issues that could potentially continue into adulthood [10]. One such health issue disproportionally faced by youth living in "health disparate" environments, is obesity [11]. Obesity is linked to other co-morbidities such as type 2 diabetes, metabolic syndrome and some cancers [12]. Obesity in youth is strongly associated with increased risk of obesity and co-morbidities in adulthood [13–15].

In summary, health disparate populations tend to have poorer health outcomes and a deficiency of access to resources. However, what is lacking, is a mechanism to assess and identify which individuals are living in "health disparate" situations, through demographic, food security and food behaviors. Additionally, it is unknown if interventions can potentially improve or attenuate health behavior declines (through knowledge and access to health information) and whether they can ameliorate health disparities.

The hypothesis of this subproject was to test if participation in a childhood obesity prevention intervention, based on youth-adult dyads cooking, eating and playing together, would impact health disparities by using a "Health Disparate" (HD) score composite that was developed from the intervention's program assessments. To test the hypothesis, the control and treatment participant groups' HD scores were compared before and 4, 12 and 24 months into the childhood obesity prevention intervention.

2. Materials and Methods

iCook 4-H was a five-state (Maine, Nebraska, South Dakota, Tennessee and West Virginia) collaborative, childhood obesity prevention program that started in September of 2013. Researchers utilized a dyad approach of pairing a 9–10-year-old child and their adult primary food preparer. The iCook 4-H curriculum was developed by researchers and Extension professionals to allow youth and adults to learn-by-doing (experiential learning model) and capitalize on the social cognitive theory for behavior change [16]. Each state enrolled control and treatment dyads, with treatment dyads completing six, 2-h face-to-face iCook 4-H group sessions. The bi-weekly sessions focused on "cooking, eating and playing together." Sessions were composed of culinary skill development and recipe preparation, a physical activity component, family mealtime and communication, and ended with goal setting. More detail on the specific iCook 4-H sessions is described elsewhere [17]. Newsletters and booster sessions were used for reinforcement over the two years. Upon completion of the program, researchers aimed to improve culinary skills, mealtime experiences and goal setting, as well as decrease sedentary time within these treatment dyads. Specifically, for the subproject described in this article, researchers sought to determine whether participation in a childhood obesity prevention intervention, iCook 4-H, could reduce participant's health disparity burden by using a Health Disparity (HD) Score.

Ethical approval was obtained by each university's Institutional Review Board prior to recruitment and the study was conducted in accordance with the Declaration of Helsinki. All subjects gave their written informed consent for inclusion before they participated in the study. This study was retrospectively registered (#54135351) on the ISRCTN online registry (www.isrctn.com).

iCook 4-H participants consisted of dyads that included a 9–10-year-old youth partnered with their primary adult meal preparer. Adult meal preparers had to be at least 19 years of age and prepare a majority of the meals in the household for the youth participant. Inclusion criteria required children to not be an age of 11 years old before 31 December 2013; have access to a computer with internet; and to be free from life-threatening illness or medical conditions, food allergies or activity-related medical restrictions that could prevent participation in a nutrition and physical activity-related intervention. Each state recruited participants from their local communities through Extension leaders, word of mouth, school mailings, and/or fliers. The data utilized will be a subproject of the main iCook 4-H intervention study.

Demographic characteristics (including gender, marital status, education level, and race/ethnicity) were collected via the baseline survey. Outcome measures were collected via survey from both control and treatment groups at baseline, 4 months, 12 months and 24 months. Outcomes from the surveys were used to develop a composite HD Score. The HD score was generated from a series of 12 questions including the USDA short form U.S. Household Food Security Survey (USHFSS) (5), participation in food assistance programs (e.g., Women, Infants and Children (WIC) or Supplemental Nutrition Assistance Program (SNAP) (1), food behavior (2), level of adult education completed (1), marital status (1), and race/ethnicity (1 adult and 1 youth question)). The USHFSS questions included HH3, HH4, AD1, AD2 and AD3, as described in the USDA survey module [18]. AD1a was excluded from the screener as not all participants were required to answer this question, as it was dependent on the response to AD1. Food behavior questions about food consumption patterns, were selected from the Expanded Food and Nutrition Education Program (EFNEP) Behavior Checklist [19]. Responses on the HD score were coded as binary variables of 0 or 1. The maximum score possible was 12 with higher scores representing increased health disparity for individuals.

All analyses were conducted using SAS (SAS®, Version 9.3) and JMP (JMP®, Version Pro 11) (SAS Institute Inc., Cary, North, CA, USA). Baseline demographic data are reported in frequencies and percentages. The difference between the control and treatment group's baseline HD scores was analyzed using an independent t-test. To fit both random and fixed effects within the data, as well as the flexibility and individual variances and covariances, a Linear Mixed Model (LMM) was used. The best fitting model was determined through Akaike Information Criterion (AIC) and other goodness-of-fit indices. Time was treated as a continuous variable in the final model. Model fit of covariance structure was determined by Model Likelihood Ratio chi-squared test (LRT). The best fitting model for HD score included only a repeated statement of time, using an autoregressive (AR1) covariance structure, correcting for the degrees of freedom using the Kenward-Roger method and Restricted Maximum Likelihood (REML) estimation, with participant ID as the subject repeated variable. Significant effects were followed up with a post-hoc Tukey test for multiple comparisons.

3. Results

3.1. Participant Characteristics

There were 228 dyads that consented and enrolled into the iCook 4-H program from all five states with 195 that continued after the first session, with mean age of youth (9.35 ± 0.67 years) and adults (38.96 ± 8.04 years), as either control dyads (n = 77) or treatment (n = 151). Table 1 shows an additional demographic breakdown. Treatment youth were primarily White (67%) and female (52%). Treatment adults were also primarily White (70%) and female (83%), with just 64% being married and about 30% with a bachelor's degree. Control youth were primarily White (61%) and male (61.0%). Control adults were also primarily White (65%) and female (81%), with about 64% being married and approximately

36% had completed some college. Based on chi-squared analysis, the only demographically significant differences were that more adults were female in the treatment group ($p = 0.019$). Over the 24 months there were 102 dropouts. Dropouts were more likely to be non-white ($p = 0.03$), not married ($p = 0.001$), have no post high school degree ($p = 0.002$), and use government food assistance programs ($p = 0.005$).

Table 1. Baseline demographics of children and adults enrolled in the iCook 4-H program.

Demographics	Treatment		Control		p-Value
	N	%	N	%	
Total Population					
Dyads	151	66.2	77	33.8	
Child gender					
Male	73	48.3	30	61.0	0.1782
Female	78	51.7	47	39.0	
Child race					
White	96	63.6	47	61.0	
Black	16	10.6	9	11.7	
Hispanic	19	12.6	11	14.3	
Native American	5	3.3	1	1.3	0.5237
Asian	0	0	2	2.6	
Other	3	2.0	2	2.6	
NA	12	7.9	5	6.5	
Adult gender					
Male	9	6.0	12	15.6	0.0190 *
Female	126	83.4	62	80.5	
Adult Race					
White	106	70.2	50	64.9	
Black	13	8.6	5	6.5	
Hispanic	16	10.6	13	16.9	
Native American	3	2.0	0	0	0.1301
Asian	1	0.6	1	1.3	
Other	0	0	3	3.9	
NA	12	7.9	5	6.5	
Marital Status					
Married	97	64.2	50	64.9	
Single	17	11.3	9	11.7	
Divorced	11	7.3	10	13.0	
Committed	13	8.6	5	6.5	0.5387
Widowed	2	1.3	0	0	
NA	11	7.3	3	3.9	
Educational Level					
Elementary	7	4.6	2	2.6	
Some High School	1	0.6	2	2.6	
High School	22	14.6	5	6.5	
Some College	31	20.5	28	36.4	
Associates	20	13.2	8	10.4	0.1952
Bachelors	45	29.8	21	27.3	
Graduate	18	11.9	7	9.1	
Doctoral	5	3.3	2	2.6	
NA	2	1.3	2	2.6	

Demographic data represented in frequency and percentages. * $p < 0.05$, Chi-squared analysis.

3.2. Pre- and Post-Intervention Health Disparity Score Composite

Complete data from 195 dyads were used at baseline to calculate control ($n = 67$) and treatment ($n = 128$) HD scores, with those missing any HD score variables removed. Baseline HD scores between groups were not statistically different (3.00 ± 2.56 control vs. 2.97 ± 2.91 treatment; $p = 0.6632$). In contrast, significant declines were found among the treatment from baseline to 12 months ($p = 0.0047$) and again from baseline to 24 months ($p = 0.0354$) (Table 2).

Table 2. HD scores among groups across time.

Time	Control				Treatment			
	HD Score				HD Score			
	N	Mean	SD	p-Value	N	Mean	SD	p-Value
Baseline	67	3.00	2.56	—	128	2.97	2.91	—
4 months	51	3.04	3.04	0.9997	109	2.16	2.49	0.4265
12 months	48	2.75	2.91	1.0000	93	1.78	2.31	0.0047*
24 months	33	2.15	2.97	0.5742	81	1.41	2.14	0.0354*

Baseline was used as the reference group for each control and treatment comparison. HD scores across time within control and treatment groups reported in mean and standard deviation (SD). Tukey adjustment for group * time p-values.

In Table 3 are the results of Linear Mixed Modeling (LMM) of HD scores across group (control and treatment) and time (baseline, 4, 12 and 24 months). HD score null model LRT was significant: ($X^2(1) = 496.12$, $p < 0.0001$). The type 3 test for fixed effects of group interaction was not significant: $F(1221) = 0.78$, $p = 0.3774$, whereas the type 3 test for time interaction was significant: $F(3394) = 3.67$, $p = 0.0124$, and approaching significance for the type 3 group by time interaction: $F(3394) = 2.58$, $p = 0.0533$. After the Tukey post-hoc comparison test, significance was found in a treatment of 12-month time interaction (baseline mean = 2.97 ± 2.91, 12-month mean = 1.78 ± 2.31, $p = 0.0406$).

Table 3. Mixed Regression Models for HD Score.

Variable	Category	Estimate	SE	t-Value	p-Value
HD Score					
Intercept		3.01	0.32	9.31	<0.0001 *
Group (referent: control):	Treatment	−0.10	0.40	−0.25	0.8047
	4 months	−0.97	0.19	−0.50	0.6190
Time	12 months	−0.04	0.26	−0.15	0.8845
	24 months	−0.63	0.34	−1.87	0.0624
	Treatment * 4 months	−0.18	0.24	−0.78	0.4369
Time*Role (referent: control; baseline):	Treatment * 12 months	0.66	0.32	−2.05	0.0406 *
	Treatment * 24 months	−0.09	0.41	−0.21	0.8299

Linear Mixed Model used to analyze the main effects of group and time on HD score. Significant effects were followed by multiple comparisons using Tukey adjustment. p-values for main effects and interactions are indicated. * $p < 0.05$.

4. Discussion

Researchers found that after a 6-session childhood obesity prevention program, treatment dyads' HD score was reduced significantly from baseline, at 12 and 24 months (Table 2). Upon further analyses, it was found that a significant interaction occurred between the treatment group and the 12-month time point for reduction in HD score after the intervention (Table 3). Compared to the treatment group, the control group had no significant decrease in their HD score (Table 2).

Although no definition has been universally agreed upon for Health Disparities [1,2,4,5], this study provided a formative look into health disparities by utilizing a series of demographic, food security and behavior questions, to capture and describe an individual's level of health disparity into one composite score. Various measures were used to determine health disparities among this population; however, many previous researchers have used epidemiological approaches to define and capture health disparity changes [2,20,21]. However, to our knowledge, this is the first study to capture a composite score that encompasses numerous factors in an intervention setting. Braveman et al. (2006) stated that "Public health surveillance is certainly not sufficient to reduce health disparities", showing a need for interventions such as iCook 4-H. Through this preliminary work, there is evidence for the importance of lifestyle interventions to decrease health disparities.

The utilization of a childhood obesity prevention program designed with a focus on behavior change for individuals and communities, aligns with the proposed recommendations of CPHHD [8]. It appears that CPHHD's vision and recommendations for improving health disparities in populations through a community-based childhood obesity curriculum, can be successful. In the future, researchers should examine whether this intervention approach can be successfully utilized with diverse populations to address health disparities [22,23].

Although a broad range of health disparity factors were included in the composite score, some limitations of the current study include the validity and comprehensiveness of the tool. This current analysis provided a pilot analysis of the score and further testing and content validity needs to be conducted. It is acknowledged that this tool is largely focused on demographics and food security characteristics. Demographic variables such as marital status and race/ethnicity would not change as a result of an intervention. Future work to include knowledge and perceptions of health disparities in populations is warranted and validates this score as a measure of health disparities. For future analysis, a larger sample size and the use of cognitive interviews should be included to ensure that the components used in the score are representative of factors that determine health disparity. Future research projects designed to examine the effect of these interventions on health disparities should include a focus on rural communities. Although health disparities exist across the U.S., these disparities are pronounced in rural areas [22].

5. Conclusions

Overall, the dyads in the treatment group in this study had a decrease in their health disparities score after being provided with a lifestyle intervention focused on families cooking, eating and playing together. Although reducing health disparities was not the main outcome of the iCook 4-H intervention, this subproject aimed to provide an initial insight and understanding to developing a health disparities score. Health disparities may potentially be reduced after providing health information; thus, specifically understanding the perceptions of health disparities in a health intervention cohort is warranted for targeting interventions to improve these scores [24].

Author Contributions: Conceptualization, A.A.W., M.D.O., K.K.K., L.F.-C., and S.E.C.; Methodology, A.A.W., M.D.O., K.K.K., L.F.-C., and S.E.C.; Data Curation, M.D.O., M.L.B., K.K.K., L.F.-C., S.E.C., and A.A.W.; Formal Analysis, M.L.B.; Writing-Original Draft Preparation, M.D.O., M.L.B., and R.L.H.; Writing-Review & Editing, M.D.O., M.L.B., R.L.H., L.F.-C., K.K.K., S.E.C., and A.A.W.; Project Administration, A.A.W., M.D.O., K.K.K., L.F.-C., and S.E.C.; Funding Acquisition, A.A.W., M.D.O., K.K.K., L.F.-C., and S.E.C.

Funding: This material is based upon work that is supported by the National Institute of Food and Agriculture, U.S. Department of Agriculture, under award number 2012-68001-19605. The third author of this work was supported by a National Institute of General Medical Sciences T32 grant (GM081741). Other funding is from the West Virginia University Hatch WVA00641 and the state experiment stations for the South Dakota State University, the University of Maine and the University of Nebraska-Lincoln.

Acknowledgments: Author's thank USDA Extension 4-H partners and participants, our multistate collaborators (University of Nebraska-Lincoln, University of Tennessee, South Dakota State University, West Virginia University, University of Maine), and the participants who enrolled in the research project. Also, a thank you to Jon Moyer for his statistical support.

References

1. Office of Disease Prevention and Health Promotion. Healthy People 2020. 2017. Available online: https://www.healthypeople.gov/ (accessed on 3 March 2017).

2. Braveman, P. Health disparities and health equity: Concepts and measurement. *Annu. Rev. Public Health* **2006**, *27*, 167–194. [CrossRef] [PubMed]

3. Shavers, V.L. Measurement of socioeconomic status in health disparities research. *J. Natl. Med. Assoc.* **2007**, *99*, 1013–1023. [PubMed]

4. Braveman, P. What are health disparities and health equity? We need to be clear. *Public Health Rep.* **2014**, *129*, 5–8. [CrossRef] [PubMed]

5. Singh, G.K.M.; van Dyck, P. A Multilevel Analysis of State and Regional Disparities in Childhood and Adolescent Obesity in the United States. *J. Community Health* **2008**, *33*, 90–102. [CrossRef] [PubMed]

6. Braveman, P.A.; Kumanyika, S.; Fielding, J.; LaVeist, T.; Borrell, L.N.; Manderscheid, R.; Troutman, A. Health disparities and health equity: the issue is justice. *Am. J. Public Health* **2011**, *101*, S149–S155. [CrossRef] [PubMed]

7. Office of Disease Prevention and Health Promotion. Healthy People 2020. Nutrition, Physical Activity, and Obesity. 2016. Available online: wwwhealthypeoplegov/2020/leading-health-indicators/2020-lhi-topics/Nutrition-Physical-Activity-and-Obesity/data (accessed on 3 March 2017).

8. Cooper, L.A.; Ortega, A.N.; Ammerman, A.S.; Buchwald, D.; Paskett, E.D.; Powell, L.H.; Thompson, B.; Tucker, K.L.; Warnecke, R.B.; McCarthy, W.J. *Calling for a Bold New Vision of Health Disparities Intervention Research*; American Public Health Association: Washington, DC, USA, 2015.

9. Braveman, P.; Barclay, C. Health Disparities Beginning in Childhood: A Life-Course Perspective. *Pediatrics* **2009**, *124*, S163–S175. [CrossRef] [PubMed]

10. Schreier, H.M.; Chen, E. Health disparities in adolescence. In *Handbook of Behavioral Medicine*; Springer: Berlin, Germany, 2010; pp. 571–583.

11. Koplan, J.P.; Liverman, C.T.; Kraak, V.I. Preventing childhood obesity: Health in the balance: Executive summary. *J. Am. Diet. Assoc.* **2005**, *105*, 131–138. [CrossRef] [PubMed]

12. Wilson, D.K. New Perspectives on Health Disparities and Obesity Interventions in Youth. *J. Pediatr. Psychol.* **2017**, *34*, 231–244. [CrossRef] [PubMed]

13. Dietz, W.H. Health consequences of obesity in youth: Childhood predictors of adult disease. *Pediatrics* **1998**, *101*, 518–525. [PubMed]

14. Sahoo, K.; Sahoo, B.; Choudhury, A.K.; Sofi, N.Y.; Kumar, R.; Bhadoria, A.S. Childhood obesity: Causes and consequences. *J. Fam. Med. Prim. Care* **2015**, *4*, 187–192.

15. Wright, C.M.; Parker, L.; Lamont, D.; Craft, A.W. Implications of childhood obesity for adult health: Findings from thousand families cohort study. *Br. Med. J.* **2001**, *323*, 1280–1284. [CrossRef]

16. Bandura, A. *Social Foundations of Thought and Action: A Social Cognitive Theory*; Prentice-Hall, Inc.: Englewood Cliffs, NJ, USA, 1986.

17. Miller, A.; Franzen-Castle, L.; Aguirre, T.; Krehbiel, M.; Colby, S.; Kattelmann, K.; Olfert, M.D.; Mathews, D.; White, A. Food-related behavior and intake of adult main meal preparers of 9–10 year-old children participating in iCook 4-H: A five-state childhood obesity prevention pilot study. *Appetite* **2016**, *101*, 163–170. [CrossRef] [PubMed]

18. Bickel, G.; Nord, M.; Price, C.; Hamilton, W.; Cook, J. *Guide to Measuring Household Food Security—Revised*; United States Department of Agriculture: Washington, DC, USA, 2000.

19. Wardlaw, M.K.; Hanula, G.; Burney, J.; Snider, S.; Jones, L.; Adler, A.; Zoumenou, V. *EFNEP Behavior Checklist Review*; United States Department of Agriculture: Washington, DC, USA, 2012.

20. Galal, O.M.; Qureshi, A.K. Dispersion index: Measuring trend assessment of geographical inequality in health—The example of under-five mortality in the Middle East/North African region, 1980–1994. *Soc. Sci. Med.* **1997**, *44*, 1893–1902. [CrossRef]

21. Manor, O.; Matthews, S.; Power, C. Comparing measures of health inequality. *Soc. Sci. Med.* **1997**, *45*, 761–771. [CrossRef]

22. Galambos, C.M. Health care disparities among rural populations: Aneglected frontier. *Health Soc. Work* **2005**, *30*, 179–181. [CrossRef] [PubMed]

23. Krieger, N.; Chen, J.T.; Waterman, P.D.; Rehkopf, D.H.; Subramanian, S.V. Race/Ethnicity, Gender, and Monitoring Socioeconomic Gradients in Health: A Comparison of Area-Based Socioeconomic Measures—The Public Health Disparities Geocoding Project. *Am. J. Public Health* **2003**, *93*, 1655–1671. [CrossRef] [PubMed]
24. Fredriksen-Goldsen, K.I.; Kim, H.-J.; Barkan, S.E.; Muraco, A.; Hoy-Ellis, C.P. Health Disparities among Lesbian, Gay, and Bisexual Older Adults: Results from a Population-Based Study. *Am. J. Public Health* **2013**, *103*, 1802–1809. [CrossRef] [PubMed]

17

Have Studies that Measure Lumbar Kinematics and Muscle Activity Concurrently during Sagittal Bending Improved Understanding of Spinal Stability and Sub-System Interactions?

Alister du Rose

Faculty of Life Sciences and Education, University of South Wales, Treforest, Pontypridd, Wales CF37 1DL, UK; alister.durose@southwales.ac.uk

Abstract: In order to improve understanding of the complex interactions between spinal sub-systems (i.e., the passive (ligaments, discs, fascia and bones), the active (muscles and tendons) and the neural control systems), it is necessary to take a dynamic approach that incorporates the measurement of multiple systems concurrently. There are currently no reviews of studies that have investigated dynamic sagittal bending movements using a combination of electromyography (EMG) and lumbar kinematic measurements. As such it is not clear how understanding of spinal stability concepts has advanced with regards to this functional movement of the spine. The primary aim of this review was therefore to evaluate how such studies have contributed to improved understanding of lumbar spinal stability mechanisms. PubMed and Cochrane databases were searched using combinations of the keywords related to spinal stability and sagittal bending tasks, using strict inclusion and exclusion criteria and adhering to PRISMA guidelines. Whilst examples of the interactions between the passive and active sub-systems were shown, typically small sample sizes meant that results were not generalizable. The majority of studies used regional kinematic measurements, and whilst this was appropriate in terms of individual study aims, the studies could not provide insight into sub-system interaction at the level of the spinal motion segment. In addition, the heterogeneity in methodologies made comparison between studies difficult. The review suggests that since Panjabi's seminal spinal control papers, only limited advancement in the understanding of these theories has been provided by the studies under review, particularly at an inter-segmental level. This lack of progression indicates a requirement for new research approaches that incorporate multiple system measurements at a motion segment level.

Keywords: spinal stability; spinal motion; electromyography; low back pain; flexion

---

1. Introduction

Spinal stability was interpreted by Panjabi (1992) to be dependent on the highly co-ordinated and optimised interactions between three sub-systems, the passive (ligaments, discs, fascia and bones), the active (muscles and tendons) and the neural control systems. According to this theory, if there is dysfunction within a specific system, compensation may be provided by adaptations in the other systems [1,2]. Panjabi suggested that abnormally increased muscle activation is a stabilisation mechanism compensating for a loss of spinal stability, a theory repeatedly supported in the subsequent literature. It has also been suggested that extended periods of myoelectrical silence (i.e., flexion relaxation) during prolonged flexion can result in a loss of spinal stability [3], and that such prolonged flexion also results in a transfer of extension moment between passive tissues and spinal muscles [4]. Such adaptations have been proposed as possible precipitators of low back pain (LBP), and it has been shown that trunk muscle recruitment patterns can be different between healthy and low back pain populations [5]. Investigations addressing the role of the active system are frequently limited however due to the inherent heterogenity of electromyography (EMG) signal data [6].

In order to improve understanding of the complex interactions between sub-systems, and possible biomechanical relationships with LBP, it is necessary to take an approach that incorporates the measurement of both lumbar kinematic and trunk muscle activation data [7]. Studies that do so include investigations into sub-system changes in response to pertubation [8], how such responses are influenced by paraspinal muscle fatigue [9–11] and the effect of spinal creep deformation [12]. A recent systematic review of such studies however, suggests that whilst a mechanism to achieve spinal stability may be for the central nervous system (CNS) to generate early postural muscle activity, this occurs regardless of the level of fatigue [13]. It was also concluded that spinal tissue creep likely does not influence spinal stability in the context of purtubation, and that in both cases, the high methodological heterogeneity between studies meant that comparison between studies was difficult [13]. In addition, as controlled pertubation studies investigate responses around a neutral spine position, no insight can be gained into possible sub-system interactions during the entire range of spinal movement.

In terms of the investigation of movements in the sagittal plane, the study of the Flexion Relaxation Phenomenon (FRP) [14] is another possible way in which insight into sub-system interaction can be gained. The deactivation of paraspinal muscle activity during the final stages of forward flexion has been interpreted as the transfer of moment between the active and passive sub-systems [15], and feasibly provides an insight into sub-system interaction. It has therefore been extensively studied [16–19], however the majority of studies only incorporate the measurement of regional kinematics, and therefore do not provide any insight from the level of the motion segment [20]. It could be argued that investigations at the inter-vertebral level are important, as inter-system feedback mechanisms are believed to act at this level [21].

It has also been common for studies to focus on individual systems in isolation, in an attempt to relate changes within each system to conditions such as LBP. Indeed, in terms of the active system, LBP has been associated with changes in paraspinal muscle cross sectional size [22], activation timings [23,24] and muscle activation amplitudes [5,25–28]. Focus on the passive system has shown potential links between LBP and lumbar range of motion (ROM) [7,29–33], and postural parameters [34], however such investigations, by considering kinematic or muscle activity parameters in isolation, can only speculate as to how such changes may relate to adapatations in the other sub-systems.

In addition, many of these studies have produced conflicting results, and there is therefore an argument that attempts should first be made to improve understanding of normal (i.e., spinal biomechanical behaviours of non-LBP populations), so as to better understand what is abnormal [35]. Investigations of the kinematics of normal controls has shown how regional spinal ranges of motion may be associated with the ranges achieved in another spinal region (i.e., as one region moves more there may be less movement in another region) [36,37], however again, such adaptations again cannot be explained in terms of sub-system adaptation, as only a single system was considered.

The complexity and inaccessability of investigating spinal control mechanisms makes the interpretation of study findings difficult. A key problem is that sub-system interaction is dynamic, and therefore the study of two or more systems concurrently in living humans requires instrumentation that can do so dynamically and concurrently. Physical activities involving sagittal bending are commonplace activities of daily living [38], and as the most widely investigated functional task, an improved knowledge of sub-system interactions during sagittal bending would be of clinical interest. Currently there are no reviews of studies that have investigated dynamic sagittal bending movements using a combination of EMG and lumbar kinematic measurements, and as such it is not clear how understanding of in vivo spinal stability concepts has advanced as a result of investigations into this functional movement of the spine. It is also of interest how the findings of such studies have helped distinguish between low back pain and non-low back pain populations.

This review addressed two fundamental questions. (1) How have studies that combine concurrent lumbar kinematic and muscle activity measurements during sagittal bending improved understanding of lumbar spinal stability mechanisms (i.e., sub-system interactions)? (2) Are studies that combine concurrent lumbar kinematic and muscle activity measurements during sagittal bending able to distinguish between groups of healthy controls (i.e., no low back pain) and those with low back pain?

2. Methods

2.1. Literature Search Strategy

PubMed and the Cochrane library were searched in March and April 2017. The systematic search was performed using combinations of the following keywords: (Electromyography or EMG or Flexion Relaxation or FRP and Kinematics or Range of Motion or ROM and Low Back Pain or Lumbar Spine and Flexion or Bending and Stability or Stabilization). Article screening was conducted by the author and was restricted to English publications between 1992 and 2017 in order to only include articles post Panjabi's seminal papers that originally explored the theory of sub-system interactions [1,2].

2.2. Inclusion and Exclusion Criteria

Articles were included for review if they met the following inclusion and exclusion criteria. Inclusion criteria consist of (1) Studies must be in vivo using adult participants (2) Weight-bearing movement in the sagittal plane (3) Include both EMG (including the lumbar paraspinal muscles) and lumbar kinematic measurements (4) Relate study findings to stability theories or spinal stabilisation. Exclusion criteria included (1) Pertubation studies (as the articles of interest were to include active movement (2) Studies measuring creep or fatigue (as single cycles of dynamic tasks will unlikely result in either) (3) Studies not investigating the lumbar spine specifically (i.e., cervical, thoracic or shoulder) (4) Studies investigating lateral flexion, axial rotation or gait (i.e., not including sagittal flexion) (5) Non-human studies (e.g., feline studies) (6) Repeatability trials. A flowchart outlining the citation selection process is shown in Figure 1. Other reasons for study exclusion included manipulation by design (e.g., investigations into the effects of noxious stimuli, high heels, taping, and exercise).

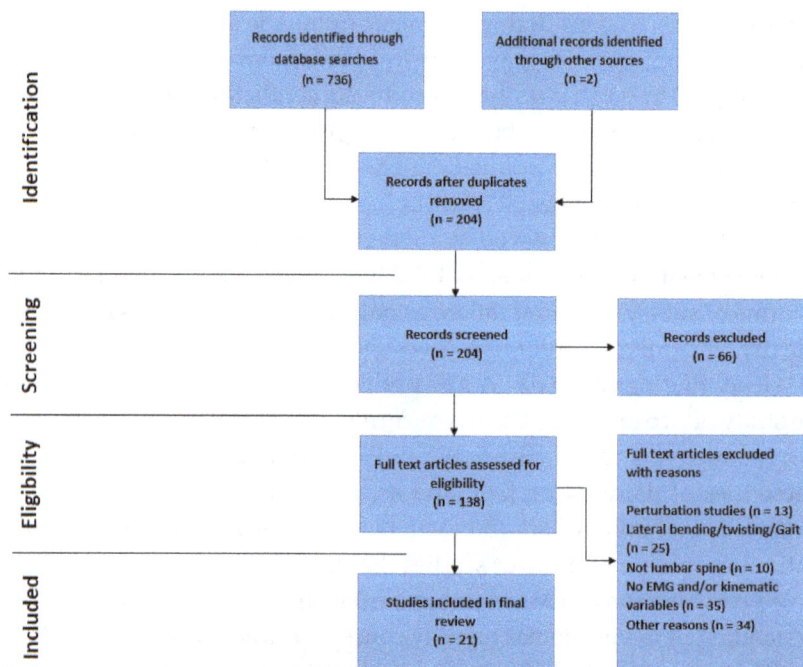

Figure 1. Prisma flowchart. Note: Additional articles (n = 2) were sourced via a manual search through the reference lists of the articles identified in the database search.

2.3. PRISMA (Preferred Reporting Items for Systematic Reviews and Meta-Analyses)

This systematic review adheres to the PRISMA guildeines.

2.4. Study Quality Assessment

This review uses a quality assessment tool developed by Abboud et al. [13] that was adapted from the Quality Index of Downs and Black [39]. Abboud et al. also created an assessment designed to specifically interpret the quality of studies incorporating EMG, which was based on Surface ElectroMyoGraphy for the Non-Invasive Assessment of Muscles (SENIAM) [40] and International Society of Electrophysiology and Kinesiology (ISEK) guidelines. This novel assessment was also incorporated. The quality assessment of each paper was performed twice (approximately 12 months apart) by a single reviewer ($r = 0.98$).

2.4.1. Overall Quality Assessment

The original quality index developed by Downs and Black (1998) has been shown to have good test-retest ($r = 0.88$) and inter-rater observability ($r = 0.75$) [13]. The adapted tool consists of 10 items that were deemed appropriate for the purpose of this review. The items included the following questions (1) Is the hypothesis/aim/objective of the study clearly described? (2) Are the main outcomes to be measured clearly described in the Introduction or Methods section? (3) Are the characteristics of the patients included in the study clearly described? (4) Are the interventions of interest clearly described? (5) Are the main findings of the study clearly described? (6) Does the study provide estimates of the random variability in the data for the main outcomes? (7) Have actual probability values been reported (e.g., 0.035 rather than <0.05) for the main outcomes except where the probability value is less than 0.001? (8) Were those subjects who were prepared to participate representative of the entire population from which they were recruited? (9) If any of the results of the study were based on "data dredging", was this made clear? (10) Were the statistical tests used to assess the main outcomes appropriate? All items were scored either 0 or 1. This produced a total quality score out of 10 for each study, with the exception of those articles that did not require population comparison, and so were scored out of 9 (Table 1). Final scores were converted into percentages and combined with the EMG quality scores, providing an overall impression of study quality (Table 2).

Table 1. Quality index assessment scores (* Studies that did not compare healthy controls to a low back pain group were rated using a 9 point scale instead of 10).

Quality Check	Category										Score	
Authors (year)	1	2	3	4	5	6	7	8	9	10	Score (/9 * or /10)	Score (%)
Arjmand et al. (2010) [41]	0	1	0	1	1	0	0	N/A	1	0	4 *	44
Burnett et al. (2004) [42]	1	1	0	1	1	1	1	1	1	1	9	90
Callaghan and Dunk 2002 [43]	1	0	0	1	1	0	1	N/A	1	1	6*	67
Cholewicki et al. (1997) [44]	1	1	0	1	1	1	0	N/A	1	1	7 *	78
Dankaerts et al. (2009) [7]	1	1	1	1	1	1	1	1	1	1	10	100
Hashemirad et al. (2009) [45]	1	1	0	1	1	1	0	N/A	1	1	7 *	78
Hay et al. (2016) [46]	0	1	0	1	1	0	0	1	1	1	6	60
Kaigle et al. (1998) [20]	1	1	1	1	1	1	0	0	1	1	8	80
Kienbacher et al. (2016) [47]	1	1	1	1	1	1	1	1	1	1	10	100
Lariviere et al. (2000) [6]	1	1	1	1	1	1	1	0	1	1	9	90
Liu et al. (2011) [48]	1	1	0	1	1	1	0	0	1	1	7	70
Luhring et al. (2015) [16]	1	1	1	1	1	1	0	N/A	1	1	8 *	89
Mayer et al. (2009) [49]	1	1	0	1	1	1	0	1	0	1	7	70
McGill and Kippers 1994 [15]	1	1	0	1	1	1	0	N/A	1	1	7 *	78
Nairn et al. (2013) [50]	1	1	0	1	1	0	1	N/A	1	1	7 *	78
Neblett et al. (2003) [51]	1	1	1	1	1	1	0	N/A	1	1	8 *	89
Ning et al. (2012) [52]	1	1	0	1	1	0	0	N/A	1	1	6 *	67
O'Sullivan et al. (2006) [17]	1	1	1	1	1	1	1	N/A	1	1	9 *	100
Paquet et al. (1994) [53]	1	1	1	1	1	1	0	1	1	1	9	90
Peach et al. (1998) [35]	1	1	0	1	1	1	0	N/A	1	1	7 *	78
Sanchez-Zuriaga et al. (2015) [26]	1	1	1	1	1	1	0	1	1	1	9	90

Table 2. Electromyography (EMG) quality assessment scores (* Studies that did not require normalisation were rated using a 3 point scale instead of 4) as per Abboud et al. (2017) [13].

EMG Quality Check	Category												Score	
Authors (year)	1.1	1.2	1.3	2.1	2.2	2.3	2.4	3.1	3.2	3.3	3.4	4	score (/3 * or /4)	score (%)
Arjmand et al. (2010) [41]	0	1	0	0	1	0	0	1	1	1	0	1	2	50
Burnett et al. (2004) [42]	1	1	0	1	1	0	0	1	1	1	0	1	4	100
Callaghan and Dunk 2002 [43]	0	1	0	0	1	0	0	1	1	1	0	1	2	50
Cholewicki et al. (1997) [44]	0	1	0	0	1	0	0	1	1	1	1	1	2	50
Dankaerts et al. (2009) [7]	1	1	1	0	1	1	1	1	1	1	1	1	4	100
Hashemerad et al. (2009) [45]	1	1	1	0	1	1	1	1	1	1	1	1	4	100
Hay et al. (2016) [46]	0	1	1	0	0	0	0	1	1	1	1	N/A	2 *	67
Kaigle et al. (1998) [20]	0	0	0	0	1	1	0	1	1	1	1	N/A	2 *	67
Kienbacher et al. (2016) [47]	1	1	1	0	1	1	1	1	1	1	1	1	4	100
Lariviere et al. (2000) [6]	0	1	0	1	0	1	0	1	1	1	0	N/A	2 *	67
Liu et al. (2011) [48]	0	0	N/A	1	0	1	0	1	1	1	1	1	3 *	100
Luhring et al. (2015) [16]	1	1	1	0	1	0	0	1	1	1	1	1	3	75
Mayer et al. (2009) [49]	0	0	0	0	0	0	0	1	1	1	0	0	1	25
McGill and Kippers 1994 [15]	1	1	1	0	1	0	0	1	1	1	1	1	3	75
Nairn et al. (2013) [50]	1	0	1	1	1	0	1	1	1	1	1	1	4	100
Neblett et al. (2003) [51]	1	1	0	1	1	0	0	0	0	0	1	N/A	2 *	67
Ning et al. (2012) [52]	0	0	1	0	1	0	0	1	1	1	1	1	2	50
O'Sullivan et al. (2006) [17]	1	1	1	1	1	1	1	1	1	1	1	1	4	100
Paquet et al. (1994) [53]	0	0	0	1	0	0	0	0	1	1	1	0	1	25
Peach et al. (1998) [35]	1	1	1	0	1	0	0	1	1	1	1	1	3	75
Sanchez-Zuriaga et al. (2015) [26]	1	1	1	0	1	1	1	1	1	1	1	1	4	100

2.4.2. Specific EMG Quality Assessment

The checklist developed by Abboud et al. (2017) [13] consists of 12 items divided into 4 sections (Table 2). The first section considers the use of surface electromyography (sEMG) electrodes (as all studies reviewed used sEMG and none used needle EMG, despite the inclusion of both terms in the literature search) and comprises a score for inter-electrode distance, electrode material and construction (i.e., bipolar). The second section considers participant skin preparation, the use of reference electrodes and electrode placement and fixation. The third section considers signal processing and includes items regarding the use of filters, rectification methodology, sampling and processing. The final section considers the appropriate use of normalisation. Each item was scored 0 or 1, and a score of 1 was attributed to a section if the item totals reached 2 or more. This produced an EMG quality score out of 4 for each study, with the exception of those articles where normalisation was not deemed necessary, and so were scored out of 3. These scores were also converted into percentages and combined with the study quality assessment scores above (Table 3).

Table 3. Combined quality index and EMG quality scores.

Authors (Year)	Quality Index Score (%)	EMG Quality Score (%)	Combined Score (%)
Arjmand et al. (2010) [41]	44	50	47
Burnett et al. (2004) [42]	90	100	95
Callaghan and Dunk 2002 [43]	67	50	58.5
Cholewicki et al. (1997) [44]	78	50	64
Dankaerts et al. (2009) [7]	100	100	100
Hashemerad et al. (2009) [45]	78	100	89
Hay et al. (2016) [46]	60	67	63.5
Kaigle et al. (1998) [20]	80	67	73.5
Kienbacher et al. (2016) [47]	100	100	100
Lariviere et al. (2000) [6]	90	67	78.5
Liu et al. (2011) [48]	70	100	85
Luhring et al. (2015) [16]	89	75	82
Mayer et al. (2009) [49]	70	25	47.5
McGill and Kippers 1994 [15]	78	75	76.5
Nairn et al. (2013) [50]	78	100	89
Neblett et al. (2003) [51]	89	67	78
Ning et al. (2012) [52]	67	50	58.5
O'Sullivan et al. (2006) [17]	100	100	100
Paquet et al. (1994) [53]	90	25	57.5
Peach et al. (1998) [35]	78	75	76.5
Sanchez-Zuriaga et al. (2015) [26]	90	100	95

3. Results

Out of a total of 736 articles identified through the literature search, 21 satisfied the inclusion/exclusion criteria. The screening process is outlined in the PRISMA flowchart (Figure 1).

3.1. Overall and EMG Quality Assessment

The overall quality assessment scores ranged from 44–100% with a mean total score of 80% (Table 1). All of the selected studies scored a 1 for their descriptions of methodology and study findings. The studies also performed well in terms of the quality of hypothesis and outcome descriptions (19/21 and 20/21 respectively), and their use of appropriate statistics and absence of data dredging (both 20/21). Areas in which the studies generally scored poorly included the description of participant characteristics (9/21) and the reporting of actual probability values (7/21). The EMG quality assessment showed scores ranging from 25–100% with a mean total score of 73% (Table 2). The assessment showed that the majority of EMG studies adequately reported the normalisation and signal processing elements, however it also highlighted a mixture of study quality when considering the detail of electrode use. The combined overall and EMG quality index scores ranged from 47–100% with a mean total score of 77% (Table 3).

3.2. General Characteristics of the Reviewed Studies

All of the studies reviewed could be placed into one of 4 categories, the majority being studies relating in some way to the flexion relaxation phenomenon (FRP): [15–17,20,26,43,45,47,49,51–53], or comparisons between LBP and healthy control participant groups: [6,7,17,20,26,42,48,49,51,53]. There was a degree of crossover however as some comparison studies also incorporated the FRP. Other study areas included EMG activation studies (other than FRP) [6,7,26,35,42,44,46,48,50,53], and spinal modelling [6,15,41,52].

Table 4 shows that typically regional kinematics were measured, with the exception of the inter-vertebral methodology used by Kaigle et al. (1998) [20]. Indeed the methods used to measure regional ROM varied between studies. This trend was also apparent in terms of electrode positioning, with many different sites being used to record activity from the same designated muscle. The table also highlights the generally small sample sizes used in this type of study, with the majority using fewer than 30 participants. The only exceptions were the studies of Mayer et al. (2009) [49], Kienbacher et al. (2016) [47], Lariviere et al. (2000) [6] and Neblett et al. (2003) [51] with participant numbers of 134, 216, 33 and 66 respectively.

Whilst the reliability of kinematic measurements was not established in all of the reviewed studies, in those that did, reliability was typically found to be excellent, however different approaches to determine reliability were evident. Dankaert et al. (2009) for example determined the inter-trial reliability of the 3 Space Fastrak system (Polhemus Navigation Science Division, Kaiser Aerospace, VT), using intraclass correlation coefficients (ICC)(3,1) [7]. Inter-trial reliability was shown with ICC's of 0.85 or greater and standard error of measurement (SEM) was also included. This was in contrast to Neblett et al. (2003) who used Pearson's product moment correlations, showing inter and intra examiner reliability of the inclinometers used to be $r = 0.92$ or greater [51].

Table 4. Study characteristics ($N = 21$).

Authors	Study Aim	EMG Variable and Lumbar Paraspinal Muscles Recorded (LMU = Lumbar Multifidus, LES = Lumbar Erector Spinae, TES = Thoracic Erector Spinae)	Lumbar Kinematic Measurements	Study Findings	Participants	Analysis
Arjmand et al. (2010) [41]	To compare a single joint model to kinematic driven model during trunk flexion.	Normalised EMG activity. Muscles Longissimus (3 cm lateral to L1) Iliocostalis (3 cm lateral to L3) Multifidus (2 cm lateral to L5).	Optotrak 4 camera system (regional) Lumbar region LED's placed on pelvis and T12.	In both models, global extensor activity peaked around 30° of flexion, due to the increase in contribution of passive structures at this point. Extensors became silent between 50–70°.	$N = 1$ A male participant with no recent history of LBP.	Quantitative comparison was not performed.
Burnett et al. (2004) [42]	To determine whether differences exist in spinal kinematics and trunk muscle activity in cyclists with and without NSCLBP.	EMG activity was quantified by obtaining the mean activation, during a 5 crank revolution period. Muscles TES (5 cm lateral to T9) LMU (2–3 cm lateral to L4–L5).	3-Space Fastrak (regional) Lower lumbar L3 relative to S2 Upper lumbar T12 relative to L3.	The LBP group demonstrated greater lower lumbar flexion than controls associated with a loss of multifidus co-contraction.	$N = 18$ mean age 37.6 years 9 non low back pain 9 NSCLBP.	Independent sample t-tests.
Callaghan and Dunk 2002 [43]	To determine if FRP occurs in seated and slumped postures.	Ensemble average normalised EMG activity. Muscles TES (5 cm lateral to T9) LES (3 cm lateral to L3).	3-Space ISOTRAK (regional) Lumbar region Sacrum relative to L1.	FRP was shown in the TES, but not the LES during Slumped sitting. TES silence during sitting also happened at earlier angle of lumbar flexion than during standing.	$N = 22$ low back pain free participants 11 males mean age 21.3 years 11 females mean age 21.9 years.	Three way ANOVA, and Tukey's post hoc multiple comparisons.
Cholewicki et al. (1997) [44]	To test the hypothesis that the flexors and extensors of the trunk are co-activated around a neutral spine posture.	Normalised EMG activity. Muscles TES (5 cm lateral to T9) LES (3 cm lateral to L3) LMU (2 cm lateral to L5–L5).	The use of 2 pieces of string attached to a chest harness and two potentiometers (regional).	Co-activation of trunk flexors and extensors was shown in healthy participants around a neutral posture.	$N = 10$ low back pain free participants 8 males and 2 females mean age 27 years.	A two factor repeated measures ANOVA.
Dankaerts et al. (2009) [7]	To test the ability of a model to distinguish between flexion pattern (FP) and active extension pattern (AEP) subgroups and healthy controls using lumbar kinematics and trunk muscle activity.	Normalised EMG activity. Superficial LMU (at the level of L5 orientated by a line between the PSIS and the L1–L2 interspace. Iliocostalis lumborum pars thoracis (lateral to L1).	3-Space Fastrak (regional) Upper lumbars T12 relative to L3 Lower lumbars L3 relative to S2.	Differences in muscle activity and spinal kinematics during flexion suggest that 2 distinct motor control patterns can exist in CNSLBP patients.	$N = 67$ participants 34 low back pain free controls, mean age 32 20 Flexion pattern NSLBP patients, mean age 36 13 Extension pattern NSLBP patients, mean age 40.	ANOVA and post hoc Bonferroni.
Hashemirad et al. (2009) [45]	To investigate the relationship between lumbar spine flexibility and LES activity during sagittal flexion and return.	Normalised EMG amplitude and signal onset/offset. Muscle LES (4 cm lateral to L3–L4).	Estimated using a camera and markers placed at the spinous processes of T12, L3 and S2 (regional).	During bending the ES of participants with high toe touch score deactivated at greater trunk and hip angles. Those with high modified Schober scores deactivated later and reactivated sooner in accordance with lumbar angle.	$N = 30$ low back pain free participants.	Pearson correlations and multiple linear regression analysis.
Hay et al. (2016) [46]	To show that wavelet coherence and phase plots can be used to provide insight into how muscle activation relates to kinematics.	EMG amplitude (linear envelope). Muscle Lumbar erector spinae (no details of positioning).	Oqus 400 motion capture system (regional) Reflective markers placed over T12 and S1.	The study showed good agreement between lumbar kinematics and linear enveloped sEMG. Validating the use of the wavelet coherence technique.	$N = 14$ low back pain free male participants.	The coefficient of determination (R^2).

Table 4. *Cont.*

Authors	Study Aim	EMG Variable and Lumbar Paraspinal Muscles Recorded (LMU = Lumbar Multifidus, LES = Lumbar Erector Spinae, TES = Thoracic Erector Spinae)	Lumbar Kinematic Measurements	Study Findings	Participants	Analysis
Kaigle et al. (1998) [20]	To concurrently quantify muscle activation of LES with the kinematics of lumbar motion segments, in low back patients and controls.	Root mean square (RMS) sEMG amplitude. Muscle LES (3 cm lateral to L3–L4).	A linkage transducer system secured by interosseous pins to L2-L3, L3-4 and L4-L5 motion segments (inter-vertebral).	ROM was less in low back pain patients and FRP occurred in participants when IV-ROM was complete before full trunk flexion	N = 13 6 low back pain free participants, mean age 40. 7 low back pain patients with suspected lumbar instability, mean age 51.	Wilcoxon rank-sum test and Wilcoxon matched-pairs signed rank test.
Kienbacher et al. (2016) [47]	To determine whether lumbar extensor activity and flexion relaxation ratios could differentiate low back pain patients (of various age groups) during flexion-extension task.	Normalised RMS sEMG amplitudes. Muscle LMU (lateral to L5) a line joining the iliac crests, and 2–3 cm bilateral and distal from their middle).	3-D accelerometers placed at the levels of T4 and L5. Used to calculate hip, lumbothoracic and gross trunk regions. (regional).	The sEMG activation was highest in over 60's and female groups during standing. This possibly relates to why this group showed minimal changes during flexion. This group also demonstrated the highest hip, and lowest lumbothoracic angle changes.	N = 216 low back pain patients. 62 (60–90 year olds) 84 (40–59 year olds) 70 (18–39 year olds).	ANOVA and bootstrap confidence intervals.
Lariviere et al. (2000) [6]	To evaluate the sensitivity of trunk muscle EMG waveforms to trunk ROM and low back pain status during flexion-extension tasks.	Mean normalised EMG activity. Muscles LES and TES (exact locations not specified).	Video cameras and reflective markers. Trunk angles relative to the vertical plane were used to determine trunk flexion (A line between the hips and the centre of C7-T1) (regional).	Principal component analysis (PCA) distance measures were sensitive to trunk ROM but not low back status. The usefulness of PCA as an effective clinical tool was not established.	N = 33 15 low back pain patients, mean age 40 18 low back pain free participants, mean age 39.	ANOVA and ICC's.
Liu et al. (2011) [48]	To develop a new test based on lumbar sEMG activity (the sEMG coordination network analysis approach) during flexion-extension, to distinguish between healthy control and low back pain groups.	Normalised RMS sEMG activity. Muscles An sEMG electrode array placed over the lumbar region (16 electrodes, target muscles not specified).	30° of trunk flexion, measured by a protractor (no further details) (regional).	Group network analysis shows a loss of global symmetric patterns in the low back pain group.	N = 21 11 low back pain patients, mean age 40. 10 low back pain free participants, mean age 28.	Did not specify. (However, groups comparison statistics and symmetry scores were used).
Luhring et al. (2015) [16]	To determine a kinematic measurement that best determines the onset and offset of the FRP.	Normalised sEMG onset and cessation. Muscle LES (4 cm lateral to L3).	Vicon MX motion capture camera system. Reflective markers placed at various locations throughout the spine including T12, L5 and pelvis (regional).	Lumbar kinematic measurements are preferential when the FRP is considered clinically.	N = 20 low back pain free participants, mean age 24.	Coefficients of Variation (CV) and ICC's.
Mayer et al. (2009) [49]	To determine when FRP occurs in patients and to correlate the findings with lumbar ROM.	Mean RMS sEMG with pre-determined cut-off values. Muscles Not identified within paper.	Gross lumbar, hip/pelvic ROM using an inclinometer (no further details provided) (regional).	After a functional restoration program, both normal FRP and normal lumbar ROM were restored in the majority of patients.	N = 134 30 low back pain free participants, mean age 38. 104 low back pain patients (mean age not provided).	Descriptive statistics including mean and SD. Sensitivity and specificity. P-values and Odds ratios (not specified).

Table 4. *Cont.*

Authors	Study Aim	EMG Variable and Lumbar Paraspinal Muscles Recorded (LMU = Lumbar Multifidus, LES = Lumbar Erector Spinae, TES = Thoracic Erector Spinae)	Lumbar Kinematic Measurements	Study Findings	Participants	Analysis
McGill and Kippers 1994 [15]	To examine the tissue loading during the period of transition between active and passive tissues during flexion.	Normalised sEMG activity. Muscles TES (5 cm lateral to T9) LES (3 cm lateral to L3).	3-Space Isotrak (regional) with sensors placed over the sacrum and T10.	The deactivation of lumbar extensor muscles during FRP occurs only in an electrical sense as they still provide force elastically.	$N = 8$ low back pain free participants, mean age 26.	Dynamic modelling.
Nairn et al. (2013) [50]	To quantify slumped sitting both in terms of spinal kinematics and sEMG.	Mean normalised sEMG activity. Muscles Lower TES (5 cm lateral to T9) LES (4 cm lateral to L3) LMU (Adjacent to L5 orientated along a line between the PSIS and the L1–L2 interspinous space.	Vicon motion capture camera system. Reflective markers placed at various locations throughout the spine including T12, L1 and bilateral PSIS's (regional).	During slumped sitting lower sEMG activity was found in the thoracic and lumbar erector spinae compared to upright sitting. Patterns varied depending on the degree of bending at each area of the spine. Thoracic kinematic and EMG information is therefore useful in these type of studies	$N = 12$ low back pain free participants, mean age 23.	ANOVA and Bonferroni correction.
Neblett et al. (2003) [51]	To assess EMG activity in terms of the FRP during dynamic flexion and to determine whether abnormal FRP patterns in NSLBP patients can be normalised.	RMS sEMG cut-off values. Muscles LES (2 cm lateral to L3).	Inclinometers at T12 and the sacrum (regional).	In asymptomatic participants, the flexion relaxation (FR) angle was always less than the maximal voluntary flexion (MVF) angle. Of the patients that completed a functional restoration program, 94% achieved FR compared to 30% pre-treatment.	$N = 66$ 12 low back pain free participants, mean age 34. 54 chronically disabled work-related spinal disorder (CDWRSD) patients	Descriptive statistics for ROM and FRP
Ning et al. (2012) [52]	To determine a boundary at which the passive tissues begin to take a significant role in trunk extensor moment (and therefore at what point EMG assisted modelling is no longer valid).	Normalised EMG activity. Muscles LES at two levels (3 cm lateral to L3 and 4 cm lateral to L4).	A magnetic-field based motion tracking system with sensors placed at T12 and S1. Lumbar flexion calculated as the pitch of T12 relative to S1 (regional).	EMG-assisted models should consider the action of the passive tissues at lower flexion angles than previously thought.	$N = 11$ low back pain free participants, mean age 26.	ANOVA and Tukey–Kramer post-hoc testing
O'Sullivan et al. (2006) [17]	To investigate the FRP of spinal muscles in healthy participants during slumped sitting from an upright position.	Normalised EMG activity offset. Muscles TES (5 cm lateral to T9) LMU (Adjacent to L5 orientated along a line between the PSIS and the L1–L2 interspinous space.	3-Space Fastrak with sensors placed over T6, T12 and S2. (regional).	LMU is active during neutral sitting and demonstrates FRP when moving from upright to slumped sitting. FRP of these muscles is also different to when standing. More variation was found in EMG patterns of the TES.	$N = 24$ low back pain free participants, mean age 32.	ANOVA and ICC's

Table 4. *Cont.*

Authors	Study Aim	EMG Variable and Lumbar Paraspinal Muscles Recorded (LMU = Lumbar Multifidus, LES = Lumbar Erector Spinae, TES = Thoracic Erector Spinae)	Lumbar Kinematic Measurements	Study Findings	Participants	Analysis
Paquet et al. (1994) [53]	To compare healthy controls and low back pain patients in terms of hip-spine movement interaction and EMG, and to verify the relationships between kinematics and EMG in these groups.	Raw EMG envelope. Area under the curve and ratio of activity at different parts of the flexion-extension cycle (not-specified). Muscles LES (at the level of L3, distance not-specified).	Electro goniometers measured angular displacements at the hip and lumbar spine using landmarks of T8 and S1 (regional).	LES activation patterns were found to be significantly different between groups when flexion was performed at the same rate and range. Abnormal hip-spine movement related to an absence of the FRP at full flexion.	N = 20 10 low back pain free participants, mean age 34. 10 low back pain patients, mean age 38.	Mann-Whitney U test and Kruskal-Wallis test
Peach et al. (1998) [35]	To document the lumbar kinematics and trunk EMG activation patterns of healthy controls during tasks including sagittal flexion	Mean normalised EMG. Muscles TES (5 cm lateral to T9) LES (3 cm lateral to L3) LMU (1–2 cm lateral to L5).	3-Space Isotrak with sensors placed over T12 and Sacrum. (regional).	A database of normal lumbar spinal kinematics and EMG patterns was created for future reference against LBP groups.	N = 24 low back pain free participants, mean age 22.	Descriptive statistics, ANOVA and Tukey's honestly significant difference (HSD) post-hoc testing
Sanchez-Zuriaga et al. (2015) [26]	To compare healthy controls and LBP patients in terms of lumbopelvic kinematics and erector spinae activity	Mean normalised EMG activity, and start and end of FRP. Muscle LES (3 cm lateral to L3).	A 3-dimensional videophotogrammetric system, with markers placed at T12, L3, L5 and the sacrum (regional).	During pain free periods, recurrent LBP patients showed significantly greater LES activity during flexion and extension. Lumbar ROM and FRP were not found to be useful to distinguish between groups.	N = 30 15 low back pain free participants, mean age 41. 15 patients with recurring low back pain (currently in a pain free stage), mean age 45.	Mann-Whitney U test

3.3. Comparing Healthy Control and Low Back Pain Groups

Of the studies above comparing LBP and healthy control groups, the majority found objective differences between the groups. Burnett et al. (2004) [42]: showed that the LBP group had greater lower lumbar flexion and reduced multifidus activity compared to controls, whilst controls showed greater upper lumbar flexion. In Dankaerts et al.'s study 2009 [7], differences were found in terms of multifidus activity and spinal kinematics between both flexion pattern (FP) and active extension pattern (AEP) provocation sub-groups and healthy controls. In summary, multifidus activity was increased in the AEP group relative to the FP at the end of flexion, and the FP group demonstrated increased activity compared to the healthy controls. These patterns were attributed to the maintenance of the lumbar lordosis during flexion in the AEP group, and the similar spinal curvature between FP and healthy control groups. The Kaigle study provided the only inter-vertebral insight into active and passive system interactions, using intra-osseous pins connected to a sliding linkage transducer system to measure inter-vertebral angular rotation [20]. The study showed that inter-vertebral angular range was significantly smaller in the LBP group, and that the majority of patients showed no reduction in paraspinal muscle activity at the end ranges of flexion. Indeed, the FRP was only present in participants who demonstrated near complete inter-vertebral rotation before maximum global trunk flexion was attained.

Two of the studies were linked and provided similar conclusions. Neblett et al. (2003) [51] showed that in terms of the FRP and patients, all LBP patients that underwent a rehabilitation program achieved normal ROM, and subsequently demonstrated the FRP, whilst Mayer et al., 2009 [49] likewise concluded that normal lumbar ROM appears to correlate with the FRP and was therefore absent in many LBP participants. However, both FRP and ROM measurements responded well after a generic rehabilitation program.

Using a network modelling and analysis approach, Liu et al. (2011) [48] claimed to be able to clearly distinguish LBP and healthy control participants using symmetric patterns and network features, and Paquet et al. (1994) [53] showed that when flexion was performed over the same rate and range, LES activity was significantly greater in the LBP group. Participants in the study with an absent FRP also demonstrated increased ROM of the hip around full flexion.

Not all studies demonstrated an ability to differentiate between LBP and control groups however. Lariviere et al. (2000) [6] for example used a novel principal component analysis (PCA) technique to investigate whether EMG and kinematics could distinguish between the two. Their PCA analysis consisted of two steps. Firstly using EMG activity envelopes from control subjects, a reference model was developed (i.e., a criteria for normal). Secondly 'distance measures' were calculated relative to the reference model. The EMG waveform of a participant was labelled as abnormal if the 'distance value' was outside a 95% confidence interval calculated from the control subjects. Whilst being sensitive to trunk ROM, the distance measures were not sensitive to low back pain status. The authors argued that this was likely due to the relatively small sample size, and therefore inadequate considering the large heterogeneity control populations. In conclusion it was considered that the tool developed was not useful in terms of distinguishing between LBP patients and controls. Sanchez-Zuriaga et al. (2015) [26] also demonstrated contrasting results, as the authors found no significant difference between LBP and healthy groups, in either FRP or lumbar ROM. The study did however show significantly greater LES activity in LBP participants during the flexion-extension task, and the LBP patients were participating during a pain free period.

3.4. Flexion Relaxation Studies

The results of some of the FRP studies [15,20,49,51,53] have already been mentioned. Callaghan and Dunk (2002) showed that during slumped sitting the TES exhibited the FRP, but the LES did not. The authors also demonstrated that this deactivation occurred earlier (i.e., at a smaller lumbar flexion angle) than LES deactivation during flexion from standing [43]. In contrast to these findings, O'Sullivan et al. (2006) showed that although LMU activity decreased (i.e., FRP was present) when going from a neutral to a slumped seated position, there were varying patterns in TES activity, as approximately half the participants showed an increase in activity and half a decrease [17]. Hashemirad et al. showed that trunk flexibility can influence FRP, with greater flexibility relating to FRP onset at larger flexion angles [45], and Luhring et al. (2015) [16] chose to address the problem of using different methodologies to measure regional kinematics in FRP studies (by acknowledging a wide range of normalised and un-normalised FRP onset angles), investigated whether lumbar (i.e., T12-L5) or trunk (i.e., shoulders and hips) angles were more consistent in terms of EMG cessation and onset. The study found that lumbar kinematic measurements were more consistent.

Finally, the study conducted by Ning et al. (2012) [52] suggested that passive tissues can produce significant loads at earlier trunk flexion angle than previously believed i.e., those suggested by Kaigle et al. (1998) [20] where erector spinae deactivation was shown to begin at between 71° and 77° of grouped inter-vertebral level flexion, or Peach et al. (1998) [35] where FRP was shown to occur between 60° and 70°.

3.5. Models

Arjmand et al. (2010) [41] compared EMG-driven (EMGAO) and multi-joint Kinematics-driven (KD) models in terms of muscle force and spinal load estimation. During a flexion task the KD model predicted greater paraspinal muscle activity compared to the EMGAO model and therefore shear and compression forces were also higher. Predictions made using the EMGAO model were also found to be level specific (i.e., L5-S1), and could not be an accurate representation of other lumbar levels (Arjmand et al. (2010) [41]). Ning et al. (2012) [52] as discussed above, determined at what trunk flexion angle the passive tissues were able to generate a significant extensor moment during forward bending (Ning et al. (2012) [52]), and McGill and Kippers 1994 [15] showed that although paraspinal muscles are electrically silent at the end range of forward flexion, these muscle continue to provide elastic resistance via passive stretching.

4. Discussion

4.1. Quality Assessment

The mean of the combined quality check and EMG scores was 77%, suggesting that the overall quality of the studies reviewed was generally good. Of particular note were the studies of Dankaerts et al. (2009) [7], Kienbacher et al. (2016) [47] and O'Sullivan et al. (2006) [17], which all scored 100%. The majority of studies used muscle activity amplitude as their key EMG parameter, and it was apparent that the majority also reported the relevant normalisation technique. The high percentage of good scores in this area, therefore makes it easier to compare amplitude results between studies. Other areas of apparent good quality reporting included the descriptions of the hypothesis, aims, and objectives of the studies, the main outcomes to be measured, the interventions of interest and the main findings. In terms of EMG quality, relevant signal processing information was also usually well reported.

This high standard of reporting was not evident throughout the review however, and trends in areas that were weaker emerged. In terms of the Quality Index assessment scores, the reporting of participant characteristics (including inclusion and exclusion criteria) and actual probability values was poor, with over half of all studies included scoring zero for these categories. Regarding the EMG quality assessment scores there was notably poor reporting of skin preparation techniques, the placement and fixation of electrodes and details regarding the use of reference electrodes, information that would be important if these studies were to be replicated. Sample sizes were also generally small, with 17/21 studies using samples of <30 participants. This potentially weakens the statistical power of these studies and increases the chance of Type II errors.

4.2. Spinal Stability and Sub-System Interaction

Whilst the studies under review do consider spinal control mechanisms, with only a single study providing inter-vertebral information, discussions concerning possible mechanisms at the motion segment level were limited. In addition, as objectives were so varied, making comparisons between studies was difficult. The studies did however consider spinal stabilisation, at least in a broad sense, and the following insights were provided.

McGill and Kippers (1994) [15] suggested that an insight into interaction between sub-systems can be found by examining the transfer of moment from active to passive tissues at the limits of forward bending. Their investigation concluded that although electrically silent during full flexion, paraspinal muscles continue to provide elastic resistance via passive stretching. They suggest that this silence is an indication of the cessation of input from the central nervous system, likely as a result of some sort of active or passive tissue feedback. As the study was based on regional spinal measurements, nothing more than generalised theories could be extrapolated. In agreement with McGill and Kippers and again highlighting a requirement for inter-vertebral data, Arjmand et al. (2010) [41] showed that in both models, increased abdominal coactivity was predicted at the end of forward flexion. This mechanism is proposed by both studies to counterbalance moments in addition to the contributions of paraspinal muscles (i.e., passive resistance) and spinal ligaments.

In agreement with these studies, Paquet et al. (1994) [53] suggested that increased paraspinal activity permits the transmission of forces via these muscles, and is a mechanism to protect damaged passive structures. It was proposed that the alteration in hip-spine movement pattern in those with an absent FRP, may be a strategy to protect the lumbar spine near its maximum range (i.e., near its peak bending moment). This raises the importance of being able to measure kinematics in different regions of a chain (i.e., not just the lumbar region). Callaghan and Dunk (2002) [43] found that FRP was not present in the TES muscle during bending. As the study did not measure thoracic angular ROM however, and assuming cascading segmental flexion, some thoracic movement will have been expected to occur before the onset of movement in the lumbar region. It is therefore difficult to comment on deactivation mechanisms. However, the results do support the common conclusion in FRP studies that as passive tissues are stretched, they eventually reach a point at which they can counter the moment produced by bending the lower back. In this case, as flexion moment may be expected to be less during slumped sitting than standing flexion, the passive tissues are able to support the moment produced at a smaller lumbar angle. This is as much detail as the authors provided, and so it was not possible to relate their findings to interactions between systems or feedback mechanisms.

The study of Hashemirad et al. (2009) [45] was based on the idea that flexibility is linked to characteristics of the active and passive tissues. The authors suggested that in agreement with Panjabi's hypotheses, when the CNS contends with increased flexibility in the passive tissues, it responds by increasing the contribution of the active system. This mechanism is represented in the study by the increased paraspinal activity associated with increased participant flexibility. The authors go on to suggest that such a mechanism is likely a spinal stabilisation strategy, however without inter-vertebral information this claim is difficult to support.

Generally speaking therefore, increased muscle activity is proposed as a mechanism that increases spinal stability, the review did however provide some contrasting findings. Peach et al. (1998) [35] investigating healthy controls, found a lack of co-contraction of abdominal and paraspinal muscles during flexion. This could suggest therefore that this may be an optimal stabilisation strategy employed by healthy spines, and that different activation strategies seen in LBP groups could represent adaptation mechanisms. In this case no speculation was provided regarding sub-system interactions. This is in contrast to the findings of Cholewicki et al. (1997) [44], who showed that trunk flexor and extensor co-activation was present during dynamic sagittal movement in participants with no history of low back pain. The study however only considered approximately 20° of flexion (i.e., around the neutral position) and cannot be compared directly with studies such as Peach et al. (1998) [35] where full flexion was performed. The authors again conclude that the co-activation is a neuromuscular activation strategy to increase stability of the lumbar spine. As a regional kinematic study, it was not possible to extrapolate insights into system interactions at the motion segment level, however the results do support the theory that any loss of spinal stiffness as a result of passive tissue damage, can be compensated by an overall increase in trunk muscle activation. As such, muscle activity may be useful as a clinical indicator. Further work was suggested which would benefit from investigations at the inter-vertebral level.

The findings of Sanchez-Zuriaga et al. (2015) [26] suggested that paraspinal activity was increased irrespective of the lumbar range of flexion achieved and may therefore indicate that deactivation mechanisms are not purely related to mechanisms such as the degree of ligament deformation as suggested elsewhere [21]. Burnett et al. (2004) [42] suggested that the LBP group in their study may have an underlying motor control dysfunction, either as a response to, or predisposing factor to a lumbar strain associated with the increased lower lumbar flexion and decreased local stabiliser activity. This is of course in direct contrast to the results of FRP studies considered in this review, which suggest that LBP is reflexively related to the increased activity of the paraspinals (i.e., the absence of the FRP). The authors also suggest that examining regions of the lumbar spine (e.g., upper and lower lumbar spine) is more revealing than measuring ranges of motion over the entire lumbar spine, given the contrast in kinematic behaviours found between groups in terms of lumbar regions. In agreement Dankaerts et al. (2009) [7] who also divided the lumbar spine into regions, concluded that increased muscle activity (examples found in both FP and AEP groups) likely represent maladaptive motor control strategies that potentially act as catalysts for ongoing strain and pain production, increase spinal load and result in impeded recovery. No detail about the proposed mechanisms were provided, however the value of further dividing kinematic regions (i.e., upper and lower lumbar spine) was demonstrated as the measurement of lumbar spine angles (i.e., T12-S2) and regional lumbar spine angles (e.g., lower lumbar spine L3-S2) produced distinctly different results.

The study by Kaigle et al. (1998) [20] was unique in that it was the only study reviewed with the capacity to comment on subsystem interactions at a motion segment level. In agreement with the theory that ligaments stretched in full flexion provide afferent impulses that then inhibit paraspinal muscles (Floyd and Silver 1955) [14], the authors conclude that as the patient group showed comparatively reduced inter-vertebral movement, the ligamentous mechanoreceptors were not sufficiently stimulated to provoke muscular inhibition. Unfortunately, due to a small sample size, even this study may not provide an inter-vertebral insight that can be generalizable to the wider population, which arguably is required to advance understanding in this area. Indeed, whilst the study of Arjmand was only small (n = 1), one of the key conclusions was that multi-joint kinematics combined with paraspinal EMG recordings would improve modelling accuracy.

Alternatively, O'Sullivan et al. (2006) [17] discussed their findings in relation to global and local paraspinal activity. The study showed that TES activity was extremely variable in participants during bending, a finding the authors suggested may be as a result of its role as a global muscle. As a globally acting muscle, it was argued to have more potential for variation in motor pattern, as it is was not directly responsible for local stabilisation as is the case for LMU. It may also be that the increase in TES activity is a strategy to maintain stability when LMU activity decreases, a mechanism perhaps employed to avoid excessive loading as a result of contraction Granata and Orishimo (2001) [9], or as additional resistance to the moment of flexion provided by the passive structures. In addition, Lariviere et al. (2000) [6] showed that TES muscles likely compensate for LES muscles when less active (such as during FRP). The authors suggest therefore it is likely that TES muscles have an important role to play in LBP patient motor control strategies, and so consideration of thoracic muscle activity should perhaps be given, even when investigations are focussed on dynamic movement within the lumbar spine.

4.3. Can the Information Aquired by Combining Lumbar Kinematic and Muscle Activity Measurements during Functional Movements Assist in Distinguishing between Groups of Healthy Controls and Those with Low Back Pain?

The review would suggest that there are many studies that have found distinguishing features in LBP populations (e.g., increased paraspinal muscle activity; decreased sagittal ROM), however, generally the study populations were small, and the large variations in methodology (particularly EMG placement and kinematic recordings) makes further analysis (including meta-analysis) difficult. There were also studies however that showed contrasting findings, or that were not able to distinguish between LBP and non-LBP groups. The wide range of methodological approaches makes it difficult to generalise such findings beyond the specific populations involved, which is a major limitation of research in this field. Whilst recommendations for EMG recordings and processing have been standardised [40,54], it would be of value if the muscles selected for these types of study were measured consistently from the same anatomical reference point. Likewise, in terms of the measurement of regional kinematics, it would be beneficial if such measurements were also standardised (i.e., between universally agreed landmarks such as L1-S1 to represent the lumbar region for example). Table 4, shows that in no two studies were the EMG electrode locations the same, and likewise all kinematic measurements differered in some way. The review does however highlight the potential of some variables for this purpose. As an example, Kienbacher et al. (2016) [47] using root mean square EMG amplitude, and regional measurements, showed that neuromuscular activation and kinematics can distinguish between CNSLBP patients with impaired or unimpaired muscle activation strategies. They suggest that the aging process is a stronger facilitator of this neuromuscular activity (i.e., increased paraspinal activity) than the pain associated with the condition. This the authors attribute to a likely increased excitability of the motor neurone pool associated with increased age [47].

The influence of pain on EMG and kinematic measurements is not well understood. It could be argued therefore that studies should either focus on healthy participants to gain a better understanding of what is normal [35], or use LBP groups that are pain free at the time of study, in order to remove for the influence of pain. In the O'Sullivan et al. (2006) [17] and Callaghan and Dunk (2002) [43] studies, both investigated low back pain free populations, and therefore the disagreement in their results (i.e., the existence or absence of the FRP in the TES) is most likely explained by methodological differences. The authors also suggest however that as TES activity is highly variable between individuals, this could possible represent inherently different motor control strategies. In addition to O'Sullivan's findings (where no thoracic kinematic data was available), Nairn et al. (2013) [50] measured thoracic movement and showed that the deactivation of the TES during slumped sitting was related to increased angles of the thoracic segment movement. This supports the view that the decrease in activity is somehow related to stretch feedback of the ligaments, and the authors concluded that regional information was therefore important. In agreement, Luhring et al. (2015) [16] argued that the global approach (i.e., global trunk angle) was less preferable to the local approach (i.e., lumbar angle) as the mechanism of FRP is proposed to be dependent on local lumbar structures. This is a logical conclusion to make, and in continuation it is likely preferable still to obtain inter-vertebral information that relates directly to the lumbar structures involved.

4.4. Are There Opportunities to Improve Understanding of Sub-System Interactions and Low Back Pain Using Studies That Utilise Kinematic and EMG Measurements Concurrently?

The argument for the increased utilisation of inter-vertebral measurements when measuring spinal ROM and muscle activity concurrently, was alluded to frequently in this review. Inter-vertebral measurements would be important in this field, as this is the level at which spinal control feedback mechanisms are believed to be initiated [21]. Whilst regional kinematics are valuable, their measurements may best be related to globally acting musculature (e.g., muscles that span between the thoracic cage and the pelvis) [55], and so insights into stabilisation mechanisms resulting from ligamentous stress, or muscle spindle activation (i.e., related to segmentally acting tissues) would arguably be best provided by inter-vertebral data.

To collect kinematic information at this level however, presents some methodological problems. Whilst skin surface markers can be used to measure inter-vertebral motion, skin movement artifacts have been shown to result in poor reliability [56,57]. Reliable segmental data therefore typically requires more invasive techniques such as x-rays [58,59] or fluoroscopy [60–64], or as shown in this review the surgical insertion of intra-osseous pins [20]. Of these, fluoroscopy perhaps stands out, as it has been repeatedly demonstrated to be accurate and reliable [33,60,65–67], and as such may be the preferable option for future studies investigating interactions between sub-systems at the motion segment level.

The term nonspecific low back pain (NSLBP) by its definition, alludes to the fact that heterogeneity in LBP causes, can make it difficult to explain with any accuracy why kinematic or muscle activity parameters may differ between and within low back pain and non-low back pain groups. The key reason for increased muscle activity and decreased spinal ROM of motion provided by this review were likely adaptive mechanisms, related to spinal stabilisation. It is however difficult to demonstrate definite links between these parameters and LBP, due to the large number of possible pathoanotomical causes. A possible next step could be to investigate ROM and muscle activity in LBP populations that have been sub classified in some way. O'Sullivan et al. (2005) used a multidimensional classification system (MDCS) which included sub-groups of patients whose LBP was aggravated by flexion or extension [68]. An opportunity therefore, would be to investigate muscle activity and kinematic patterns at the motion segment level in LBP in patients who have been allocated to such groups, possibly providing new insight into the biomechanical origins of LBP at this level.

4.5. Key findings and recommendations

- Increased muscle activity and co-contraction are strategies adopted to stabilise the lumbar spine.
- Whilst generalised conclusions regarding spinal stabilisation were seen throughout the literature, insights into the understanding of spinal sub-system interactions at the motion segment level were limited.
- Parameters shown to distinguish between non-LBP and LBP populations include spinal ROM and trunk muscle activation, including the FRP. Typically, LBP groups demonstrated comparatively reduced ROM, increased muscle activity and an absent FRP.
- Future studies should consider more frequent use of sub-divided regional or inter-vertebral kinematic measurements, and would benefit from methodological standardisation.
- More extensive exploration of thoracic kinematic and muscle activity parameters may be beneficial in order to enhance understanding of lumbar spinal stabilisation mechanisms.

4.6. Limitations

Whilst the review focused on studies that investigated bending in the sagittal plane, it is acknowledged that other planes of movement (i.e., coronal and transverse) and different tasks may also provide important insights into spinal stabilisation mechanisms. In addition, as the quality assessment of each paper was performed by one individual, the repeatability between separate reviewers was not known. It is also acknowledged that the small number of data bases used to search for articles (i.e., PubMed and the Cochrane library) may be considered a limitation.

5. Conclusions

Many studies found differences in kinematic or EMG variables capable of distinguishing between LBP and healthy control groups, however the differences in methodology between studies mean that only broad generalisations can be made.

No one study set out with the explicit objective to explore sub-system interaction, however many did attempt to relate their findings to such mechanisms. A common weakness in study design was that studies used regional kinematic measurements, which can only ever at best provide a broad interpretation of sub-system interaction. It was therefore unsurprising that conclusions relating to sub-system interaction were limited. The studies that did were those that investigated sub-divided spinal regions or inter-vertebral kinematic measurements [7,20], and even these did not use truly inter-vertebral data, as the data was pooled from several inter-vertebral levels.

There is an apparent unmet need to better understand spinal stability and the assertion that the passive, active and motor control systems need to act in concert for function to be optimal [1]. An enhanced understanding could feasibly result in improved sub-grouping and diagnosis of LBP patients, and the development of more targeted therapeutic interventions, and therefore represents an important area of research. Whilst this review provides many examples of how changes in one sub-system may result in changes in another to compensate, the investigations have typically focused on regions of the spine and not at the motion segment level. In order to improve understanding of such interactions and the mechanisms behind them, it could be argued therefore that more emphasis could be placed on research focusing at the segmental level, the level at which communication between sub-systems is believed to be initiated. Improved understanding may also be hindered due to the fact that studies either focus on sub-systems individually or that it has not been possible to study their interactions during dynamic tasks.

It has been shown that although it is possible to measure numerous variables relating to spinal function, until one can measure in vivo inter-vertebral dynamic kinematics and relate it to one of the other sub-systems in detail, it will not be possible to make significant progress in this area. This lack of progression was reflected in this review and highlights the requirement for new approaches to research that incorporate these elements. Future studies should consider technologies that enable inter-vertebral measurements, not just in the lumbar spine but ideally throughout the thoracic, pelvic, hip and cervical regions too. It has been shown that stabilisation during sagittal bending can be influenced by the paraspinal muscle activity of both lumbar flexors and extensors, and abdominals, and that the TES may play an important role in lumbar stabilisation [5,25]. Measurement of these muscles, including activation timings and amplitudes, should therefore be included in studies whenever possible. Standardisation of investigation methodologies is also recommended, as the current heterogeneity in approaches makes any comparison between studies difficult.

Funding: This research received no external funding.

Acknowledgments: The author would like to thank the University of South Wales for allocating sufficient time for the author to conduct the review.

References

1.   Panjabi, M.M. The stabilising system of the spine—Part 1: Function, dysfunction, adaptation and enhancement. *J. Spinal Disord.* **1992**, *5*, 383–389. [CrossRef] [PubMed]

2.   Panjabi, M.M. The stabilising system of the spine—Part 2: Neutral zone and instability hypothesis. *J. Spinal Disord.* **1992**, *5*, 390–397. [CrossRef] [PubMed]

3.   Olson, M.W.; Li, L.; Solomonow, M. Flexion-relaxation response to cyclic lumbar flexion. *Clin. Biomech.* **2004**, *19*, 769–776. [CrossRef] [PubMed]

4.   Shin, G.; Mirka, G.A. An in vivo assessment of the low back response to prolonged flexion: Interplay between active and passive tissues. *Clin. Biomech.* **2007**, *22*, 965–971. [CrossRef] [PubMed]

5.   Van Dieen, J.H.; Cholewicki, J.; Radebold, A. Trunk Muscle Recruitment Patterns in Patients With Low Back Pain Enhance the Stability of the Lumbar Spine. *Spine* **2003**, *28*, 834–841. [CrossRef] [PubMed]

6.   Lariviere, C.; Gagnon, D.; Loisel, P. The comparison of trunk muscles EMG activiation between subjects with and without chronic low back pain during flexion-extension and lateral bending tasks. *J. Electromyogr. Kinesiol.* **2000**, *10*, 79–91. [CrossRef]

7. Dankaerts, W.; O'Sullivan, P.B.; Burnett, A.F.; Straker, L.M.; Davey, P.; Gupta, R. Discriminating Healthy Controls and Two Clinical Subgroups of Nonspecific Chronic Low Back Pain Patients Using Trunk Muscle Activation and Lumbosacral Kinematics of Postures and Movements. *Spine* **2009**, *34*, 1610–1618. [CrossRef] [PubMed]

8. Silfies, S.P.; Mehta, R.; Smith, S.S.; Karduna, A.R. Differences in Feedforward Trunk Muscle Activity in Subgroups of Patients With Mechanical Low Back Pain. *Arch. Phys. Med. Rehabil.* **2009**, *90*, 1159–1169. [CrossRef] [PubMed]

9. Granata, K.P.; Orishimo, K.F. Response of trunk muscle coactivation to changes in spinal stability. *J. Biomech.* **2001**, *34*, 1117–1123. [CrossRef]

10. Sanchez-Zuriaga, D.; Adams, M.A.; Dolan, P. Is Activation of the Back Muscles Impaired by Creep or Muscle Fatigue? *Spine* **2010**, *35*, 517–525. [CrossRef] [PubMed]

11. Abboud, J.; Nougarou, F.; Descarreaux, M. Muscle Activity Adaptations to Spinal Tissue Creep in the Presence of Muscle Fatigue. *PLoS ONE* **2016**, *11*, e0149076. [CrossRef] [PubMed]

12. Hendershot, B.; Bazrgari, B.; Muslim, K.; Toosizadeh, N.; Nussbaum, M.A.; Madigan, M.L. Disturbance and recovery of trunk stiffness and reflexive muscle responses following prolonged trunk flexion: Influences of flexion angle and duration. *Clin. Biomech.* **2011**, *26*, 250–256. [CrossRef] [PubMed]

13. Abboud, J.; Lardon, A.; Boivin, F.; Duga, C.; Descarreaux, M. Effects of Muscle Fatigue, Creep, and Musculoskeletal Pain on Neuromuscular Responses to Unexpected Perturbation of the Trunk: A Systematic Review. *Front. Hum. Neurosci.* **2017**, *10*, 667. [CrossRef] [PubMed]

14. Floyd, W.F.; Silver, P.H.S. The function of the erectores spinae muscles in certain movements and postures in man. *J. Physiol.* **1955**, *129*, 184–203. [CrossRef] [PubMed]

15. McGill, S.M.; Kippers, V. Transfer of loads between lumbar tissues during the flexion-relaxation phenomenon. *Spine* **1994**, *19*, 2190–2196. [CrossRef] [PubMed]

16. Luhring, S.; Schinkel-Ivy, A.; Drake, J.D.M. Evaluation of the lumbar kinematic measures that most consistently characterize lumbar muscle activation patterns during trunk flexion: A cross-sectional study. *J. Manip. Physiol. Ther.* **2015**, *38*, 44–50. [CrossRef] [PubMed]

17. O'Sullivan, P.P.; Dankaerts, W.P.; Burnett, A.P.; Chen, D.M.; Booth, R.M.; Carlsen, C.M.; Schultz, A.M. Evaluation of the Flexion Relaxation Phenomenon of the Trunk Muscles in Sitting. *Spine* **2006**, *31*, 2009–2016. [CrossRef] [PubMed]

18. Sarti, M.A.; Lison, J.F.; Monfort, M.; Fuster, M.A. Response of the Flexion-Relaxation Phenomenon Relative to the Lumbar Motion to Load and Speed. *Spine* **2001**, *26*, E421–E426. [CrossRef] [PubMed]

19. Descarreaux, M.; Lafond, D.; Jeffrey-Gauthier, R.; Centomo, H.; Cantin, V. Changes in the flexion relaxation response induced by lumbar muscle fatigue. *BMC Musculoskelet. Disord.* **2008**, *9*, 10. [CrossRef] [PubMed]

20. Kaigle, A.M.; Wesberg, P.; Hansson, T.H. Muscular and kinematic behavior of the lumbar spine during flexion-extension. *J. Spinal Disord.* **1998**, *11*, 163–174. [CrossRef] [PubMed]

21. Solomonow, M.; Zhou, B.H.; Harris, M.; Lu, Y.; Baratta, R.V. The ligamento-muscular stabilizing system of the spine. *Spine* **1998**, *23*, 2552–2562. [CrossRef] [PubMed]

22. Fortin, M.; Macedo, L.G. Multifidus and Paraspinal Muscle Group Cross-Sectional Areas of Patients With Low Back Pain and Control Patients: A Systematic Review with a Focus on Blinding. *Phys. Ther.* **2013**, *93*, 873–888. [CrossRef] [PubMed]

23. Williams, J.M.; Haq, I.; Lee, R.Y. An Investigation Into the Onset, Pattern, and Effects of Pain Relief on Lumbar Extensor Electromyography in People with Acute and Chronic Low Back Pain. *J. Manip. Physiol. Ther.* **2013**, *36*, 91–100. [CrossRef] [PubMed]

24. Nelson-Wong, E.; Alex, B.; Csepe, D.; Lancaster, D.; Callaghan, J.P. Altered muscle recruitment during extension from trunk flexion in low back pain developers. *Clin. Biomech.* **2012**, *27*, 994–998. [CrossRef] [PubMed]

25. Reeves, N.P.; Cholewicki, J.; Silfies, S.P. Muscle activation imbalance and low-back injury in varsity athletes. *J. Electromyogr. Kinesiol.* **2006**, *16*, 264–272. [CrossRef] [PubMed]

26. Sanchez-Zuriaga, D.; Lopez-Pascual, J.; Garrido-Jaen, D.; Garcia-Mas, M.A. A Comparison of Lumbopelvic Motion Patterns and Erector Spinae Behavior Between Asymtomatic Subjects and Patients with Recurrent Low Back Pain During Pain-Free Periods. *J. Manip. Physiol. Ther.* **2015**, *38*, 130–137. [CrossRef] [PubMed]

27. Ahern, D.K.; Follick, M.J.; Council, J.R.; Laserwolston, N.; Litchman, H. Comparison of lumbar paravertebral Emg patterns in chronic low back pain patients and non-patient controls. *Pain* **1988**, *34*, 153–160. [CrossRef]

28. Kuriyama, N.; Ito, H. Electromyographic Functional Analysis of the Lumbar Spinal Muscles with Low Back Pain. *J. Nippon. Med Sch.* **2005**, *72*, 165–173. [CrossRef] [PubMed]

29. McGregor, A.H.; McCarthy, I.D.; Dore, C.J.; Hughes, S.P. Quantitative assessment of the motion of the lumbar spine in the low back pain population and the effect of different spinal pathologies on this motion. *Eur. Spine J.* **1997**, *6*, 308–315. [CrossRef] [PubMed]

30. Abbott, J.; Fritz, J.; McCane, B.; Shultz, B.; Herbison, P.; Lyons, B.; Stefanko, G.; Walsh, R. Lumbar segmental mobility disorders: Comparison of two methods of defining abnormal displacement kinematics in a cohort of patients with non-specific mechanical low back pain. *BMC Musculoskelet. Disord.* **2006**, *7*, 45. [CrossRef] [PubMed]

31. Kulig, K.; Powers, C.; Landel, R.; Chen, H.; Fredericson, M.; Guillet, M.; Butts, K. Segmental lumbar mobility in individuals with low back pain: In vivo assessment during manual and self-imposed motion using dynamic MRI. *BMC Musculoskelet. Disord.* **2007**, *8*, 8. [CrossRef] [PubMed]

32. Teyhen, D.S.; Flynn, T.W.; Childs, J.D.; Kuklo, T.R.; Rosner, M.K.; Polly, D.W.; Abraham, L.D. Fluoroscopic Video to Identify Aberrant Lumbar Motion. *Spine* **2007**, *32*, E220–E229. [CrossRef] [PubMed]

33. Mellor, F.E.; Thomas, P.; Thompson, P.; Breen, A.C. Proportional lumbar spine inter-vertebral motion patterns: A comparison of patients with chronic non-specific low back pain and healthy controls. *Eur. Spine J.* **2014**, *23*, 2059–2067. [CrossRef] [PubMed]

34. Mehta, V.A.; Amin, A.; Omeis, I.; Gokaslan, Z.L.; Gottfried, O.N. Implications of Spinopelvic Alignment for the Spine Surgeon. *Neurosurgery* **2012**, *70*, 707–721. [CrossRef] [PubMed]

35. Peach, J.P.; Sutarno, C.G.; McGill, S.M. Three-Dimensional Kinematics and Trunk Muscle Myoelectric Activity in the Young Lumbar Spine: A Database. *Arch. Phys. Med. Rehabil.* **1998**, *79*, 663–669. [CrossRef]

36. Mitchell, T.; O'Sullivan, P.B.; Burnett, A.F.; Straker, L.; Smith, A. Regional differences in lumbar spinal posture and the influence of low back pain. *BMC Musculoskelet. Disord.* **2008**, *9*, 152. [CrossRef] [PubMed]

37. Hemming, R.; Sheeran, L.; van Deursen, R.; Martin, R.W.; Sparkes, V. Regional spinal kinematics during static postures and functional tasks in people with non-specific chronic low back pain. *Int. J. Ther. Rehabil.* **2015**, *22*, S8. [CrossRef]

38. Colloca, C.J.; Hinrichs, R.N. The biomechanical and clinical significance of the lumbar erector spinae flexion-relaxation phenomenon: A review of literature. *J. Manip. Physiol. Ther.* **2005**, *28*, 623–631. [CrossRef] [PubMed]

39. Downs, S.; Black, N. The feasibility of creating a checklist for the assessment of the methodological quality both of randomised and non-randomised studies of health care interventions. *J. Epidemiol. Community Health* **1998**, *52*, 377–384. [CrossRef] [PubMed]

40. Hermens, H.J.; Freriks, B.; Merletti, R.; Stegeman, D.; Blok, J.; Rau, G.; Disselhorst-Klug, C.; Hagg, G. *European Recommendations for Surface Electromyography: Results of the SENIAM Project*; Roessingh Research and Development: Enschede, The Netherlands, 1999.

41. Arjmand, N.; Gagnon, D.; Plamondon, A.; Shirazi-Adl, S.; Lariviere, C. A comparative study of two trunk biomechanical models under symmetric and asymmetric loadings. *J. Biomech.* **2010**, *43*, 485–491. [CrossRef] [PubMed]

42. Burnett, A.F.; Cornelius, M.W.; Dankaerts, W.; O'Sullivan, P.B. Spinal kinematics and trunk muscle activity in cyclists: A comparison between healthy controls and non-specific chronic low back pain subjects—A pilot investigation. *Man. Ther.* **2004**, *9*, 211–219. [CrossRef] [PubMed]

43. Callaghan, J.C.; Dunk, N.M. Examination of the flexion relaxation phenomenon in erector spinae muscles during short duration slumped sitting. *Clin. Biomech.* **2002**, *17*, 353–360. [CrossRef]

44. Cholewicki, J.; Panjabi, M.M.; Khachatryan, A. Stabilizing function of trunk flexor-extensor muscles around a neutral spine posture. *Spine* **1997**, *22*, 2207–2212. [CrossRef] [PubMed]

45. Hashemirad, F.; Talebian, S.; Hatef, B.; Kahlaee, A.H. The relationship between flexibility and EMG activity pattern of the erector spinae muscles during trunk flexion-extension. *J. Electromyogr. Kinesiol.* **2009**, *19*, 746–753. [CrossRef] [PubMed]

46. Hay, D.; Wachowiak, M.P.; Graham, R.B. Evaluating the relationship between muscle activation and spine kinematics through wavelet coherence. *J. Appl. Biomech.* **2016**, *32*, 526–531. [CrossRef] [PubMed]

47. Kienbacher, T.; Ferhmann, E.; Habenicht, R.; Koller, D.; Oeffel, C.; Kollmitzer, J.; Mair, P.; Ebenbichler, G.R. Age and gender related neuromuscular pattern during trunk flexion-extension in chronic low back pain patients. *J. NeuroEng. Rehabil.* **2016**, *13*, 16. [CrossRef] [PubMed]

48. Liu, A.; Wang, J.; Hu, Y. Network modeling and analysis of lumbar muscle surface EMG signals during flexion–extension in individuals with and without low back pain. *J. Electromyogr. Kinesiol.* **2011**, *21*, 913–921. [CrossRef] [PubMed]

49. Mayer, T.; Neblett, R.; Brede, E.; Gatchel, R.J. The Quantified Lumbar Flexion-Relaxation Phenomenon Is a Useful Measurement of Improvement in a Functional Restoration Program. *Spine* **2009**, *34*, 2458–2465. [CrossRef] [PubMed]

50. Nairn, B.; Chisholm, S.; Drake, J.D.M. What is slumped sitting? A kinematic and electromyographical evaluation. *Man. Ther.* **2013**, *18*, 498–505. [CrossRef] [PubMed]

51. Neblett, R.; Mayer, T.G.; Gatchel, R.J.; Keeley, J.; Proctor, T.; Anagnostis, C. Quantifying the Lumbar Flexion-Relaxation Phenomenon: Theory, Normative Data, and Clinical Applications. *Spine* **2003**, *28*, 1435–1446. [CrossRef] [PubMed]

52. Ning, X.; Jin, S.; Mirka, G.A. Describing the active region boundary of EMG-assisted biomechanical models of the low back. *Clin. Biomech.* **2012**, *27*, 422–427. [CrossRef] [PubMed]

53. Paquet, N.; Malouin, F.; Richards, C.L. Hip-Spine Movement Interaction and Muscle Activation Patterns During Sagittal Trunk Movements in Low Back Pain Patients. *Spine* **1994**, *19*, 596–603. [CrossRef] [PubMed]

54. Hermens, H.J.; Freriks, B.; Disselhorst-Klug, C.; Rau, G. Development of recommendations for SEMG sensors and sensor placement procedures. *J. Electromyogr. Kinesiol.* **2000**, *10*, 361–374. [CrossRef]

55. Bergmark, A. Stability of the lumbar spine: A study in mechanical engineering. *Acta Orthop. Scand.* **1989**, *60*, 1–54. [CrossRef]

56. Cerveri, P.; Pedotti, A.; Ferrigno, G. Kinematical models to reduce the effect of skin artifacts on marker-based human motion estimation. *J. Biomech.* **2005**, *38*, 2228–2236. [CrossRef] [PubMed]

57. Zhang, X.; Xiong, J. Model-guided derivation of lumbar vertebral kinematics in vivo reveals the difference between external marker-defined and internal segmental rotations. *J. Biomech.* **2003**, *36*, 9–17. [CrossRef]

58. Ogston, N.G.; King, G.J.; Gertzbein, S.D.; Tile, M.M.D.; Kapasouri, A.; Rubenstein, J.D. Centrode Patterns in the Lumbar Spine: Baseline Studies in Normal Subjects. *Spine* **1986**, *11*, 591–595. [CrossRef] [PubMed]

59. Pearcy, M.J.; Portek, I.; Shepherd, J. Three dimensional x-ray analysis of normal movement in the lumbar spine. *Spine* **1984**, *9*, 294–297. [CrossRef] [PubMed]

60. Ahmadi, A.; Maroufi, N.; Behtash, H.; Zekavat, H.; Parnianpour, M. Kinematic analysis of dynamic lumbar motion in patients with lumbar segmental instability using digital videofluoroscopy. *Eur. Spine J.* **2009**, *18*, 1677–1685. [CrossRef] [PubMed]

61. Breen, A.C.; Teyhen, D.S.; Mellor, F.E.; Breen, A.C.; Wong, K.W.N.; Deitz, A. Measurement of inter-vertebral motion using quantitative fluoroscopy: Report of an international forum and proposal for use in the assessment of degenerative disc disease in the lumbar spine. *Adv. Orthop.* **2012**, *2012*, 802350. [CrossRef] [PubMed]

62. Du Rose, A.; Breen, A. Relationships between lumbar inter-vertebral motion and lordosis in healthy adult males: A cross sectional cohort study. *BMC Musculoskelet. Disord.* **2016**, *17*, 121. [CrossRef] [PubMed]

63. Du Rose, A.; Breen, A. Relationships between Paraspinal Muscle Activity and Lumbar Inter-Vertebral Range of Motion. *Healthcare* **2016**, *4*, 4. [CrossRef] [PubMed]

64. Wong, K.; Luk, K.; Leong, J.; Wong, S.; Wong, K. Continuous dynamic spinal motion analysis. *Spine* **2006**, *31*, 414–419. [CrossRef] [PubMed]

65. Breen, A.; Muggleton, J.; Mellor, F. An objective spinal motion imaging assessment (OSMIA): Reliability, accuracy and exposure data. *BMC Musculoskelet. Disord.* **2006**, *7*, 1–10. [CrossRef] [PubMed]

66. Teyhen, D.S.; Flynn, T.W.; Bovik, A.C.; Abraham, L.D. A new technique for digital fluoroscopic video assessment of sagittal plane lumbar spine motion. *Spine* **2005**, *30*, E406–E413. [CrossRef] [PubMed]

67. Yeager, M.S.; Cook, D.J.; Cheng, B.C. Reliability of computer-assisted lumbar intervertebral measurement using a novel vertebral motion analysis system. *Spine J.* **2014**, *14*, 274–281. [CrossRef] [PubMed]

68. O'Sullivan, P. Diagnosis and classificiation of chronic low back pain disorders: Maladaptive movement and motor control impairments as underlying mechanism. *Man. Ther.* **2005**, *10*, 242–255. [CrossRef] [PubMed]

18

Bereaved Family Members' Satisfaction with Care during the Last Three Months of Life for People with Advanced Illness

Anna O'Sullivan [1,*] [iD], Anette Alvariza [1,2], Joakim Öhlen [3,4,5] and Cecilia Håkanson [1,6,*]

[1] Department of Health Care Sciences, Palliative Research Centre, Ersta Sköndal Bräcke University College, P.O. Box 11189, SE-100 61 Stockholm, Sweden; anette.alvariza@esh.se

[2] Capio Palliative Care Unit, Dalen Hospital, Åstorpsringen 6, Enskededalen, SE-121 87 Stockholm, Sweden

[3] Institute of Health and Care Sciences, Sahlgrenska Academy at the University of Gothenburg, 41346 Gothenburg, Sweden; joakim.ohlen@fhs.gu.se

[4] Centre for Person-Centered Care, Sahlgrenska Academy at the University of Gothenburg, 40530 Gothenburg, Sweden

[5] The Palliative Centre, Sahlgrenska University Hospital, P.O. Box 457, SE-405 30 Gothenburg, Sweden

[6] Department of Nursing Science, Sophiahemmet University, P.O. Box 5605, SE-114 86 Stockholm, Sweden

* Correspondence: anna.osullivan@esh.se (A.O.); cecilia.hakanson@shh.se (C.H.)

Abstract: Background: Studies evaluating the end-of-life care for longer periods of illness trajectories and in several care places are currently lacking. This study explored bereaved family members' satisfaction with care during the last three months of life for people with advanced illness, and associations between satisfaction with care and characteristics of the deceased individuals and their family members. Methods: A cross-sectional survey design was used. The sample was 485 family members of individuals who died at four different hospitals in Sweden. Results: Of the participants, 78.7% rated the overall care as high. For hospice care, 87.1% reported being satisfied, 87% with the hospital care, 72.3% with district/county nurses, 65.4% with nursing homes, 62.1% with specialized home care, and 59.6% with general practitioners (GPs). Family members of deceased persons with cancer were more likely to have a higher satisfaction with the care. A lower satisfaction was more likely if the deceased person had a higher educational attainment and a length of illness before death of one year or longer. Conclusion: The type of care, diagnoses, length of illness, educational attainment, and the relationship between the deceased person and the family member influences the satisfaction with care.

Keywords: end-of-life care; palliative care; Sweden; quality of health care; proxy measurement

1. Introduction

Societal needs for palliative care have increased, due to improved living conditions and enhanced treatments for advanced illnesses, resulting in global ageing populations with a high prevalence of long-term illness [1,2]. Palliative care is a person-centered interdisciplinary approach to care with the aim of improving quality at the end of life and the wellbeing of all patients and their family members facing issues associated with life-limiting illness. The provision of palliative care should, if needed, be provided in all care places and to all patients in need thereof [3], and can accordingly be provided on a general level at home, in nursing homes or hospitals, and through services with palliative expertise (e.g., specialized home care and hospice care) [4]. Central aspects of importance for palliative care are the prevention and relief of suffering, early identification and assessment, treatment of symptoms and other problems (i.e., physical, psychosocial, psychological, and spiritual), communication about end-of-life issues with patients and family members, shared decision-making, and support to family members. Hence, these are also central aspects of importance when evaluating quality in palliative care.

Studies show that individual and socioeconomic factors influence where people are cared for at the end of life and die, and that such factors also may affect the quality of the care within the care places. For example, age is a factor associated with the access to and quality of palliative care, with a higher age resulting in lower access and quality [5–7]. Another factor relevant to access to palliative care and adequate end-of-life care interventions is educational attainment, with less well-educated people appearing to be disadvantaged regarding the use of specialist and general palliative care [5,8]. Several studies have also pointed to the diagnosis influencing access to palliative care. For example, people with diseases other than cancer (e.g., COPD (chronic obstructive pulmonary disease), heart disease, and dementia) have poorer access than those with cancer, resulting in less symptom control and less communication about end-of-life issues [9–11].

Studies about the quality of care in places where most people are cared for during their last months of life, in the Swedish context, are relatively sparse. Assessments of quality have traditionally been based on the health care providers' perspective, and this has also been the case for palliative care. However, in the past few years, giving a voice to patients' and family members' perspectives has been increasingly emphasized [12]. Family members are important sources of knowledge for evaluating care during the last period of life [13,14], and a recognized way to measure the care quality is to evaluate the satisfaction of patients and their family members with the care received.

Even though the care trajectory in advanced illness usually entails care in several care places, previous studies about family members' satisfaction with care have often focused only one or two care places. In addition, they usually only focus on the last days/week in life and only specific patient groups (e.g., cancer patients). These studies have shown that several factors are rated as important for a high level of satisfaction with the care provided: information/communication, emotional support, and a healthcare professional pointed out to the family members as overseeing the individual's care [15,16].

The place of care is also important for family satisfaction. Specialized palliative care units have been rated with higher satisfaction than hospitals, nursing homes, and primary health care [17–20]. However, several studies have also shown that bereaved family members' satisfaction with care during the terminal phase has been high [15,21,22]. People with advanced illness often have experiences from various care settings during their last period of life. One common care place is the hospital [23]. In studies about care at the end of life in hospitals, shortcomings have been reported regarding palliative care efforts such as symptom relief and timely communication about palliative treatment, death, and dying [6,24–26]. Inadequate symptom relief and lack of timely communication have also been reported in studies about palliative care in nursing homes [22,27–29].

In summary, the relevant international literature indicates that individual and socio-economic factors, diagnosis, and the care place/type of care service are factors that can influence the type of care received, the quality of the care, and the satisfaction thereof. Studies on the evaluation of and satisfaction with care at the end of life do exist for different patient groups in different care places, but the majority present the health care professionals' perspective of the last days or week of life of the ill person. Hence, there is a need for more comprehensive studies evaluating the care at the end of life for all patient groups in potential need of palliative care, in several care places, for a longer period of the illness trajectory, and based on the perspective of patients and/or their family members. The objectives of this study were to explore bereaved family members' satisfaction with care during the last three months of life for people with advanced illness, and to investigate associations between satisfaction with care and the characteristics of deceased individuals and family members.

2. Materials and Methods

This study had a cross-sectional survey design and was approved by the Regional Ethical board in Stockholm, Sweden: Approval number: 2017/265-31.

2.1. Study Context and Sample

Care at the end of life in Sweden can be provided at home, in hospitals, in nursing homes, and in specialized palliative care units (e.g., hospices). The sample consisted of adult bereaved family members of individuals who died in four different hospitals in two Swedish health care regions, between August 2016 and April 2017. The hospitals included from the two regions are general county hospitals. None of the hospitals have specialized high-end care or cancer centers, but all hospitals have oncological clinics. The sample consisted of bereaved family members of individuals who died in a wide range of clinics in the different hospitals. The study participants' deceased family members had received care from several different types of care services in different care places, besides the care they received before death in one of the hospitals.

The regions chosen for this study were based on a previous population-based place of death study showing regional variations regarding where people are likely to die [30]. The inclusion criteria were: aged 18 years or older (both bereaved family members and deceased individuals), underlying/contributory causes of death (ICD-10 codes) according to the Murtagh et al. [1] model, and death occurring no less than four and no more than twelve months before recruitment to the study. The direct cause of death and the underlying causes of death were based on the physician's documentation in the patient's medical records. Murtagh and co-workers' model includes the following disease categories: HIV/AIDS; Malignant Neoplasm; Alzheimer's, dementia and senility; Neurodegenerative disease; Heart disease inclusive cerebrovascular disease; Respiratory diseases; Liver disease; and Renal disease. The time period of four to twelve months was based on experiences in previous studies using the VOICES (SF) and the VOICES manual [17,18,31,32]. An additional inclusion criterion was that the deceased individual had an identifiable bereaved family member. The person listed as primary contact in the patient's data record was invited to participate in the study.

2.2. Recruitment and Data Collection

Of all patients who died in the recruitment hospitals during the study period, 74% ($n = 1277$) met the inclusion criteria. They were identified by hospital administrators based on the inclusion criteria. One health care professional at each hospital (assigned to assist one of the researchers—Anna O'Sullivan) identified the deceased patients' bereaved family members ($n = 1277$) via the hospital's patient records. One of the researchers (Anna O'Sullivan) sent written information about the study including the contact information of one of the researchers (Anna O'Sullivan), the VOICES (SF) questionnaire, and a pre-paid return envelope to the included bereaved family members. This written information also indicated that they could withdraw from the study at any time without any explanation or consequence. Furthermore, the participants were assured that the data would be confidential. The participants consented by returning the questionnaire. This was a single-postal survey, meaning that no reminder was sent out. This lack of reminder was for ethical reasons (i.e., being sensitive towards the receivers possibly not wishing to participate).

The VOICES (SF) Questionnaire

The VOICES (SF) questionnaire—Views of Informal Carers–Evaluation of Services (Short Form)—is a questionnaire designed to retrospectively evaluate bereaved family members' experiences of the quality of care during the last three months of life of an ill family member. VOICES (SF) evaluates the care received in several care places and provides information about both the processes and structures of the care as well as patient outcomes.

The questionnaire has previously been used for different patient groups and in various healthcare settings, both at population level and in cross-sectional studies, mainly in the United Kingdom, where it was developed [18]. The complete version of VOICES (SF) has been translated and validated into other languages [33,34]. The Swedish culturally adapted and validated version [35] of the questionnaire contains 75 items divided into several domains: Care at home; Care homes; Hospital care; Specialized palliative care units/hospice care. The items are about individual and demographic characteristics (e.g., age, sex, educational attainment, country of birth, relationship to the deceased person), symptom relief, communication, support, collaboration, caregivers' approaches, and satisfaction with both the care in different care places as well as with the overall care. At the end of the questionnaire, there are three open-ended questions.

For this study, we used the items regarding care satisfaction and items on individual and demographic characteristics. The items regarding care satisfaction were on a Likert scale of possible responses: excellent, good, fair, poor, and don't know. One item—"Overall, and taking all services into account, how would you rate his/her care in the last three months of life?"—also had the additional response option "outstanding". This item is in this study referred to as "overall satisfaction with care". VOICES (SF) aims to cover as many of the various care places and care services that an individual may have had during the last three months of life, and hence not all items are relevant for all the participating bereaved family members. The items regarding care places or care services not relevant were therefore not answered. The item "overall satisfaction with care" was however answered by all.

2.3. Statistical Analysis

For the quantitative data, explorative descriptive and logistic regression analyses were performed. Descriptive statistical analyses were used to explore the characteristics of the bereaved family members and the deceased individuals, and for the satisfaction with the care in different care places, provided by different caregivers. Multivariable logistic regression analyses were performed to explore associations between overall satisfaction with care and the characteristics of the deceased individuals and their bereaved family members. For these analyses, the forced entry method was initially used, and all co-variables were entered simultaneously. Co-variables were considered to have a significant association with the outcome if $p < 0.05$. The analyses were then also performed as step-wise forward to confirm the significance of the co-variables, by adding the co-variables one by one. The significant co-variables remained significant throughout the whole analysis process, and no other co-variables were significant at any point during the analyses.

The dependent variable was overall satisfaction with care during the last three months of life, in all care settings. The independent variables were age, sex, and educational attainment for both the deceased individuals and the family members. Additional independent variables were diagnosis; length of illness before death; health care region; and relationship between the deceased person and the family member. Due to the small sample size, the dependent and independent variables were dichotomized and merged to permit logistic regression analyses. The dependent variable was merged into two categories—high or all other—with high including the response categories outstanding/excellent/good, and all other consisting of the categories fair/poor/unknown. This dichotomization of the variable "overall satisfaction" has also been applied in previous studies using VOICES (SF) [22,31,32]. Missing data were excluded from the analyses. The age variable for the deceased individuals was dichotomized into two age categories: "under 85 years old" (<85 years) and "85 years old and over" (>85 years). The age variable for the bereaved family members was dichotomized into two age categories, "18–59 years old" and "60+". The variable educational attainment was dichotomized into two categories (lower education and higher secondary/higher), and length of illness before death was categorized into "less than 1 year" or "1 year and over". The variable for cancer/non-cancer was created based on the underlying causes of death and dichotomized, with individuals dying from an illness ICD coded as C00–C99 categorized as cancer and all other diagnoses non-cancer. The non-malignant neoplasms were not represented in the sample.

Therefore, the term "cancer" was applied. The variable "relationship between the deceased person and the bereaved family member" was categorical: spouse (including partner), child, and other (e.g., sibling, parent, friend). Two models for analyses were performed, one for associations with the deceased individuals' characteristics, and one for associations with the bereaved family members' characteristics.

Statistical Package for the Social Sciences (SPSS) version 22.0 (IBM Corp., Armonk, NY, USA) was used for all statistical computations.

2.4. Qualitative Descriptive Analysis

In the final part of the questionnaire, three open-ended questions ask the responder if there is anything else they would like to add about the care received, and if there is anything they regard to have been particularly good or bad about the care. For these three questions, a qualitative descriptive analysis was performed [36] to enhance understanding of the quantitative results and to explore aspects of the care that are potentially important for the care satisfaction from the perspective of bereaved family members. The analysis was based on a total of 425 comments made by 220 participants. The number of comments per participant varied between one to three, and some comments comprised several aspects. Initially, all open-ended answers were read closely to get an overview. The answers were then read again to identify and code, with as little interpretation as possible, the statements that represented diverse (positive and negative) experiences of the care, and a quantitative count of the frequencies of statements was made. Finally, the statements were categorized into aspects expressed as particularly positive or negative parts of the care, presented in the Results section.

3. Results

In total, 485 (response rate = 37.9%) bereaved family members participated in the study. The individual characteristics of the non-responding family members were not available. For the deceased individuals linked to the non-responding family members, only age, sex, and diagnosis were available, and there were no differences regarding these from the sample.

3.1. Deceased Individuals' Characteristics

Of the deceased individuals, 50.3% were men, with ages ranging between 40 years old to 90 years or older. The direct causes of death were heart diseases including cerebrovascular diseases (42.5%), respiratory diseases (32.4%), and cancer (20.2%). Heart disease (56.3%) was also the largest underlying cause of death (Table 1). Out of the total 485 deceased individuals, 45.2% received care from district- and county nurses; general practitioners (GPs), 58.7%; specialized home care, 23.8%; hospital care, 90.7%; nursing home care, 28.5%; and hospice care, 16.1%.

3.2. Participant Characteristics—Family Members

Of the 485 participating family members, 70.7% were women. Ages ranged between 18 years old and 90 years or older. Of the participants, 51.4% were children of the deceased person and 34.3% were spouses or partners. See Table 1 for further details.

Table 1. Characteristics of deceased individuals and family members.

Characteristics	Deceased Individuals		Family Members	
	% [a]	*n*	% [a]	*n*
Sex (Missing = x/485)	-	(0/485)	-	(0/485)
Male	50.3	(244)	29.3	(142)
Female	49.7	(241)	70.7	(343)
Age (Missing = x/485)	-	(1/485)	-	(8/485)
18–29	-	-	0.8	(4)
30–39	-	-	1.6	(8)
40–49	1.2	(6)	6.8	(33)

Table 1. *Cont.*

Characteristics	Deceased Individuals		Family Members	
	% [a]	*n*	% [a]	*n*
50–59	2.3	(11)	22.3	(108)
60–69	8.9	(43)	31.3	(152)
70–79	23.1	(112)	22.9	(111)
80–89	36.7	(178)	11.3	(55)
90+	27.6	(134)	1.2	(6)
Educational attainment (Missing = x/485)	-	(5/485)	-	(3/485)
Lower secondary education	72.4	(351)	29.5	(143)
Higher secondary education	11.1	(54)	30.5	(148)
Higher education	15.5	(75)	39.4	(191)
Direct cause of death [b]	-	-	-	-
Cancer	20.2	(66)	-	-
Heart diseases (incl. cerebrovascular)	42.5	(139)	-	-
Alzheimer's	0	(0)	-	-
Respiratory diseases	32.4	(106)	-	-
Renal diseases	3.1	(10)	-	-
Neurodegenerative diseases	0.6	(2)	-	-
Liver diseases	1.2	(4)	-	-
Underlying cause of death 1 [b]	-	-	-	-
Cancer	15.8	(64)	-	-
Heart diseases (incl. cerebrovascular)	56.3	(228)	-	-
Alzheimer's	1.0	(4)	-	-
Respiratory diseases	15.1	(61)	-	-
Renal diseases	9.4	(38)	-	-
Neurodegenerative diseases	1.0	(4)	-	-
Liver diseases	1.5	(6)	-	-
Underlying cause of death 2 [b]	-	-	-	-
Cancer	15.2	(52)	-	-
Heart diseases (incl. cerebrovascular)	64.3	(220)	-	-
Alzheimer's	3.5	(12)	-	-
Respiratory diseases	10.2	(35)	-	-
Renal diseases	4.4	(15)	-	-
Neurodegenerative diseases	0.9	(3)	-	-
Liver diseases	1.2	(4)	-	-
HIV/Aids	0.3	(1)	-	-
Length of illness before death (Missing = x/485)	-	(6/485)	-	-
Sudden	5.4	(26)	-	-
<24 h	2.1	(10)	-	-
>24 h–1 week	10.7	(52)	-	-
>1 week–1 month	13.0	(63)	-	-
>1 month–6 months	14.8	(72)	-	-
>6 months–1 year	10.3	(50)	-	-
1 year or more	42.5	(206)	-	-
Relationship (Missing = x/485)	-	(4/485)	-	-
Spouse	34.5	(166)	-	-
Child	51.8	(249)	-	-
Other [c]	13.7	(66)	-	-

[a] Column percentage displayed; [b] Underlying causes of death according to Murtagh's (2014) model for potential palliative care needs; [c] Other = e.g., sibling, friend, parent.

3.3. Satisfaction with Care

3.3.1. Ratings

Of the participants, 78.7% rated the overall care, taking all care during the last three months into account, as high. For the specific care places/services, 87.1% of the participants reported being satisfied with the care received by the deceased person in a hospice, 87% with the hospital care, 72.3% with district/county nurses, 65.4% with nursing homes, 62.1% with specialized home care, and 59.6% with general practitioners (GPs). See Figure 1 for the detailed distribution of the specific categories of satisfaction.

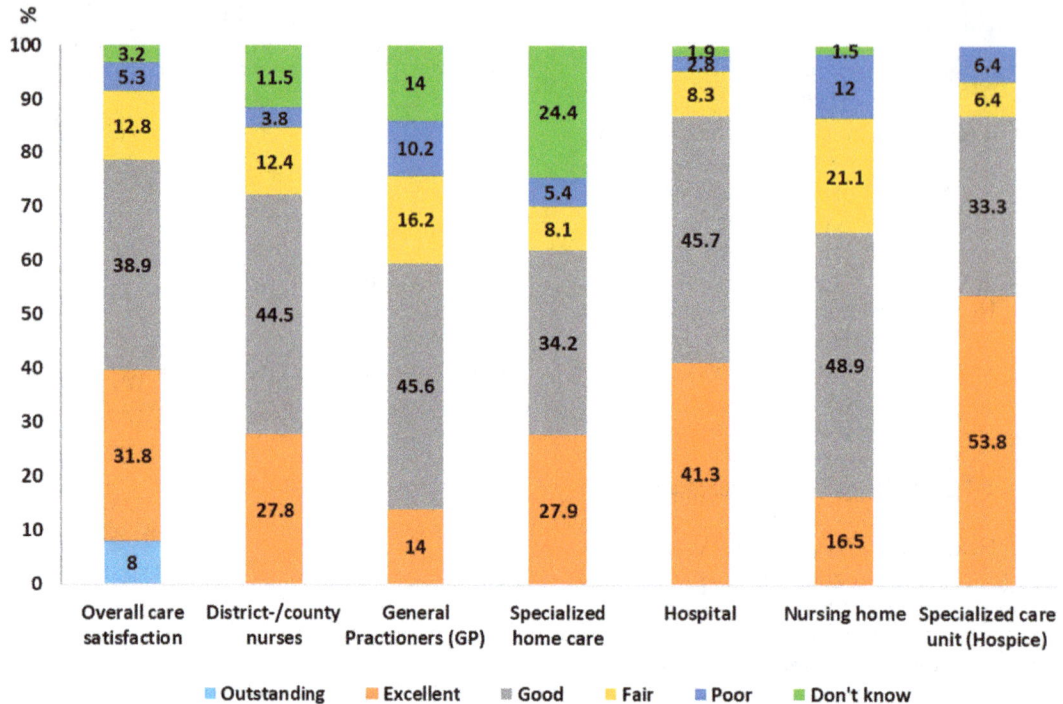

Figure 1. Distribution of bereaved family members' satisfaction with care, the overall care, and different care places/types of care services. * Percentage of satisfaction is to be seen in proportion of the sample receiving different types of care/services, not as a percentage of the total sample. Missing: Overall care satisfaction 2%; District/county nurses 4.6%; General Practitioners (GPs) 6.7%; Specialized home care 3.5%; Hospital 1.6%; Nursing home 3.6%; Specialized care unit (Hospice) 0%.

3.3.2. Descriptive Responses

The descriptive analysis of the open-ended questions revealed aspects of satisfaction with care related to information and communication, staff performance, and care place/type of care service. Some aspects were reported as particularly positive or as particularly negative, while some aspects were reported as positive when fulfilled and as negative when unmet.

Information and Communication

Aspects of care related to information and communication about the disease, prognosis, and treatments were reported both in the context of particularly positive and particularly negative. Well-functioning communication (i.e., being continuously updated and informed in a sensitive way about the prognosis and about the point at which death was to be expected soon) was reported as positive. A lack of information of a crucial nature, such as prognosis or a rapid decrease in health status and imminent death, were reported as negative aspects for satisfaction with care: "The staff didn't call us when he got worse during the night. He would have surely appreciated having his close family nearby when he was feeling poorly."

Staff Performance

Satisfaction with care related to staff performance, such as their approach, competence, and commitment was frequently reported. Being treated with respect and dignity by the health care staff was reported as particularly positive. "The staff in the emergency room looked after dad in a professional and nice manner, and us the family members." The staff's lack of commitment (e.g., not giving the patient the time needed, being uncaring or uninterested, and revealing a lack of knowledge) was reported as particularly negative. Support from the staff for the family during the illness trajectory, at death, and after the death, as well as the staff's ability to relieve pain were aspects of satisfaction with care reported as positive when fulfilled, and as negative when unmet.

Care Places and Types of Care Services

Frequently reported aspects of care being particularly negative, related to different care places and care services, were poor co-operation between caregivers and internally between the staff, too long a wait in the emergency room, too many emergency room visits or too many care places, as well as the wait to receive or even access certain care: "It took way too long before we got any kind of help, when we finally got him into a short-term nursing home, then he died after two weeks, in a hospital after two days. Alone."

Specific care places were reported as highly satisfactory and others as not: "The care in the intensive care unit was very good and the contact with and information to us family members was good. The care in the hospital ward was poor. Understaffed, no continuity, very little surveillance and poor information to us family members." Reported satisfaction with care related to the care places and types of care services also included the availability of the health care provider, the possibility of a single room, and of staying with the dying person.

3.4. Associations between Satisfaction with Care and Co-Variables

Regression analyses for associations between satisfaction with care and co-variables showed significant associations between diagnoses (cancer/non-cancer), length of illness, and educational attainment, as well as the relationship to the deceased person. Bereaved family members that were spouses of deceased individuals were more likely to be satisfied with the care than children or other relatives (OR = 2.86; CI: 1.40–5.80). Furthermore, bereaved family members of deceased individuals with cancer were more likely to express higher satisfaction with the care (OR = 2.10; CI: 1.19–3.73). By contrast, they were more likely to have a lower satisfaction with the overall care if (i) the illness duration (before death) was one year or longer (OR = 1.75; CI: 1.09–2.79); (ii) the deceased person had a higher educational attainment (OR = 2.03; CI: 1.14–3.61); or (iii) the bereaved family member had a higher educational attainment (OR = 2.02; CI 1.08–3.76). There were no significant associations for bereaved family members' age or sex, nor for the deceased individuals' age, sex, or the health care region (Table 2).

Table 2. Associations between the deceased individuals' and bereaved family members' characteristics, and the bereaved family members' overall satisfaction with care during the last three months of life in all care places.

Co-Variables	Overall High Satisfaction OR [a] 95% CI [b]	p-Value [c]
Deceased individuals	-	-
Sex	-	-
Male	1 [d]	
Female	0.98 (0.62–1.56)	0.95
Age	-	-
<85	1	-
>85	1.54 (0.94–2.51)	0.08
Underlying cause of death	-	-
Non-cancer	1	-
Cancer	2.10 (1.19–3.73)	0.01
Length of illness before death	-	-
Less than 1 year	1	

Table 2. *Cont.*

Co-Variables	Overall High Satisfaction OR [a] 95% CI [b]	*p*-Value [c]
1 year or more	0.57 (0.35–0.91)	0.01
Health Care region	-	-
Southeast	1	-
Stockholm	1.29 (0.81–2.07)	0.27
Bereaved family members	-	-
Sex	-	-
Male	1	-
Female	0.84 (0.49–1.43)	0.53
Age	-	-
18–59	1	-
60+	1.05 (0.37–1.93)	0.85
Relationship	-	-
Spouse	2.86 (1.40–5.80)	0.00
Child	1.98 (1.07–3.69)	0.03
Other [e]	1	-
Educational attainment	-	-
Lower/elementary	1	-
Higher secondary/higher	0.49 (0.26–0.92)	0.02

[a] Odds ratio; [b] Confidence interval; [c] Regression coefficient significant if $p < 0.05$ for Chi-square; [d] Categories with the value 1 are the reference category; [e] Other = e.g., sibling, friend, parent.

4. Discussion

The results show that the level of satisfaction with care was associated with the bereaved family member's relationship to the deceased individual and the length of the deceased individual's illness before death, as well as whether the death was caused by cancer or another illness. The results also show significant associations between satisfaction with care and the deceased individual's and the bereaved family member's educational attainment. Satisfaction with care varied for different care places and types of care services, but indicated that the overall satisfaction with the care was relatively high.

The association between level of satisfaction with the care and the bereaved family member's relationship to the deceased individual was somewhat unexpected, and sheds light on an area that has been the focus of relatively few studies. Ringdal et al. [37] found that children of the deceased individuals were likely to be less satisfied with the care than spouses, in a study measuring bereaved family members' satisfaction with end of life care. By contrast, Ozcelik et al. [38] found in their study on the satisfaction with care of family members of patients with advanced cancer that the relationship between the bereaved family member and the deceased individual had no significant association for care satisfaction. One possibility is that the relationship has no association with satisfaction of the care when it comes to patients with a cancer diagnosis. It could also be that children of the deceased individuals have been included in the care in different ways compared to spouses, perhaps leading to children being less satisfied with the care.

The results show that both the length of illness before death and the type of diagnosis influenced the degree of care satisfaction. The importance of diagnosis for access to palliative care has previously been shown in several studies, in which individuals with a cancer diagnosis had greater access to palliative care than non-cancer patients [9,10,39]. This is in line with other studies on access to specialist palliative care for non-cancer patients [40–42]. The importance of the care place/type of care services for family satisfaction as well as the quality of the care at the end of life has been shown in previous studies, where specialized palliative care units have been rated with higher satisfaction than hospitals, nursing homes, and primary health care [17–20,25,26,43,44]. The higher satisfaction with the care received in specialized palliative care units may be explained by the fact that specialized palliative care units are expected to provide palliative care to all their patients, compared to general care units that have both a curative and palliative aim with their care. Hence, the care in specialized palliative care units is also provided by staff with a higher knowledge of and a specialization in palliative care. Studies have shown that several aspects are important to improve palliative care in care places not specialized in palliative care (e.g., knowledge and awareness of palliative care, the staff and time to provide palliative care, as well as the organizational structure for it) [45–47].

In this study, the bereaved family members with a higher educational attainment were more likely to have a *lower* satisfaction with care, as were family members of the deceased individuals with a higher educational attainment. To the best of our knowledge, this finding has not been confirmed in other published studies. In fact, previous research has more commonly suggested the opposite—that the higher the educational attainment, the greater the access to information and healthcare in general [5,8]. One assumption is that bereaved family members of deceased individuals with a higher educational attainment (or indeed family members with a higher educational attainment themselves) might expect better health care in general.

The results of the analyses of the answers to the open-ended questions in this study confirmed the importance of the care place/type of care service. Further, the qualitative results showed that communication and information as well as the performance of the staff were valued parts of the care. Several studies have shown the importance of adequate and timely communication regarding the illness, prognosis, and imminent death [20,21,48], as well as the importance of being treated with dignity and respect [20,49,50]. The importance of care place/care services—and differences in care satisfaction related to these—might be especially prominent in this study because of the construction of the VOICES (SF) questionnaire itself.

Methodological Considerations

This study's response rate was at the lower end (37.9%), and could potentially have been improved by using reminders and repeated mail outs. However, this was not done for ethical reasons —to respect and avoid upsetting participants who did not wish to take part. Some of the deceased persons had several different care places and care services during the last three months of life. Unfortunately, we do not know the reason for care admissions or the length of care in each care place, or if anything particularly crucial occurred in a certain care place, because this information is not included in the questionnaire items. Hence, we do not know if and how this affected the overall satisfaction with care during the last three months, and this must be regarded as a limitation of the study results. Hence, the VOICES (SF) questionnaire has the benefit of enabling the evaluation of most care services received during the last three months of life, but it does have limits regarding the possibilities for analyses of the answers for the care trajectories, since it does not provide information on the length, reason for, or order of the different care events.

None of the participants have contacted the researchers to report any negative reactions towards the request for participation or towards the questionnaire itself. A few stated that they did not wish to participate because they did not feel well or because they were still grieving, whereas others very much appreciated the opportunity to share their experiences and found answering the questions beneficial for their bereavement.

The results from this study can make no claim of generalization on a population level, since the sample consists of the bereaved family members of individuals who died in four hospitals in two Swedish health care regions and should be understood in that context. A further limitation is that the sample consisted mainly of native Swedes, and the very small part of the sample with other origin was mainly from other Scandinavian countries, which is not representative of the pluralism of Sweden. Still, the study does provide new and important knowledge about bereaved family members' satisfaction with the care received during the last three months of life.

5. Conclusions

This study shows that most of the bereaved family members reported being highly satisfied with the care received during the last three months of life. However, almost one-fifth ($n = 86$) of the participants rated their satisfaction with the overall care as low. Factors seemingly influencing the bereaved family members' care satisfaction were the relationship to the deceased person, a cancer diagnosis, educational attainment, and the length of illness prior to death. The results also show that the bereaved family members had the highest satisfaction with the care provided in specialized palliative care units and the lowest with the care from general practitioners. Hence, it is plausible that the type of care services and care place are important for the satisfaction with the care. However, further studies are needed to explore in more depth the quality of and satisfaction with care in different care places and to further investigate the factors that are crucial for a high/low satisfaction with care at the end of life.

Author Contributions: Conceptualization: A.O., C.H., A.A., J.Ö. were involved in the conception and design of the study. Methodology: A.O. carried out the data collection and data cleaning. Formal Analysis: Statistical analyses were carried out by A.O. and C.H. and were critically revised by A.A. and J.Ö. The qualitative descriptive analysis was carried out by A.O. and was critically revised by C.H, A.A. and J.Ö. Writing—Original Draft Preparation: the manuscript was drafted by A.O. with critical input from all other authors. All authors read, revised, and approved the final manuscript.

Funding: The study was funded by Ersta Sköndal Bräcke University College, Sven and Dagmar Salén's foundation and The Swedish Society of Nursing's foundation.

Acknowledgments: We would like to thank the hospitals involved as well as the study participants for all their co-operation.

References

1. Murtagh, F.E.; Bausewein, C.; Verne, J.; Groeneveld, E.I.; Kaloki, Y.E.; Higginson, I.J. How many people need palliative care? A study developing and comparing methods for population-based estimates. *Palliat. Med.* **2014**, *28*, 49–58. [CrossRef] [PubMed]

2. Morin, L.; Aubry, R.g.; Frova, L.; MacLeod, R.; Wilson, D.M.; Loucka, M.; Csikos, A.; Ruiz-Ramos, M.; Cardenas-Turanzas, M.; YongJoo, R.; et al. Estimating the need for palliative care at the population level: A cross-national study in 12 countries. *Palliat. Med.* **2017**, *21*, 526–536. [CrossRef] [PubMed]

3. World Health Organization (WHO) Definition of Palliative Care. Geneva. World Health Organization. Available online: http://www.who.int/cancer/palliative/definition/en/ (accessed on 20 September 2018).

4. Radbruch, L. White Paper on standards and norms for hospice and palliative care in Europe: Part 1 Recommendations from the European Association for Palliative Care. *Eur. J. Palliat. Care* **2010**, *17*, 22–33.

5. Payne, M. Inequalities, end-of-life care and social work. *Prog. Palliat. Care* **2010**, *18*, 221–227. [CrossRef]

6. Gardiner, C.; Cobb, M.; Gott, M.; Ingleton, C. Barriers to providing palliative care for older people in acute hospitals. *Age Ageing* **2011**, *40*, 233–238. [CrossRef] [PubMed]

7. Lindskog, M.; Tavelin, B.; Lundström, S. Old age as risk indicator for poor end-of-life care quality— A population-based study of cancer deaths from the swedish register of palliative care. *Eur. J. Cancer* **2015**, *51*, 1331–1339. [CrossRef] [PubMed]

8. Bossuyt, N.; Van den Block, L.; Cohen, J.; Meeussen, K.; Bilsen, J.; Echteld, M.; Deliens, L.; Van Casteren, V. Is individual educational level related to end-of-life care use? Results from a nationwide retrospective cohort study in belgium. *J. Palliat. Med.* **2011**, *14*, 1135–1141. [CrossRef] [PubMed]

9. Ahmadi, Z.; Lundström, S.; Janson, C.; Strang, P.; Emtner, M.; Currow, D.C.; Ekström, M. End-of-life care in oxygen-dependent copd and cancer: A national population-based study. *Eur. Respir. J.* **2015**, *46*, 1190–1193. [CrossRef] [PubMed]

10. Romem, A.; Tom, S.E.; Beauchene, M.; Babington, L.; Scharf, S.M. Pain management at the end of life: A comparative study of cancer, dementia, and chronic obstructive pulmonary disease patients. *Palliat. Med.* **2015**, *29*, 464–469. [CrossRef] [PubMed]

11. Eriksson, H.; Milberg, A.; Hjelm, K.; Friedrichsen, M. End of life care for patients dying of stroke: A comparative registry study of stroke and cancer. *PLoS ONE* **2016**, *11*, e0147694. [CrossRef] [PubMed]

12. Bausewein, C.; Daveson, B.A.; Currow, D.C.; Downing, J.; Deliens, L.; Radbruch, L.; Defilippi, K.; Lopes Ferreira, P.; Costantini, M.; Harding, R.; et al. Eapc white paper on outcome measurement in palliative care: Improving practice, attaining outcomes and delivering quality services—Recommendations from the european association for palliative care (eapc) task force on outcome measurement. *Palliat. Med.* **2016**, *30*, 6–22. [CrossRef] [PubMed]

13. McPherson, C.J.; Addington-Hall, J.M. Judging the quality of care at the end of life: Can proxies provide reliable information? *Soc. Sci. Med.* **2003**, *56*, 95–109. [CrossRef]

14. Henoch, I.; Lövgren, M.; Wilde-Larsson, B.; Tishelman, C. Perception of quality of care: Comparison of the views of patients' with lung cancer and their family members. *J. Clin. Nurs.* **2012**, *21*, 585–594. [CrossRef] [PubMed]

15. Erin, S.; Brigette, H.; Blair, H.; Wei, X.; Jeff, M.; Lesia, W.; Ru, T.; Daren, H.; Robert, F. Factors affecting family satisfaction with inpatient end-of-life care. *PLoS ONE* **2014**, *11*, e110860.

16. Virdun, C.; Luckett, T.; Davidson, P.M.; Phillips, J. Dying in the hospital setting: A systematic review of quantitative studies identifying the elements of end-of-life care that patients and their families rank as being most important. *Palliat. Med.* **2015**, *29*, 774–796. [CrossRef] [PubMed]

17. Addington-Hall, J.M.; O'Callaghan, A.C. A comparison of the quality of care provided to cancer patients in the uk in the last three months of life in in-patient hospices compared with hospitals, from the perspective of bereaved relatives: Results from a survey using the voices questionnaire. *Palliat. Med.* **2009**, *23*, 190–197. [CrossRef] [PubMed]

18. Hunt, K.J.; Shlomo, N.; Richardson, A.; Addington-Hall, J. *Voices Re-Design and Testing to Inform a National End-of-Life Care Survey*; Final report for the department for health; University of South Hampton: Southampton, UK, 2011.

19. Roza, K.A.; Lee, E.J.; Meier, D.E.; Goldstein, N.E. A survey of bereaved family members to assess quality of care on a palliative care unit. *J. Palliat. Med.* **2015**, *18*, 358–365. [CrossRef] [PubMed]

20. Ong, J.; Brennsteiner, A.; Chow, E.; Hebert, R.S. Correlates of family satisfaction with hospice care: General inpatient hospice care versus routine home hospice care. *J. Palliat. Med.* **2016**, *19*, 97–100. [CrossRef] [PubMed]

21. Kaarbø, E. End-of-life care in two norwegian nursing homes: Family perceptions. *J. Clin. Nurs.* **2011**, *20*, 1125–1132. [CrossRef] [PubMed]

22. Andersson, S.; Lindqvist, O.; Fürst, C.J.; Brännström, M. End-of-life care in residential care homes: A retrospective study of the perspectives of family members using the voices questionnaire. *Scand. J. Caring Sci.* **2016**, *31*, 72–84. [CrossRef] [PubMed]

23. Pivodic, L.; Pardon, K.; Morin, L.; Addington-Hall, J.; Miccinesi, G.; Cardenas-Turanzas, M.; Onwuteaka-Philipsen, B.; Naylor, W.; Ruiz Ramos, M.; Van den Block, L.; et al. Place of death in the population dying from diseases indicative of palliative care need: A cross-national population-level study in 14 countries. *J. Epidemiol. Community Health* **2016**, *70*, 17–24. [CrossRef] [PubMed]

24. Al-Qurainy, R.; Collis, E.; Feuer, D. Dying in an acute hospital setting: The challenges and solutions. *Int. J. Clin. Pract.* **2009**, *63*, 508–515. [CrossRef] [PubMed]

25. Woo, J.; Lo, R.; Cheng, J.O.Y.; Wong, F.; Mak, B. Quality of end-of-life care for non-cancer patients in a non-acute hospital. *J. Clin. Nurs.* **2011**, *20*, 1834–1841. [CrossRef] [PubMed]

26. Reyniers, T.; Houttekier, D.; Cohen, J.; Pasman, H.R.; Deliens, L. The acute hospital setting as a place of death and final care: A qualitative study on perspectives of family physicians, nurses and family carers. *Health Place* **2014**, *27*, 77–83. [CrossRef] [PubMed]

27. Penders, Y.W.; Van den Block, L.; Donker, G.A.; Deliens, L.; Onwuteaka-Philipsen, B.; Euro, I. Comparison of end-of-life care for older people living at home and in residential homes: A mortality follow-back study among gps in the netherlands. *Br. J. Gen. Pract.* **2015**, *65*, e724–e730. [CrossRef] [PubMed]

28. Morin, L.; Johnell, K.; Van den Block, L.; Aubry, R.g. Discussing end-of-life issues in nursing homes: A nationwide study in france. *Age Ageing* **2016**, *45*, 395–402. [CrossRef] [PubMed]

29. Smedbäck, J.; Öhlen, J.; Årestedt, K.; Alvariza, A.; Fürst, C.J.; Håkanson, C. Palliative care during the final week of life of older people in nursing homes: A register-based study. *Palliat. Support. Care* **2017**, *15*, 417–424. [CrossRef] [PubMed]

30. Håkanson, C.; Öhlen, J.; Morin, L.; Cohen, J. A population-level study of place of death and associated factors in sweden. *Scand. J. Public Health* **2015**, *43*, 744–751. [CrossRef] [PubMed]

31. Young, A.J.; Rogers, A.; Addington-Hall, J.M. The quality and adequacy of care received at home in the last 3 months of life by people who died following a stroke: A retrospective survey of surviving family and friends using the views of informal carers evaluation of services questionnaire. *Health Soc. Care Community* **2008**, *16*, 419–428. [CrossRef] [PubMed]

32. Young, A.J.; Rogers, A.; Dent, L.; Addington-Hall, J.M. Experiences of hospital care reported by bereaved relatives of patients after a stroke: A retrospective survey using the voices questionnaire. *J. Adv. Nurs.* **2009**, *65*, 2161–2174. [CrossRef] [PubMed]

33. Hughes, R.; Saleem, T.; Addington-Hall, J. Towards a culturally acceptable end-of-life survey questionnaire: A bengali translation of voices. *Int. J. Palliat. Nurs.* **2005**, *11*, 116–123. [CrossRef] [PubMed]

34. Ross, L.; Neergaard, M.A.; Petersen, M.A.; Groenvold, M. Measuring the quality of end-of-life care: Development, testing, and cultural validation of the danish version of views of informal carers' evaluation of services–short form. *Palliat. Med.* **2018**, *32*, 804–814. [CrossRef] [PubMed]

35. O'Sullivan, A.; Öhlen, J.; Alvariza, A.; Håkanson, C. Adaptation and validation of the voices (sf) questionnaire—For evaluation of end-of-life care in sweden. *Scand. J. Caring Sci.* **2017**, *32*, 1254–1260. [CrossRef] [PubMed]

36. Krippendorff, K. *Content Analysis: An Introduction to Its Methodology*, 3rd ed.; SAGE: Los Angeles, CA, USA, 2013.

37. Ringdal, G.I.; Jordhøy, M.S.; Kaasa, S. Family satisfaction with end-of-life care for cancer patients in a cluster randomized trial. *J. Pain Symptom Manag.* **2002**, *24*, 53–63. [CrossRef]

38. Ozcelik, H.; Cakmak, D.E.; Fadiloglu, C.; Yildirim, Y.; Uslu, R. Determining the satisfaction levels of the family members of patients with advanced-stage cancer. *Palliat. Support. Care* **2015**, *13*, 741–747. [CrossRef] [PubMed]

39. Brown, C.E.; Jecker, N.S.; Curtis, J.R. Inadequate palliative care in chronic lung disease. An issue of health care inequality. *Ann. Am. Thorac. Soc.* **2016**, *13*, 311–316. [CrossRef] [PubMed]

40. Hess, S.; Stiel, S.; Hofmann, S.; Klein, C.; Lindena, G.; Ostgathe, C. Trends in specialized palliative care for non-cancer patients in germany—Data from the national hospice and palliative care evaluation (hope). *Eur. J. Intern. Med.* **2014**, *25*, 187–192. [CrossRef] [PubMed]

41. Lundström, S.; Fransson, G.; Axelsson, B. Specialized Palliative Care in Sweden, for Whom and How Well? *Palliat. Med.* **2016**, *30*, NP173.

42. Rosenwax, L.; Spilsbury, K.; McNamara, B.; Semmens, J. *A Retrospective Population Based Cohort Study of Access to Specialist Palliative Care in the Last Year of Life: Who Is Still Missing out a Decade on?* BioMed Central Ltd.: London, UK, 2016.

43. Witkamp, F.E.; van Zuylen, L.; Borsboom, G.; van der Rijt, C.C.; van der Heide, A. Dying in the hospital: What happens and what matters, according to bereaved relatives. *J. Pain Symptom Manag.* **2015**, *49*, 203–213. [CrossRef] [PubMed]

44. de Boer, D.; Hofstede, J.M.; de Veer, A.J.E.; Raijmakers, N.J.H.; Francke, A.L. Relatives' perceived quality of palliative care: Comparisons between care settings in which patients die. *BMC Palliat. Care* **2017**, *16*, 41. [CrossRef] [PubMed]

45. National board of Health Care. Palliative Care Ath the End of life: Summary and Improvement Areas. (In Swedish: Palliativ vård i livets slutskede: Sammanfattning med förbättringsområden). Available online: http://www.socialstyrelsen.se/Lists/Artikelkatalog/Attachments/20396/2016-12-3.pdf (accessed on 30 October 2018).

46. Mousing, C.A.; Timm, H.; Lomborg, K.; Kirkevold, M. Barriers to palliative care in people with chronic obstructive pulmonary disease in home care: A qualitative study of the perspective of professional caregivers. *J. Clin. Nurs.* **2018**, *27*, 650–660. [CrossRef] [PubMed]

47. Van Riet Paap, J.; Vernooij-Dassen, M.; Brouwer, F.; Meiland, F.; Iliffe, S.; Davies, N.; Leppert, W.; Jaspers, B.; Mariani, E.; Sommerbakk, R.; et al. Improving the organization of palliative care: Identification of barriers and facilitators in five European countries. *Implement Sci.* **2014**, *9*, 130. [CrossRef] [PubMed]

48. Lundquist, G.; Rasmussen, B.H.; Axelsson, B. Information of imminent death or not: Does it make a difference? *J. Clin. Oncol.* **2011**, *29*, 3927–3931. [CrossRef] [PubMed]

49.   Robinson, J.; Gott, M.; Ingleton, C. Patient and family experiences of palliative care in hospital: What do we know? An integrative review. *Palliat. Med.* **2014**, *28*, 18–33. [CrossRef] [PubMed]
50.   De Santo-Madeya, S.; Safizadeh, P. Family satisfaction with end-of-life care in the intensive care unit: A systematic review of the literature. *Dimens. Crit. Care Nurs.* **2017**, *36*, 278–283. [CrossRef] [PubMed]

Permissions

All chapters in this book were first published in HEALTHCARE, by MDPI; hereby published with permission under the Creative Commons Attribution License or equivalent. Every chapter published in this book has been scrutinized by our experts. Their significance has been extensively debated. The topics covered herein carry significant findings which will fuel the growth of the discipline. They may even be implemented as practical applications or may be referred to as a beginning point for another development.

The contributors of this book come from diverse backgrounds, making this book a truly international effort. This book will bring forth new frontiers with its revolutionizing research information and detailed analysis of the nascent developments around the world.

We would like to thank all the contributing authors for lending their expertise to make the book truly unique.

They have played a crucial role in the development of this book. Without their invaluable contributions this book wouldn't have been possible. They have made vital efforts to compile up to date information on the varied aspects of this subject to make this book a valuable addition to the collection of many professionals and students.

This book was conceptualized with the vision of imparting up-to-date information and advanced data in this field. To ensure the same, a matchless editorial board was set up. Every individual on the board went through rigorous rounds of assessment to prove their worth. After which they invested a large part of their time researching and compiling the most relevant data for our readers.

The editorial board has been involved in producing this book since its inception. They have spent rigorous hours researching and exploring the diverse topics which have resulted in the successful publishing of this book. They have passed on their knowledge of decades through this book. To expedite this challenging task, the publisher supported the team at every step. A small team of assistant editors was also appointed to further simplify the editing procedure and attain best results for the readers.

Apart from the editorial board, the designing team has also invested a significant amount of their time in understanding the subject and creating the most relevant covers. They scrutinized every image to scout for the most suitable representation of the subject and create an appropriate cover for the book.

The publishing team has been an ardent support to the editorial, designing and production team. Their endless efforts to recruit the best for this project, has resulted in the accomplishment of this book. They are a veteran in the field of academics and their pool of knowledge is as vast as their experience in printing. Their expertise and guidance has proved useful at every step. Their uncompromising quality standards have made this book an exceptional effort. Their encouragement from time to time has been an inspiration for everyone.

The publisher and the editorial board hope that this book will prove to be a valuable piece of knowledge for researchers, students, practitioners and scholars across the globe.

List of Contributors

Julie Lewis, Corinne R. Boudreau, JamesW. Patterson, Jonathan Bradet-Legris and Vett K. Lloyd
Department. Biology, Mount Allison University, Sackville, NB E4L 1G7, Canada

Sissi Palma Ribeiro, Jessica M. LaCroix, Fernanda De Oliveira, Laura A. Novak, Su Yeon Lee-Tauler, Charles A. Darmour, Kanchana U. Perera and Marjan Ghahramanlou-Holloway
Suicide Care, Prevention, and Research Initiative, Department of Medical and Clinical Psychology, Uniformed Services University, Bethesda, MD 20814, USA

David B. Goldston
Department of Psychiatry, Duke University, Durham, NC 27708, USA

Jennifer Weaver
Inpatient Psychiatry, Fort Belvoir Community Hospital, VA 22060, USA

Alyssa Soumoff
Department of Psychiatry, Walter Reed National Military Medical Center, Bethesda, MD 20889, USA

Md Saiful Islam, Md Mahmudul Hasan, Xiaoyi Wang and Md Noor-E-Alam
Mechanical and Industrial Engineering, Northeastern University, Boston, MA 02115, USA

Hayley D. Germack
Mechanical and Industrial Engineering, Northeastern University, Boston, MA 02115, USA
National Clinician Scholars Program, Yale University School of Medicine, New Haven, CT 06511, USA
Bouvé College of Health Sciences, Northeastern University, Boston, MA 02115, USA

Brandt A. Smith
Department of Psychology, Columbus State University, Columbus, GA 31907, USA

Jihane Hajj
Department of Nursing, Widener University, One University Pl, Chester, PA 19013, USA

Natalie Blaine and Jola Salavaci
Department of Pharmacy, Penn Presbyterian Medical Center, 51 N 39th St, Philadelphia, PA 19104, USA

Douglas Jacoby
Department of Cardiology, Penn Presbyterian Medical Center, 51 N 39th St, Philadelphia, PA 19104, USA

Teresa Lesiuk
Music Therapy, University of Miami, Frost School of Music 5499 San Amaro Dr., N306, Coral Gables, FL 33146, USA

Jennifer A. Bugos
Music Education, University of South Florida, School of Music, 4202 E. Fowler Ave., MUS 101, Tampa, FL 33620, USA

Brea Murakami
Department of Music, Pacific University, Forest Grove, OR 97116, USA

Courtney L. Scherr, Amy A. Ross and Sanjana Ramesh
Center for Communication and Health, Department of Communication Studies, Northwestern University, 710 North Lake Shore Drive, 15th Floor, Chicago, IL 60611; USA

Sharon Aufox, Catherine A. Wicklund and Maureen Smith
Center for Genetic Medicine, Feinberg School of Medicine, Northwestern University, 645 N Michigan Ave, Suite 630, Chicago, IL 60611, USA

Cara L. Berkowitz, Lisa Mosconi, Olivia Scheyer, Aneela Rahman, Hollie Hristov and Richard S. Isaacson
Department of Neurology, Weill Cornell Medicine, New York, NY 10021, USA

Chia-Lun Lo
Department of Health Business Administration, Fooyin University, Daliao District, Kaohsiung 831, Taiwan

Hsiao-Ting Tseng
Department of Information Management, Tatung University, Zhongshan District, Taipei 104, Taiwan

Chi-Hua Chen
College of Mathematics and Computer Science, Fuzhou University, Minhou County, Fuzhou 350100, China

Joshua De Sipio
Department of Medicine, Gastroenterology/Liver Diseases Division, Cooper University Health, Camden, NJ 08103, USA

John Gaughan
Cooper Research Institute, Cooper University Health, Camden, NJ 08103, USA

Susan Perlis
Office of Medical Education, Cooper Medical School of
Rowan University, Camden, NJ 08103, USA

Sangita Phadtare
Department of Biomedical Sciences, Cooper Medical
School of Rowan University, Camden, NJ 08103,
USA

Niral J. Patel, Karishma A. Datye and Sarah S. Jaser
Department of Pediatrics, Vanderbilt University
Medical Center, Nashville, TN 37232, USA

Wei Gao, Sumaya Huque and Irene J. Higginson
Cicely Saunders Institute of Palliative Care, Policy
and Rehabilitation, King's College London, Bessemer
Road, Denmark Hill, London SE5 9PJ, UK

Myfanwy Morgan
Institute of Pharmaceutical Science, King's College
London, London SE1 9NH, UK

Laurie S. Abbott
College of Nursing, Florida State University,
Tallahassee, FL 32306-4310, USA

Elizabeth H. Slate
Department of Statistics, Florida State University,
Tallahassee, FL 32306-4310, USA

Lene Bjørn Jensen
Public Health Consultant, Haderslev Municipality,
Noerregade 41, 6100 Haderslev, Denmark

Irena Lukic and Gabriel Gulis
Unit for Health Promotion Research, University of
Southern Denmark, 6700 Esbjerg, Denmark

Steven G. Koven
Urban Studies Institute, University of Louisville, 426
West Bloom Street, Louisville, KY 40208, USA

Melissa D. Olfert, Makenzie L. Barr and Rebecca L. Hagedorn
Davis College of Agriculture, Natural Resources and
Design, Division of Animal and Nutritional Sciences,
West Virginia University, G016 Agricultural Science
Building, Morgantown, WV 26506, USA

Lisa Franzen-Castle
Nutrition and Health Sciences Department, University
of Nebraska-Lincoln, 110 Ruth Leverton Hall, Lincoln,
NE 68583-0806, USA

Sarah E. Colby
Department of Nutrition, University of Tennessee, 1215
W. Cumberland Avenue, 229 Jessie Harris Building,
Knoxville, TN 37996-1920, USA

Kendra K. Kattelmann
Department of Health and Nutritional Sciences, South
Dakota State University, SWG 425, Brookings, SD
57007, USA

Adrienne A. White
School of Food and Agriculture, University of Maine,
5735 Hitchner Hall, Orono, ME 04469, USA

Alister du Rose
Faculty of Life Sciences and Education, University of
South Wales, Treforest, Pontypridd, Wales CF37 1DL,
UK

Anna O'Sullivan
Department of Health Care Sciences, Palliative
Research Centre, Ersta Sköndal Bräcke University
College, SE-100 61 Stockholm, Sweden

Anette Alvariza
Department of Health Care Sciences, Palliative
Research Centre, Ersta Sköndal Bräcke University
College, SE-100 61 Stockholm, Sweden
Capio Palliative Care Unit, Dalen Hospital,
Åstorpsringen 6, Enskededalen, SE-121 87 Stockholm,
Sweden

Joakim Öhlen
Institute of Health and Care Sciences, Sahlgrenska
Academy at the University of Gothenburg, 41346
Gothenburg, Sweden
Centre for Person-Centered Care, Sahlgrenska
Academy at the University of Gothenburg, 40530
Gothenburg, Sweden
The Palliative Centre, Sahlgrenska University Hospital,
SE-405 30 Gothenburg, Sweden

Cecilia Håkanson
Department of Health Care Sciences, Palliative
Research Centre, Ersta Sköndal Bräcke University
College, SE-100 61 Stockholm, Sweden
Department of Nursing Science, Sophiahemmet
University, SE-114 86 Stockholm, Sweden

Index